Mental Health Nursing Skills

Mental Health Nursing Skills

SECOND EDITION

Edited by

Patrick Callaghan

*Professor of Mental Health Science and Academic Lead, LSBU Doctoral College,
South Bank University, London, UK*

Tommy Dickinson

*Professor of Nursing Education, Associate Dean (International Education),
and Head of the Department of Mental Health Nursing, King's College London, London, UK*

Anne Felton

Head of the Institute of Health and Allied Professions, Nottingham Trent University, Nottingham, UK

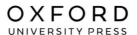

OXFORD
UNIVERSITY PRESS

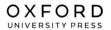

OXFORD
UNIVERSITY PRESS

Great Clarendon Street, Oxford, OX2 6DP,
United Kingdom

Oxford University Press is a department of the University of Oxford.
It furthers the University's objective of excellence in research, scholarship,
and education by publishing worldwide. Oxford is a registered trade mark of
Oxford University Press in the UK and in certain other countries

© Oxford University Press 2024

The moral rights of the authors have been asserted

First edition published in 2009
Second edition published in 2024

Published in the United States of America by Oxford University Press
198 Madison Avenue, New York, NY 10016, United States of America

British Library Cataloguing in Publication Data
Data available

Library of Congress Control Number: 2022943242

ISBN 978–0–19–286404–8

DOI: 10.1093/med/9780192864048.001.0001

Printed in the UK by
Bell & Bain Ltd., Glasgow

Dedication

Sadly, one of our authors, Dr Alan Pringle passed away during the book's production. Alan was an inspiring academic, a wonderful colleague, and a good friend to many. Our thoughts are with Alan's family, friends, and colleagues.

Foreword

It is an honour to be invited to write the foreword to what is a timely and important contribution to the expanding literature on mental health nursing. The publication of this book coincides with the centenary anniversary of the first substantial textbook for mental health nurses issued in 1923. In fact, the need for a basic textbook for nurses was first mooted by the Medico Psychological Association towards the end of the nineteenth century and *A Handbook for Attendants on the Insane* appeared in 1885. It consisted of 64 pages of distilled medical knowledge with guidance on the principles of hygiene, exercise, and the maintenance of order in mental hospitals. It was testimony to the advocacy of enlightened commissioners and doctors who had noted that relationships formed between nurses (attendants) and patients were often far more effective in bringing about improvements in patients' conditions than medical treatments. Some superintendents of asylums argued therefore that training should be provided to a nursing workforce that had much to offer but was currently ill-educated, little skilled, and undervalued; they felt that improving the education of attendants would also enhance the standing of psychiatry both within the profession of medicine and in the public mind.

The 1923 edition of the *Handbook*, now called *The Handbook for Mental Nurses*, was a far more substantial version of the original and consisted of more than 400 pages. There was a greater emphasis on nursing care even though, of the 42 contributors, only two were nurses. The role of the nurse, the *Handbook* stated, was to oversee the hygiene, nutrition, exercise, and recreation of patients. Nurses were responsible for the ventilation of wards, the administration of drugs, and the safekeeping of ward keys. They were encouraged to form therapeutic relationships with patients, using suggestion, and persuasion, while encouraging self-reflection and re-education. They were reminded that favouring certain patients over others was inappropriate and that it was important to know when to speak to patients and when to say nothing. Perhaps rather sadly, while the *Handbook* aimed to define good practice, its main purpose, as stated in the 'Introduction', was to enable nurses to pass their examinations!

The world of *The Handbook for Mental Nurses* was fundamentally impacted and ultimately diminished by the two World Wars. In the aftermath of global conflict, severe overcrowding, underfunding, deeply ingrained institutional attitudes on the part of both nurses and patients, and a pervading sense of hopelessness afflicted the hospitals. In 1948, psychiatry was absorbed into the new NHS which, together with the Mental Health Act of 1959, sought to reduce admissions, establish outpatient clinics, and relocate mental health services within communities so that mental health nurses worked alongside other health care providers or were integrated into their services. By the 1980s, nurse training and education had transferred from the NHS to the university sector which remains to this day the primary credentialing agency. Within this new context of higher education, mental health nursing had to start to define its theoretical bases, its methods of intellectual inquiry, its professional parameters, and its domains of practice.

As I write, there is unprecedented demand for mental health care from people of all ages and backgrounds following the COVID-19 pandemic and during the current cost-of-living crisis. Some service users have found their access to care and social support abruptly terminated; staffing levels have been affected by COVID-19 infection and stress. The present book which, in contrast to the 1923 *Handbook*, is written predominantly by nurses, is uncompromising in its recognition of the complexity of improving care in straitened circumstances. It engages head-on with the multiple contemporary influences on mental health care, including politics, economics, culture, and the law, and confronts such vexed issues as professional territorialism, scope of practice, leadership and management, consumer rights, resource allocation, medicines management, risk management, and service user participation in care.

Each richly referenced chapter assists the reader to move from definition to explanation and, most importantly, to application. Readers are reminded that while interventions need to be evidence-based, they must also be tailored to individual needs and delivered with insight, empathy, compassion, judgement, and resilience. In the context of values, evidence, communication, health promotion, and recovery, chapters cover such topics as self-harm, dementia, neurodevelopmental disorders, substance use, and the care of children and young people.

Although this book is being published one hundred years after the 1923 *Handbook*, there is much still to do to improve mental health care. Deficits that were present a century ago persist, including stigma, abuse of human rights, power imbalances, inadequate funding, and lack of social support and effective treatments. Nonetheless, the book also makes clear how much has been achieved and can be celebrated. The ill-educated nurses of a century ago would marvel at what nursing has become, applaud those at the forefront of innovation, and commend the thirst for knowledge on the part of nurses reading this book. From one who has participated in and observed mental health nursing for over half a century, I would like to acknowledge the contributions of the editors and authors who have shared their knowledge, experiences, and wisdom in order to ensure that this book is a high watermark in the evolution of mental health nursing. Unlike the 1923 *Handbook*, this book has far more to offer than enabling readers to pass their exams. It can be read and re-read and should be a resource to be consulted frequently throughout readers' careers.

Professor Peter Nolan (Emeritus)
York, 2023

Contents

Contributors

Opeyemi Atanda, Lecturer, Division of Psychology, School of Applied, London South Bank University, London, UK

Mark J. Baker, Lecturer, Mental Health Nursing Department, King's College London, London, UK

Carmel Bond, Lecturer in Mental Health Nursing, Research Associate, Florence Nightingale Foundation, Sheffield Hallam University, Sheffield, UK

Geoff Brennan, Safewards Clinical Supervisor and Honorary Lecturer, Florence Nightingale Faculty of Nursing, Midwifery & Palliative Care, King's College London, London, UK

Simon Burrow, Senior Lecturer, Division of Nursing, Midwifery and Social Work, School of Health Sciences, University of Manchester, Manchester, UK

Debbie Butler, Advisory Group Member, Institute of Mental Health, University of Nottingham, Nottingham, UK

Patrick Callaghan, Professor of Mental Health Science and Academic Lead, Doctoral College, London South Bank University, London, UK

Tim Carter, Assistant Professor, Mental Health, School of Social Sciences, University of Nottingham, Nottingham, UK

Marie Chellingsworth, Clinical Director, The CBT Resource, UK; and Senior Lecturer, School of Psychology, Arden University, UK

Adam Chillman, Senior Lecturer in Mental Health Nursing, Nottingham Trent University, Nottingham, UK

Michael Coffey, Professor, School of Health and Social Care, Faculty of Medicine, Health and Life Science, Swansea University, Swansea, UK

Paul Crawford, Professor of Health Humanities, School of Health Sciences, University of Nottingham, UK

Tommy Dickinson, Professor of Nursing Education, Associate Dean (International Education), and Head of the Department of Mental Health Nursing, King's College London, London, UK

Wayne Ennis, Peer Support Worker and Expert by Experience, Mersey Care NHS Foundation Trust, UK

Anne Felton, Head of the Institute of Health and Allied Professions, Nottingham Trent University, Nottingham, UK

Maria Filip, Cognitive Behavioural Therapist, Nottinghamshire Healthcare NHS Foundation Trust, Nottingham, UK

Annmarie Grealish, Associate Professor in Mental Health Nursing, Department of Nursing and Midwifery, University of Limerick, Limerick, Ireland

Richard Griffith, Head of Ethics and Law, School of Health and Social Care, Swansea University, Swansea, UK

Andrew C. Grundy, Lived Experience Researcher, University of Manchester, Manchester, UK

Ben Hannigan, Professor of Mental Health Nursing, School of Healthcare Sciences, Cardiff University, Cardiff, UK

Anita Henderson, Lecturer/Practitioner in Mental Health Nursing, King's College London, London, UK

Juanita Hoe, Professor of Dementia Care, Geller Institute of Ageing and Memory (GIAM), University of West London, London, UK

Roupmatee Joggyah, Lecturer in Nursing Education, King's College London, London, UK

Christine Kakai, Senior Clinical Teaching Fellow, King's College London, London, UK

John Keady, Professor of Older People's Mental Health Nursing, Division of Nursing, Midwifery and Social Work, School of Health Sciences, University of Manchester, Manchester, UK

Rachel Lees, Trust Lead for Self-Harm and Suicide Prevention, Nottinghamshire Healthcare NHS Foundation Trust, Nottingham, UK

Roy Litvin, Lecturer in Mental Health Nursing Education, King's College London, London, UK

Stephen McKenna Lawson, Teacher, Mental Health Nursing, University of Cardiff, Cardiff, UK

Jean Morrissey, Lecturer in Mental Health Nursing, School of Nursing and Midwifery, Trinity College, University of Dublin, Ireland

Mary Munro, Clinical Effectiveness Lead Mental Health, Scottish Ambulance Service, Edinburgh, UK; and Associate Lecturer, Robert Gordon University, Aberdeen, UK

Jeanette Murray, Volunteer and Expert by Experience, Mersey Care NHS Foundation Trust, UK

Michael Nash, Associate Professor in Mental Health Nursing, Trinity College Dublin, Dublin, Ireland

Mark Pearson, Assistant Professor, Mental Health School of Health Sciences, University of Nottingham, Nottingham, UK

Alan Pringle, Assistant Professor, Mental Health Nursing, University of Nottingham, Nottingham, UK

Helen Pusey, Senior Lecturer, Division of Nursing, Midwifery and Social Work, School of Health Sciences, University of Manchester, Manchester, UK

Paula Reavey, Professor of Psychology and Mental Health, London South Bank University, London, UK

Helen Rees, Senior Lecturer in Mental Health Nursing, Nottingham Trent University, Nottingham, UK

Billy Ridler, Associate Lecturer, Robert Gordon University, Aberdeen, UK

Dave Riley, Mental Health Nurse and Quality Improvement Partner, Mersey Care NHS Foundation Trust, UK

Greg Rooney, Principal Lecturer and Professional Lead, Mental Health, University of Hertfordshire, Hatfield, UK

Jessica Sears, Doctoral Clinical Academic Fellow, RMN. King's College London and South London and Maudsley NHS Foundation Trust, London, UK

Jane Sedgwick-Müller, Associate Dean (Mental Health Nursing), Faculty of Health, Health & Community Services, Government of Jersey; Visiting Lecturer, Faculty of Nursing, Midwifery & Paliative Care, King's College London; Associate Lecturer, School of Health, Robert Gordon University; Executive Board Member, UK Adult ADHD Network (UKAAN.org)

Alan Simpson, Professor of Mental Health Nursing, King's College London, London, UK

Zaynab Yasin Sohawon, Chief Executive Officer of Emotion Dysregulation in Autism, Mental Health Charity for Autistic Young People, Birmingham, UK

Susan Sookoo, Senior Lecturer in Nursing Education, Mental Health Nursing Department, King's College London, London, UK

Gemma Stacey, Director of Academy, Florence Nightingale Foundation, London, UK

Theo Stickley, Senior Fellow, Institute of Mental Health, Nottingham, UK

Adam Sutcliffe, Manager, The Level, Framework Housing Association, Nottingham, UK

Rachel Thompson, Consultant Admiral Nurse for Lewy Body Dementia, Dementia UK/The Lewy Body Society, London, UK

Gemma Trainor, Associate Professor in Mental Health Nursing, School of Health and Society, University of Salford, Salford, UK

Isaac Tuffour, Senior Lecturer in Mental Health, College of Health Education & Life Sciences, Birmingham City University, UK

Haseem Usman, Clinical Teacher/Lecturer, Mental Health Nursing Department, King's College London, London, UK

Eleni Vangeli, Senior Lecturer in Psychology, London South Bank University, London, UK

Emma Wadey, Faculty, Department of Health and Medical Sciences, University of Surrey, Guildford, UK

Dan Warrender, Lecturer in Mental Health Nursing, School of Applied Sciences, Abertay University, Dundee, UK

Keith Waters, Honorary Research Fellow (Self-Harm/Suicide Prevention), Centre for Research and Development, Derbyshire Healthcare NHS Foundation Trust, Kingsway Hospital, Derby, UK

Nick Weaver, Lecturer in Mental Health Nursing, School of Healthcare Sciences, Cardiff University, Cardiff, UK

Andy Willis, National Suicide Prevention Alliance Influencer; Expert by Experience Lead and Personality Disorder LEAP Northamptonshire Healthcare (NHS) Foundation Trust, Northamptonshire, UK

Chris Young, Lived Experience Mental Health Activist

Companion website

Purchasers of the print version of *Mental Health Nursing Skills*, Second Edition, are also entitled to free access to the companion website. It can be accessed at: www.oup.com/mhns

Username: Mentalhealthcare
Password: Therapeutic

The companion website contains additional resources designed to accompany the chapters in this book, including questions, case studies, exercises, and audio recordings.

The reader is encouraged to consult this resource in conjunction with reading the chapters.

Service users' views and expectations of mental health nurses

Andrew C. Grundy

Debbie Butler

Learning outcomes

By the end of this chapter, you should be able to:

1 Understand why service user views and expectations of mental health nurses' matter

2 Identify the key attributes and skills of mental health nurses from service user perspectives

3 Appreciate the core qualities of mental health nursing practice from service user points of view

4 Consider the implications for improving nursing practice, education, and the services and systems in which nurses operate to benefit service users.

▼ Background

Since the early 1990s, there has been an expectation that service users (SUs) should be 'involved' in the design and evaluation of NHS mental health services in the UK, and in their own care, treatment, and planning (Bee et al., 2015). With growing evidence that SUs themselves did not feel involved, it became important to understand the notion of involvement from SU perspectives (Grundy et al., 2016).

SUs have identified nursing attributes, skills, and ways of working that could either help or hinder involvement. This chapter is based on a systematic review published in 2008 (Bee et al, 2008), which provided the broad nursing attributes identified here. Literature searches were conducted to update the evidence in each of these domains, with a narrative synthesis presented here.

▼ Nursing attributes

SUs have clear views and expectations of mental health nurses (MHNs) in terms of what attributes a good MHN possesses, and by contrast what poor mental health nursing is like. In this section, we will explore both the good and the poor, looking at each attribute from a SU point of view, and why it matters to us.

Empathy–Indifference

Empathy is often described as 'putting yourself in another's shoes' (Gerace et al., 2018). It has an emotional dimension

2016, in terms of *feeling for* the individual when acknowledging their difficult or distressing situation. It also has a cognitive dimension, focused on *knowing* another person's thoughts and feelings in their unique situation, reaching an empathic understanding (Gerace et al., 2018). Thus, empathy generates a shared understanding of the SU's experience. It involves the skill of active listening, fully concentrating on what is being said with the intent to understand (Horgan et al., 2021). It also involves genuine interest in the other person and the skill of asking exploratory questions (Horgan et al., 2021). Empathy is seen as a key nursing attribute that leads to SUs feeling heard, validated, and understood.

Compassionate–Heartless

Compassion is interrelated with empathy, and it relates to showing concern about the suffering of others and seeking to comfort and support them (Gunasekara et al., 2014). Compassion shows a warmth towards others and a motivation to relieve suffering. Uncompassionate MHNs, by contrast, are cold and unconcerned (Gerace et al., 2018). Compassion is enacted in practical acts of kindness and concern, and a helpfulness that looks to meet other people's needs. SUs expect MHNs to be nice to people, to be kind to them, to be friendly (Horgan et al., 2021), and compassion is framed as an essential aspect of 'caring' for people. Some SUs suggest that compassion fatigue is one explanation for poor care.

Sensitive–Insensitive

Sensitivity is a concept that overlaps with empathy and compassion. It shows an understanding and awareness of a SU's feelings and is accompanied by a desire to try to minimize distress and not seeking to cause undue further distress (Gunasekara et al., 2014). By contrast, insensitivity feels no consideration for others' feelings and thereby displays no such concern (Gerace et al., 2018). Sensitivity is mindful about *how* to have those difficult but necessary conversations, such as discussions around risk/safety (Culter et al., 2020). It is also a skill in managing other people's emotions well.

Available–Distant

Overall, SUs are looking for staff to be emotionally available (Horgan et al., 2021; Terry and Coffey, 2019). For SUs, this is seen in a willingness to develop meaningful connections, rather than staying removed, distant, or detached. Chit-chat or banter (phatic communication) can be important foundations for building meaningful relationships (Shattell et al., 2007; Stewart et al., 2015). SUs are seeking someone they can trust and open up to (Ganzini et al., 2013). A key barrier to this in acute settings is that staff are perceived to not have the time to develop relationships, and that that is not a priority; instead, they are physically unavailable (shut away in the nursing office) and overwhelmed with bureaucratic tasks (Terry and Coffey, 2019).

Respect–Disrespect

SUs want MHNs to treat them with respect (Gunasekara et al., 2014; Horgan et al., 2021). Respect can be conveyed in conversation by a polite and courteous manner, rather than a curt or rude one. It involves not only the content of what is said, but also the tone and feel of it. Some SUs report feeling patronized or talked to condescendingly (Gunasekara et al., 2014). Respect can also be conveyed in taking steps to protect the rights, wishes, dignity, and privacy of the SU (Horgan et al., 2021). SUs expect to be treated 'as a human being', rather than less than one, and adult SUs expect to be treated as such, and not be infantilized (Horgan et al., 2021).

Non-judgemental–Prejudicial

Being non-judgemental means avoiding moral judgements about another's background, attitudes, speech, and/or behaviour (Horgan et al., 2021). Sadly, people with so-called personality disorders still face high levels of stigma from staff *within* services (Romeu-Labayen et al., 2022). Judgemental and pathologizing language is still used by nursing staff and heard by SUs—that they are attention-seeking, manipulative, team-splitters, and it is all behavioural. Such judgements then impact the nursing 'care' of those SUs, leaving many feeling dismissed, disbelieved, and neglected (Romeu-Labayen et al., 2022). While it is increasingly acknowledged that unconscious bias is an issue, MHNs need to be challenging poor staff attitudes when they come to light (Crandlemire, 2020). Nursing practices, such as handovers, should be conducted as though the individual were present, and documentation should be written assuming the individual will access it.

✖ Being judged—a service user perspective

I have been judged many times, even someone saying I wasn't a good mum because I had mental health problems. But the worst judgement came from a mental health nurse at the depot clinic. I exercise a lot and one day when my depot was due, I decided that I would run from my house to the clinic. When I arrived, the nurse made a cutting comment about the way I was dressed. I told her that my line of work doesn't need me to dress in a formal style, and if I didn't have to dress for work why should I dress formally to attend clinic? I was left feeling as though I had just been in the headmistress's office and being spoken to as though I was 5 years old. I asked to just be given my depot and meds, and then left. I felt very upset and feared that my medical notes would now say that I was very confrontational when all I did was stand up for myself. I made a formal complaint, but I was then asked by the manager if I thought the incident was in my head. Being judged by a professional in this way is simply not okay.

Trustworthy–Unreliable

SUs are looking to MHNs to show trustworthiness, dependability, and reliability. Here they are looking for consistency (Forchuk and Reynolds, 2001). They also emphasize the importance of 'being true to your word'. All this involves key skills of organization, planning, and good time management. SUs also stress that they want MHNs to tell the truth, to admit to mistakes or to acknowledge forgetting to implement prior decisions/actions. This is related to a perception that, at times, staff seem to be more accountable to the organization and its needs, rather than being personally accountable to the individual (and their carer(s), where relevant) (Rio et al., 2020). SUs prioritize personal accountability.

Hopeful–Demoralizing

Some SUs are looking to nursing staff to instil a sense of hope about the future (Horgan et al., 2021). Being in a difficult and vulnerable position can lead to SUs feeling hopeless, and some are looking to staff to hold out the possibility of personal recovery. Hopelessness can be accompanied by a sense of powerlessness, along with a fatalism that believes that the individual is unable to change their prospects. Services can compound these problems, rather than relieve them; being treated like 'a hopeless case' can be demoralizing.

Summary

SUs have clear views of what makes a good or bad MHN, both in terms of their attributes and skills. They also have clear expectations of what makes for good nursing care and support.

▼ Nursing practice

The nursing attributes and skills outlined above are operationalized in different and interrelated *ways of working* with individuals in practice. SUs have clear views and expectations as to how they want MHNs to work with them, and the core components and qualities of those working relationships. This section will explore SU perspectives and expectations of these ways of working.

Engagement

SUs are looking to MHNs to be engaging and to facilitate engagement. Successful engagement requires both 'engaging with' a process and a state of 'being engaged in' a relationship, conceived as an internal state experienced by the individuals (e.g. desire, willingness, enthusiasm, and emotional investment), expressed in observable behaviour (e.g. verbal contributions) that exceed mere meeting attendance, and which may be visible in non-verbal cues (e.g. body language, focus, and attention) (Bright et al., 2015; McAllister et al., 2019). Importantly, professionals also need to be engaged in the relational process. Thus, disengagement is not a 'patient problem', it is not to be situated as their sole responsibility, since that ignores the role of the professional to facilitate engagement, the nature or quality of the working relationship that has been formed or otherwise, and the organizational culture in which the interactions occur (Bee et al., 2015; Bright et al., 2015; McAllister et al., 2019).

SU perspectives on engagement with MHNs have largely derived from qualitative studies focusing on patients who have been judged to be 'disengaged' from services. Wright et al. (2011), for example, stressed that SUs and MHNs in assertive outreach teams both value the importance of contact time, of dialogue (both talking and listening), and of feeling and being understood, with an emphasis upon reaching a shared understanding of issues, as key facilitators of engagement. Aspects that hinder engagement for MHNs in acute settings focus on their own experience of the ward (vicarious traumatization; violence, threats of violence, and associated fears) and difficulties facilitating engagement due to a lack of training, supervision, and confidence (Polacek et al., 2015).

Collaboration

SUs also emphasize the importance of working in collaboration with nursing staff. Collaboration describes the relationship between different parties who are working together (Storm and Edwards, 2013); it is often used synonymously with 'partnership' and particularly emphasizes a relationship of equity between involved parties (Majid and Gagliardi, 2019). SUs are looking to collaborate with MHNs in a spirit of mutual cooperation, particularly as a move away from paternalistic or tokenistic models of care where the locus of decision-making power lies with the nursing professional (Majid, 2020; Thompson, 2007). However, while MHNs in acute settings stated that they routinely collaborated with SUs, the SUs themselves reported

a lack of routine collaboration (Terry and Coffey, 2019). Thus, the success of a collaborative relationship needs to be judged by all parties involved (Reid et al., 2018).

'Shared decision-making' is a form of collaborative working in the arena of making plans and decisions (Slade, 2017). It is conceptualized as a process of joint deliberation or 'participatory deliberation' (Bee et al., 2015). Aoki (2020) has suggested that shared decision-making is a *communication process* rooted in the SU–professional relationship, involving goal-sharing, information-sharing (in an accessible form), deliberation, mutual agreement, and follow-up. Slade (2017) has called for an ethical imperative for shared decision-making approaches, arguing that SUs have the right to self-determination and, as far as possible, to be treated as a competent decision-maker, such that shared decision-making constitutes a 'values-based practice' irrespective of clinical outcomes.

Dahlqvist-Jönsson et al. (2015) explored the concept of 'participation' in decision-making from a SU perspective. They found that the SU view of participation in decision-making was that it was predicated on two key *internal factors:* SUs feeling respected as a person, and also feeling confident in their own ability. SUs furthermore needed four *external factors* in place: personal support before, during, and after attendance at a decision-making forum; access to knowledge in accessible formats; having a good dialogue (fostered by having sufficient discussion/reflection time, the ability to openly express desires and wishes, and the chance to evaluate information together); and, finally, having clarity about responsibilities by developing individual care plans (Dahlqvist-Jönsson et al., 2015). Many SUs are thus looking to be supported by MHNs in their own decision-making.

Person-centredness

SUs value a person-centred approach to nursing care and support whereby professionals aim to deliver care and support that is individualized or personalized and thus tailored to the unique person; at its core is 'the patient as a person' (Mead and Bower, 2000). It is predicated on SUs having sufficient engagement to identify and express need and on professionals eliciting, recognizing, and respecting SU-led needs (Bee et al., 2015). Person-centredness is seen to require a holistic or 'biopsychosocial' approach towards the individual (Castro et al., 2016). SUs are increasingly looking to nursing staff for socioeconomic support, particularly around applying for benefits (Recovery in the Bin, 2019). Person-centred care emphasizes nursing *knowledge* in particular—knowledge of the individual, knowledge of any carer(s), knowledge of services, knowledge of treatment and support options, and knowledge of available support/resources in different communities (Horgan et al., 2021). While not looking to services to meet all their goals and needs, SUs do look to MHNs to signpost them to other resources or groups.

Therapeutic

SUs emphasize the importance of MHNs adopting a therapeutic approach to all nursing systems and processes (McAllister et al., 2019; Molin et al., 2016). The production of a nursing care plan, for instance, should address the needs and concerns of the individual, in a process that involves the person themselves (Rio et al., 2020). In acute inpatient settings, there is also an awareness that nursing processes can be perceived to be serving custodial aims rather than therapeutic ones. For example, nursing observations can be reduced to mere surveillance with the aim of controlling behaviour, rather than as opportunities for meaningful engagement and interaction (Insua-Summerhays et al., 2018). The qualities and skills of a good MHN outlined above are thus operationalized in interactions with SUs that lead to the development of meaningful 'therapeutic relationships' (Molin et al., 2016; Rio et al., 2020; Shattell et al., 2007).

✖ Developing my care plan—a service user perspective

I had written up my care plan with my care coordinator, and it laid out my needs in my own words and from my own point of view, which was really validating. It also made clear the goals we were going to work on together, and it outlined who was responsible for what. It was reviewed every 6 months. At one review meeting I said that I really wanted to try reducing my antipsychotic medication. While my care coordinator had concerns, she supported my decision. We then drew up an advanced statement together, thinking through how I'd want to be supported should the worst happen, and that I relapse—particularly if I lost insight. I can see how these documents obviously benefit the system, but they are also beneficial and empowering to me.

Empowering

Empowerment is particularly seen in SUs having decision-making power/influence, having access to information and resources, and having a range of options from which to make choices—not just yes/no, and either/or (Castro et al., 2016; Chamberlin 1997). It impacts, and is expressed in, feelings and emotions (a feeling of assertiveness; a feeling that the individual can make a difference; not feeling alone/feeling part of a group; expressing anger) and upon one's understanding (learning to see things differently; learning about anger; understanding that people have rights; learning skills that the individual defines as important). Outcomes of empowerment are focused on *transformation*, in terms of effecting change in one's life and one's community; changing others' perceptions of one's competency and capacity to act; the ability to self-disclose; growth and change that is never ending and self-initiated; and increasing one's positive self-image and overcoming stigma (Chamberlin, 1997). Thus, MHNs providing information and choice are crucial conditions for empowerment, with survivors emphasizing a focus on emotional, cognitive, and personal and situational transformation and change. SUs are looking to MHNs to empower them (Castro et al., 2016). Many recognize power dynamics at play within services and within nursing processes ('Us versus Them' dynamics; Wyder et al., 2013) that can contribute to powerlessness.

Recovery-focused?

SUs have distinguished 'recovery from' mental illness (rooted in a biomedical model focused on overcoming symptoms and upon a cure) versus 'recovery in' mental illness (rooted more in approaches to trauma or addiction; Davidson and Roe, 2007). Various attempts to summarize recovery principles emphasize the importance of redefining self-identity in the light of experience, of having hope for the future, and having power and control. Some SUs expect MHNs to work with 'personal recovery' (as defined by the individual) as a goal or outcome of nursing care and support (Horgan et al., 2021).

Mental health services are expected to promote and facilitate recovery principles. 'Recovery competencies' for providers have been delineated, emphasizing processes of engagement, of person-centredness, and of continuity of care, particularly across care transitions (Chen et al., 2013). They also involve a process of promoting a 'trajectory of recovery' that is focused on hope, empowerment, meaning, and growth (Chen et al., 2013). Even under conditions of detention, Wyder et al. (2013) argue that offering hope, building relationships, and offering control wherever possible can promote recovery, and that detention and enforced treatment should be framed as staff 'using temporary coercion to restore power and agency' (p. 579).

There are, however, many SUs who are concerned that the concept of recovery has been co-opted by professionals to serve neoliberal/capitalist agendas—getting people off benefits, back into work, contributing to society, etc. A group called Recovery in the Bin strongly argue for the place of the unrecovered within services and wider society, and that people should not be coerced or pressured to recover (Recovery in the Bin, 2019). They assert that recovery is impossible for many due to their socioeconomic conditions, which the current recovery agenda largely ignores (Recovery in the Bin, 2019).

Summary

SUs have clear views and expectations around how they want MHNs to work with them. Nursing education should look to help aspiring MHNs develop a skill set in these key areas.

▲ Conclusion

SUs conceive of mental health nursing care primarily as the formation of an interpersonal relationship, focused upon the qualities of the working relationship that is developed between them, that can be 'therapeutic' and thus transformative. MHNs need to possess attributes, skills, and training for us to feel able to approach you, and for us to feel truly cared for and supported. These attributes and skills are put into practice in particular ways of working that can help involve us in our own treatment, care, decision-making, and planning. Nursing systems, processes, and organizational contexts can either serve to help or hinder the formation of those relationships. Thus, nursing observations can be custodial or therapeutic; nursing care planning can be merely bureaucratic or engaging and empowering for us. Nurses need to attend to both our internal state (our thoughts and feelings) and the external conditions that can help develop our working relationship, particularly around support, providing information/knowledge, and offering real choice. Nurses also need to be mindful that we will have different conceptions of recovery (some even abandoning the term), and thus different individual goals and needs.

✖ Tips from service users

1   Take time to sit down with us and really listen to our perspectives, experiences, goals, and needs.

2   Remember to maintain a holistic, person-centred, and biopsychosocial approach towards us, including consideration of our socioeconomic circumstances.

3   Continue to reflect on your values, how you put them into practice, and how you treat and speak to us.

W   Companion website

For extra resources on the topics covered in this chapter, visit the companion website at: www.oup.com/mhns

✚ References

Aoki, Y. (2020). *Shared decision making for adults with severe mental illness: a concept analysis. Japan Journal of Nursing Science 17(4), e12365.*

Bee, P., Playle, J., Lovell, K., Barnes, P., Gray, R., and Keeley, P. (2008). *Service user views and expectations of UK-registered mental health nurses: a systematic review of empirical research. International Journal of Nursing Studies 45(3), 422–457.*

Bee, P., Price, O., Baker, J., and Lovell, K. (2015). *A systematic synthesis of barriers and facilitators to service user-led care planning. British Journal of Psychiatry 207(2), 104–114.*

Bright, F. A. S., Kayes, N. M., Worrall, L., and McPherson, K. M. (2015). *A conceptual review of engagement in healthcare and rehabilitation. Disability and Rehabilitation 37(8), 643–654.*

Castro, E. M., Regenmortel, T. V., Vanhaecht, K., and Sermeus, W. (2016). *Patient empowerment, patient participation and patient-centeredness in hospital care: a concept analysis based on a literature review. Patient Education and Counselling 99(12), 1923–1939.*

Chamberlin, J. (1997). *A working definition of empowerment. Psychiatric Rehabilitation Journal 20(4), 43–46.*

Chen, S.-P., Krupa, T., Lysaght, R., McCay, E., and Piat, M. (2013). *The development of recovery competencies for in-patient mental health providers working with people with serious mental illness. Administration and Policy in Mental Health 40(2), 96–116.*

Crandlemire, L. A. (2020). *Unconscious bias and the impacts on caring: the role of the clinical nursing instructor. International Journal for Human Caring 24(2), 84–91.*

Cutler, N. A., Sim, J., Halcomb, E., Moxham, L., and Stephens, M. (2020). *Nurses' influence on consumers' experience of safety in acute mental health units: a qualitative study. Journal of Clinical Nursing 29(21–22), 4379–4386.*

Dahlqvist-Jönsson, P., Schön, U. K., Rosenberg, D., Sandlund, M., and Svedberg, P. (2015). *Service users' experiences of participation in decision making in mental health services. Journal of Psychiatric and Mental Health Nursing 22(9), 688–697.*

Davidson, L. and Roe, D. (2007). *Recovery from versus recovery in serious mental illness: one strategy for lessening confusion plaguing recovery. Journal of Mental Health 16(4), 459–470.*

Forchuk, C. and Reynolds, W. (2001). *Clients' reflections on relationships with nurses: comparisons from Canada and Scotland, Journal of Psychiatric and Mental Health Nursing, 8, 45–51.*

Ganzini, L., Denneson, L. M., Press, N., Bair, M. J., Helmer, D. A., Poat, J., and Dobscha, S. K. (2013). *Trust is the basis for effective suicide risk screening and assessment in veterans. Journal of General Internal Medicine 28(9), 1215–1221.*

Gerace, A., Oster, C., O'Kane, D., Hayman, C. L., and Muir-Cochrane, E. (2018). *Empathic processes during nurse-consumer conflict situations in psychiatric inpatient units: a qualitative study. International Journal of Mental Health Nursing 27(1), 92–105.*

Gunasekara, I., Pentland, T., Rodgers, T., and Patterson, S. (2014). *What makes an excellent mental health nurse? A pragmatic inquiry initiated and conducted by people with lived experience of service use. International Journal of Mental Health Nursing 23(2), 101–109.*

Grundy, A. C., Bee, P., Meade, O., Callaghan, P., Beatty, S., Olleveant, N., and Lovell, K. (2016). *Bringing meaning to user involvement in mental health care planning: a qualitative exploration of service user perspectives, Journal of Psychiatric and Mental Health Nursing, 23, 12–21.*

Horgan, A., O'Donovan, M., Manning, F., Doody, R., Savage, E., Dorrity, C., O'Sullivan, H., Goodwin, J., Greaney, S., Biering, P., Bjornsson, E., Bocking, J., Russell, S., Griffin, M., MacGabhann, L., van der Vaart, K. J., Allon, J., Granerud, A., Hals, E., ... Happell, B. (2021). *'Meet me where I am': mental health service users' perspectives on the desirable qualities of a mental health nurse. International Journal of Mental Health Nursing 30(1), 136–147.*

Insua-Summerhays, B., Hart, A., Plummer, E., Priebe, S., and Barnicot, K. (2018). *Staff and patient perspectives on therapeutic engagement during one-to-one observation. Journal of Psychiatric and Mental Health Nursing 25(9–10), 546–557.*

Majid, U. (2020). *The dimensions of tokenism in patient and family engagement: a concept analysis of the literature. Journal of Patient Experience 7(6), 1610–1620.*

Majid, U. and Gagliardi, A. (2019). *Clarifying the degrees, modes, and muddles of 'meaningful' patient engagement in health services planning and designing. Patient Education and Counselling 102(9), 1581–1589.*

McAllister, S., Robert, G., Tsianakas, V., and McCrae, N. (2019) Conceptualising nurse-patient engagement on acute mental health wards: An integrative review, *International Journal of Nursing Studies,* 93, 106–118.

Mead, N. and Bower, P. (2000). *Patient-centredness: a conceptual framework and review of the empirical literature. Social Science & Medicine 51(7), 1087–1110.*

Molin, J., Graneheim, U. H., and Lindgren, B.-M. (2016). *Quality of interactions influences everyday life in psychiatric inpatient care—patients' perspectives. International Journal of Qualitative Studies on Health and Well-being 11(1), 29897.*

Polacek, M. J., Allen, D. E., Damin-Moss, R. S., Schwartz, A. J. A., Sharp, D., Shattell, M., Souther, J., and Delaney, K. R. (2015). *Engagement as an element of safe inpatient psychiatric environments. Journal of the American Psychiatric Nurses Association 21(3), 181–190.*

Recovery in the Bin, Edwards, B. M., Burgess, R., and Thomas, E. (2019, 13 September). *Neorecovery: A Survivor Led Conceptualisation and Critique [Transcript]. Keynote presented at the 25th International Mental Health Nursing Research Conference, The Royal College of Nursing, London, UK. Available at: https://recoveryinthebin.org/2019/09/16/__trashed-2/*

Reid, R., Escott, P., and Isobel, S. (2018). *Collaboration as a process and an outcome: consumer experiences of collaborating with nurses in care planning in an acute inpatient mental health unit. International Journal of Mental Health Nursing 27(4), 1204–1211.*

Rio, J. H. M., Fuller, J., Taylor, K., and Muir-Cochrane, E. (2020). *A lack of therapeutic engagement and consumer input in acute inpatient care planning limits*

fully accountable mental health nursing practice. *International Journal of Mental Health Nursing 29(2), 290–298.*

Romeu-Labayen, M., Tort-Nasaree, G., Cuadra, M., Palou, R. G., and Galbany-Estragues, P. (2022). *The attitudes of mental health nurses that support a positive therapeutic relationship: the perspective of people diagnosed with BPD. Journal of Psychiatric and Mental Health Nursing 29(2), 317–326.*

Slade, M. (2017). *Implementing shared decision making in routine mental health care. World Psychiatry 16(2), 146–153.*

Shattell, M. M., Starr, S. S., and Thomas, S. P. (2007). *'Take my hand, help me out': mental health service recipients' experience of the therapeutic relationship. International Journal of Mental Health Nursing 16(4), 274–284.*

Stewart, D., Burrow, H., Duckworth, A., Dhillon, J., Fife, S., Kelly, S., Marsh-Picksley, S., Massey, E., O'Sullivan, J., Qureshi, M., Wright, S., & Bowers, L. (2015). *Thematic analysis of psychiatric patients' perceptions of nursing staff. International Journal of Mental Health Nursing 24(1), 82–90.*

Terry, J. and Coffey, M. (2019). *Too busy to talk: examining service user involvement in nursing work. Issues in Mental Health Nursing 40(11), 957–965.*

Thompson, A. G. H. (2007). *The meaning of patient involvement and participation in health care consultations: a taxonomy. Social Science & Medicine 64(6), 1297–1310.*

Wright, N., Callaghan, P., and Bartlett, P. (2011). *Mental health service users' and practitioners' experience of engagement in assertive outreach: a qualitative study, Journal of Psychiatric and Mental Health Nursing 18(9), 822–832.*

Wyder, M., Bland, R., and Crompton, D. (2013). *Personal recovery and involuntary mental health admissions: the importance of control, relationships and hope. Health 5(3), 574–581.*

② Values-based mental health nursing

Isaac Tuffour

Learning outcomes

By the end of this chapter, you should be able to:

1 Understand various concepts attributed to values

2 Know what values-based practice means in contemporary mental health nursing

3 Understand clinical skills needed to deliver values-based practice in mental health nursing.

▼ Introduction

Before we look at value-based mental health nursing in depth, let's start to explore and understand our own values and the values of those with whom we are working.

We all have distinct values. Our personal values are shaped by our culture, individual beliefs, prejudices, myths, life experiences, and societal influences which serve as a driving force (or incentive) for our actions. Despite this, explaining our values to others might be challenging. You can help to clarify your values by providing opportunities to explore and recognize them. This is true for both users and caregivers of mental health services, as well as all those seeking to provide mental health care.

Through the process of exploration, sometimes you may discover that service users, carers, or those working to help them—whether an advocate, social worker, psychologist, mental health nurse, occupational therapist, doctor, or a manager of services—share your values. However, there will be moments when you recognize that the values of other professionals involved in the care process differ and may be at odds. When this happens, you may be unsure of what to do.

Values are diverse and multifaceted. Therefore, the main purpose of this chapter is to help you develop an understanding that the core of values-based practice is mutual respect for diversity of values (Fulford, 2013). As an accountable

and responsible professional mental health nurse, who abides by a professional code of conduct, you will need to bring several skills to bear to manage the conflict of values. These skills include self-awareness, reasoning, knowledge, and, to embrace difference and resolve conflict, skills in communication, negotiation, and working in partnership respectfully, with all parties (Woodbridge and Fulford, 2004).

Because of the diversity of values, we cannot and should not try to prescribe acceptable or appropriate values outside of broad frames of shared values, such as the first category of the *Best Practice Competencies and Capabilities for Pre-Registration Mental Health Nurses in England: The Chief Nursing Officer's Review of Mental Health Nursing*—putting values into practice—that requires students, at the point of registration, to identify and demonstrate their understanding of the key values and principles, and to apply this values base 'to promote a culture that values and respects the diversity of individuals and enables their recovery' (Department of Health, 2006, p. 5). Alternatively, the values of the 'six Cs' of nursing—Care, Compassion, Communication, Courage, Competence, and Commitment—articulated in *Compassion in Practice: Nursing, Midwifery, and Care Staff: Our Vision and Strategy* (Department of Health, 2012) is for nurses to prioritize patients as individuals. Furthermore, the NHS Constitution (Table 2.1) identifies six values that all health care professionals must uphold

Table 2.1 The NHS Constitution

Working together for patients	Patients come first in everything we do
Respect and dignity	We value every person—whether patient, their families or carers, or staff—as an individual, respect their aspirations and commitments in life, and seek to understand their priorities, needs, abilities, and limits
Commitment to quality of care	We earn the trust placed in us by insisting on quality and striving to get the basics of quality of care—safety, effectiveness, and patient experience—right every time
Compassion	We ensure that compassion is central to the care we provide and respond with humanity and kindness to each person's pain, distress, anxiety, or need
Improving lives	We strive to improve health and well-being and people's experiences of the NHS
Everyone counts	We maximize our resources for the benefit of the whole community, and make sure nobody is excluded, discriminated against, or left behind

Source: data from Department of Health and Social Care (2021). *The NHS Constitution for England*. Available at: https://www.gov.uk/government/publications/the-nhs-constitution-for-england/the-nhs-constitution-for-england

to provide the best possible care to patients (Department of Health and Social Care, 2021).

Similarly, the *Mental Health Nursing Competence and Career Framework* guides qualified nurses and mental health nursing students in providing modern and transformational care to ensure that people with mental health difficulties are treated with dignity, respect, and receive the care and support they need and deserve (Higher Education England, 2020).

▼ What are values?

According to Fulford (2011), the term 'values' in health care is commonly associated with 'ethical values'. However, Morgan et al. (2016) state that the word has many different meanings, and synonyms like 'ethics', 'principles', 'morals', 'virtues', and 'standards' are sometimes used instead. As a result, the term might be criticized as a nebulous and abstract concept. Table 2.2 gives us a definition of each of these terms.

Morgan et al. (2016) tell us that values can signify different things to different people in different professional, cultural, and historical settings. This, of course, complicates the meaning of values. Table 2.3 shows lists of words/phrases associated with values by health care workers during values-based practice training workshops.

It is indeed important to remember, though, that values in health care are not only understood through the perspective of individual professions. Many essential values are shared. For example, the values of patient autonomy (freedom of choice) and acting in the person's best interests are widely shared values (as seen in Table 2.3), and it is these common values that create the foundation for ethical codes and guidelines (Fulford, 2011) like the Nursing and Midwifery Council (NMC) Code of professional standards of practice and behaviour (NMC, 2018).

Identifying your personal values

Table 2.2 shows lists of words/phrases associated with values by people with health care backgrounds during values-based practice training workshops (from Morgan et al., 2016, p. 45). Before exploring the meaning of values-based practice in mental health, it may be useful to reflect on your personal understanding of the term 'values', by going to the companion website and completing the activity in exercise 1, adapted from Morgan et al. (2016).

Table 2.2 List of words/phrases associated with values

List 1	List 2	List 3
Core beliefs	Concepts which govern ethics	What you believe in
Your perspective on the world	Right and wrong	Self-esteem
Principles—cultural, individual	Belief systems	Principles
Justice	Ideals and priorities	Integrity
Anything that's valued	Govern behaviour and decisions	Openness/honesty
Integral to being human	Community health—individuals, society, culture	Personal motivating force
Quality of life	Ideals	Primary reference point
Right to be heard	Morals	Ethics
Social values	Principles	Virtues
Self-respect	Standards	Sharing
Valuing neighbours	Conscience	Touchstones/bases
Guiding you	Fluid/changeable	Willing to sacrifice for
Core beliefs		Self-interested tenets
		Areas of negotiation in relationships

Reproduced from Morgan, A., Felton, A., Fulford, K. W. M., Kalathil, J., and Stacey, G. (2016). *Values and Ethics in Mental Health: An Exploration for Practice*. London: Palgrave Ch 4. Copyright © Alastair Morgan, Anne Felton, Bill (K. W. M.) Fulford, Jayasree Kalathil, and Gemma Stacey 2016.

Diversity of values, law, and ethics

In nursing, the NMC Code (NMC, 2018) provides codes or frameworks that inform our professional engagement with mental health users and carers. One might expect that users' and carers' values may differ from our professional values, as they are based on the unique importance each individual user (or carer) attaches to their personal wishes, desires, thoughts, feelings, needs, behaviour, and relationships. As a result, you must learn to deal sensitively with a diversity of values and make balanced judgements in different contexts (Morgan et al., 2016). However, you must always remember that values that drive practice should always take precedence over your personal values (Fulford, 2011).

You should be aware of several key pieces of anti-discrimination legislations that influence mental health care decisions and values. The Human Rights Act 1998 (Equality and Human Rights Commission, 2018), the Equality Act 2010, and the UN Convention on the Rights of Persons with Disabilities (Equality and Human Rights Commission, 2020), which the UK has ratified, are among these

Table 2.3 Words/phrases associated with values in health care

Concept	Definition
Values	Goals and beliefs that establish a behaviour and guide decision-making (Chitty and Black, 2007)
Ethics	Moral principles on how we should live (Morgan et al., 2016)
Principle	A moral rule or a strong belief that influences your actions (Oxford Learner's Dictionaries, 2022a)
Morals	The inquiry into 'norms or values, about ideas of right and wrong, good and bad, what should and what should not be done' (Raphael, 1981, p. 8)
Virtue	'An acquired human quality the possession and exercise of which tends to enable us to achieve those goods internal to practices and the lack of which effectively prevents us from achieving any such goods' (MacIntyre, 1985, p. 191)
Standards	A level of behaviour that someone considers to be morally acceptable (Oxford Learner's Dictionaries, 2022b)

Box 2.1 The four basic principles of ethics

Autonomy: respecting and supporting decisions made with autonomy.

Beneficence: relieving, lessening, or preventing harm and providing benefits balanced against risk and cost.

Non-maleficence: avoiding causing harm.

Justice: fairly distributing benefits, risks and costs.

Source: data from Beauchamp, T. L. and Childress, J. F. (2013). *Principles of Biomedical Ethics*, 7th ed. New York: Oxford University Press, p. 13.

anti-discriminatory laws and statutes. The Mental Health Act 1983 (Department of Health, 2015), and the Mental Capacity Act 2005 (Department of Constitutional Affairs, 2007) are two essential laws that are relevant to your practice.

Furthermore, remember that having a good character is important for your nursing practice (Newham, 2015). But, to make ethical decisions that protect your service users and practice, you must also have a strong awareness of ethical theories surrounding health care. Your practice must revolve around the four basic principles of ethics: respect for autonomy, beneficence, non-maleficence, and justice outlined by Beauchamp and Childress (2013) (summarized in Box 2.1).

Dignity, confidentiality, consent, competency, cooperation, accountability, and trustworthiness are some ethical issues articulated in the NMC Code (NMC, 2018) that you must also comply with in your dealings with service users.

▼ What is values-based practice?

Values-based practice can be defined as:

a personalized care, where patients' [service users'] expectations and needs are included in a holistic approach of medicine [mental health nursing] that considers physical, mental, and spiritual well-being. Physicians [mental health nurses] and patients [service users] should change their points of view, implementing a new process of care where they are actively and equally involved, each of them with their expertise: one with clinical knowledge and the other with his/her life. They are experts of different but equally important subjects. (Marzorati and Pravettoni, 2017, p. 104)

This definition implies that values-based practice is not a recipe for 'anything goes'. It is person centred. Also, the approach reflects the diversity of clinicians' and patients' values, it is evidence based, and it operates within the framework of shared values (Fulford, 2011). In this regard, values-based mental health nursing practice can be defined as an evidence-based practice that respects a person's uniqueness while demonstrating understanding, reciprocity, and shared decision-making. It is a collaborative endeavour helping to consider service users' values and preferences.

Elements of values-based practice

In Figure 2.1, Morgan et al. (2016) illustrate some elements of values-based practice in mental health. As shown in Figure 2.1, values are often complex and conflicting, so the starting point of values-based practice in mental health nursing is mutual respect of individuality. The values relevant to a given circumstance are then brought to the foreground of our thinking via crucial clinical abilities such as awareness, reasoning, knowledge, communication, professional relationships, and collaboration within frameworks of shared values, evidence, and clinical decision-making (Morgan et al., 2016). Table 2.4 also provides the same values-based practice items as Figure 2.1. As Morgan et al. (2016) point out, values-based practice is all about building on best practices. It is critical that you incorporate some of the concepts mentioned in this chapter into your own thinking about best practice.

The NIMHE values framework

The National Institute for Mental Health in England (NIMHE) (2004) created a ground-breaking values framework (Box 2.2) that is built on three principles of values-based practice—recognition, raising awareness, and

Features of values	Values-based practice
The variety of values	Starting point is... Mutual respect for differences of values
Foreground and background Complex and conflicting Shared values	Process involves... • Clinical skills • Professional relationships • Links between values and evidence • Partnership
Guide clinical decision making	Outputs are... Balanced decisions in individual situations

Figure 2.1 From values to values-based practice

Reproduced from Morgan, A., Felton, A., Fulford, K. W. M., Kalathil, J., and Stacey, G. (2016). *Values and Ethics in Mental Health: An Exploration for Practice*. London: Palgrave, Ch 4. Copyright © Alastair Morgan, Anne Felton, Bill (K. W. M.) Fulford, Jayasree Kalathil, and Gemma Stacey 2016.

Table 2.4 The clinical skills for values-based practice

Elements of values-based practice	Make brief comments next to each element
Premise of mutual respect	
Skills areas	
1 Awareness	
2 Reasoning	
3 Knowledge	
4 Communication	
Professional relationships	
5 Person-values-centred care	
6 Extended multidisciplinary team	
Values and evidence	
7 Two feet principle	
8 Squeaky wheel principle	
9 Science-driven principle	
Partnership	
10 Dissensus within frameworks of shared values`	
Balanced decisions in individual situations	

Reproduced from Morgan, A., Felton, A., Fulford, K. W. M., Kalathil, J., and Stacey, G. (2016). *Values and Ethics in Mental Health: An Exploration for Practice*. Palgrave, London, Ch 4. Copyright © Alastair Morgan, Anne Felton, Bill (K. W. M.) Fulford, Jayasree Kalathil, and Gemma Stacey 2016.

respect—and serves as the foundation for recovery practice. Even though the NIMHE is no longer in existence, it had a strong commitment to user-led service development, and its values framework remains relevant for values-based practice (Morgan et al., 2016).

Clinical skills needed for values-based practice

As outlined by Morgan et al. (2016), Table 2.5 summarizes the four clinical skills necessary for value-based practice: awareness of values, reasoning about values, knowledge of values, and communication skills.

Box 2.2 The NIMHE values framework

1 Recognition: NIMHE recognises the role of values alongside evidence in all areas of mental health policy and practice.

2 Raising awareness: NIMHE is committed to raising awareness of the values involved in different contexts, the role/s they play and their impact on practice in mental health.

3 Respect: NIMHE respects diversity of values and will support ways of working with such diversity that makes the principle of service user centrality a unifying focus for practice. This means that the values of each individual service user/client and their communities must be the starting point and key determinant for all actions by professionals.

Respect for diversity of values encompasses several specific policies and principles concerned with equality of citizenship. It is anti-discriminatory because discrimination in all its forms is intolerant of diversity. Thus, respect for diversity of values has the consequence that it is unacceptable (and unlawful in some instances) to discriminate on grounds such as gender, sexual orientation, class, age, abilities, religion, race, culture, or language. Respect for diversity within mental health is also:

- User-centred—it puts respect for the values of individual users at the centre of policy and practice.

- Recovery-oriented—it recognizes that building on the personal strengths and resiliencies of individual users, and on their cultural and racial characteristics, there are many diverse routes to recovery.

- Multidisciplinary—it requires that respect be reciprocal, at a personal level (between service users, their family members, friends, communities and providers), between different provider disciplines (such as nursing, psychology, psychiatry, medicine, social work) and between different organizations (including health, social care, local authority housing, voluntary organizations, community groups, faith communities and other social support services).

- Dynamic—it is open and responsive to change.

- Reflective—it combines self-monitoring and self-management with positive self-regard.

- Balanced—it emphasizes positive as well as negative values.

- Relational—it puts positive working relationships supported by good communication skills at the heart of practice. NIMHE will encourage educational and research initiatives aimed at developing the capabilities (the awareness, attitudes, knowledge and skills) needed to deliver mental health services that will give effect to the principles of values-based practice.

Reproduced from National Institute for Mental Health in England, Sainsbury Centre for Mental Health, and the National Health Service University (2004). The national framework of values for mental health. In: *The Ten Essential Shared Capabilities: A Framework for the Whole of the Mental Health Workforce*. London: Department of Health.

▼ Person-values-centred care

'Person-centred care' is a buzzword in modern health care that has diverse meanings depending on the context (Morgan et al., 2016). In medicine, 'personalized medicine' is frequently used to replace person-centred care (Fulford et al., 2012). In mental health settings, person-centred care refers to putting the needs of the service user, rather than the concerns of the service, at the centre of decision-making, work planning, and delivery (Morgan et al., 2016). The bedrock of your mental health nursing practice should be person-centred care. Fulford and Woodbridge (2008)

report that service users'/survivors' values can get buried in the background of clinical decision-making. Person-values-centred care is about expressing genuine interest in what matters most to the service user, rather than imposing your assumptions (Morgan et al., 2016). To do so, you must possess strong therapeutic communication skills as well as knowledge of Rogers' (1979) three basic therapeutic relationship conditions—congruence/genuineness, empathy, and unconditional positive regard—to understand their values.

Table 2.5 Four clinical skills necessary for value-based practice

Awareness of values	This includes a greater understanding of values and their variation. It includes an understanding of the often-surprising extent to which other people's values differ from our own. The first step towards wisdom in values-based practice is to acknowledge that we all make assumptions about each other's values, and that these assumptions are frequently incorrect
	It is critical that we become more aware of our own values so that they do not overshadow those of the service users/survivors with whom we are working with. It is always critical to keep the values of service users at the forefront of our minds
Reasoning about values	Values reasoning differs from other types of reasoning in that it is used to help us comprehend the values at play in a specific circumstance rather than to find answers
Knowledge of values	Knowledge, including research knowledge, can assist in predicting which values are likely to be at play in each situation
	The most important thing to remember about research understanding of values is that it should never be utilized to override or replace the individual's actual values
	Everyone is different. As a result, research can assist us by indicating the values that are likely to be present in a certain situation. However, you should never go from the general to the particular.
	For example, we run the risk of generalizing from the group to the individual in some cultural contexts. We shouldn't assume that just because someone is a Muslim, they exclusively eat Halal meat
Communication skills	Communication skills are crucial in values-based practice as well as any other area of health care, particularly for eliciting values and resolving conflicts

Source: data from Morgan, A., Felton, A., Fulford, K. W. M., Kalathil, J., and Stacey, G. (2016). *Values and Ethics in Mental Health: An Exploration for Practice*. London: Palgrave.

▼ Maintaining values in practice

You will face various challenges as a mental health nurse. For example, you will be expected to make critical decisions about service users daily; however, to be able to make the best decisions, you must be able to grasp the principles of good clinical decision-making and the choices that will benefit the service user. A seminal work by Curtis et al. (2012) revealed that students reported feeling vulnerable due the dissonance between professional ideals and practice reality. Morgan et al. (2016) state that organizational and structural constraints, conflict, compliance, and conformity are some of the challenges that will be there throughout your career.

Making ethical and legal decisions about service users' care is rarely simple in mental health nursing, especially when it comes to truth-telling (Edwards, 2014). In mental health

nursing, truth-telling is an essential component of the service user–clinician relationship; without it, the clinician risks losing the service user's trust (Varky, 2019). However, despite the emphasis on patient autonomy, a time may come that you believe that telling the service user the truth is the correct thing to do, but you may feel constrained by expectations of colleagues, or by what the patient's family have requested (Edwards, 2014). The conundrum is, while the NMC Code (NMC, 2018) is quite clear on this matter, directing you to 'act with honesty and integrity at all times' (p. 18), it also instructs you to 'work co-operatively … respect the skills, expertise, and contributions of your colleagues, referring matters to them when appropriate' (p. 10). As a novice or experienced practitioner, you may find yourself floundering in scenarios like this. However, you can rest assured that telling the truth to service users would not breach any laws or (possible) any NMC Code of professional standards and behaviour, because acting honestly implies telling the truth (Edwards, 2014).

Remember that recognizing and embracing the challenges in practice, raising awareness of values (see Morgan et al. (2016, p. 228) for a comprehensive list of the resources for raising awareness of values), teamwork, dissension processes that allow for the existence of different values, upholding of human rights, mutual respect, and embracing policies that support values-based mental health practice and recovery practice are all important impetuses for maintaining your values in practice (Morgan et al., 2016). These are important 'values journeys' that provide you with the opportunity to learn and become a competent practitioner as you are exposed to clinical practice (Callwood et al., 2019).

▲ Conclusion

This chapter has examined many different meanings and synonyms for values. It reveals that discussions of values involve many terms, such as ethics, principles, morals, virtues, and standards. Values mean different things in different contexts. As a result, the term could be interpreted as ambiguous. Despite the ambiguity, many essential health care values are shared, and professional values always take precedence over personal values.

Some general and specific laws, as well as ethical principles driving mental health care decisions and values have been explored. Words and phrases have been presented to help you identify your personal values. The definition of values-based practice has been discussed and applied to the mental health sector.

Frameworks and clinical skills required for values-based practice in mental health nursing have been explored. It has been suggested that person-centred care should be the bedrock of your mental health nursing practice.

✖ Tips from service users

1 I would like to be treated as an individual with unique values. Nurses should not assume that all people from the same ethnic group have the same values.
2 My beliefs on causes of my mental illness must be accommodated when planning my care. Also, because I am an expert on my values, I am eager to collaborate in the creation of my own unique/individual care.
3 Mental health nurses should feel free to challenge some of my values if they negatively impact my well-being.

W   Companion website

For extra resources on the topics covered in this chapter, visit the companion website at: www.oup.com/mhns

✚   References

Beauchamp, T. L. and Childress, J. F. (2013). *Principles of Biomedical Ethics*, 7th ed. New York: Oxford University Press.

Callwood, A., Groothuizen, J. E., and Allan, H. T. (2019). *The 'values journey' of nursing and midwifery students* selected using multiple mini interviews; year two findings. *Journal of Advanced Nursing 75(5), 1074–1084.*

Chitty, K. K. and Black, B. P. (2007). *Professional Nursing: Concepts and Challenges, 5th ed. St. Louis, MO: Saunders/Elsevier.*

Curtis, K., Horton, K., and Smith, P. (2012). *Student nurse socialization in compassionate practice: a grounded theory study. Nurse Education Today 32(7), 790–795.*

Department of Constitutional Affairs (2007). *The Mental Capacity Act 2005 Code of Practice. London: The Stationery Office.*

Department of Health (2006). *Best Practice Competencies and Capabilities for Pre-Registration Mental Health Nurses in England: The Chief Nursing Officer's Review of Mental Health Nursing. London: Department of Health.*

Department of Health (2012). *Compassion in Practice: Nursing, Midwifery and Care Staff: Our Vision and Strategy. Available at: https://www.england.nhs. uk/wp-content/uploads/2012/12/compassion-in-pract ice.pdf*

Department of Health (2015). *Mental Health Act 1983: Code of Practice. Available at: https://assets.pub lishing.service.gov.uk/government/uploads/system/uplo ads/attachment_data/file/435512/MHA_Code_of_Pract ice.PDF*

Department of Health and Social Care (2021). *The NHS Constitution for England. Available at: https://www.gov. uk/government/publications/the-nhs-constitution-for- england/the-nhs-constitution-for-england*

Edwards, S. (2014). *Telling the truth? Nursing Ethics 21(4), 383–384.*

Equality and Human Rights Commission (2018). *The Human Rights Act. Available at: https://www.equality humanrights.com/en/human-rights/human-rights-act*

Equality and Human Rights Commission (2020). *UN Convention on the Rights of Persons with Disabilities (CRPD). Available at: https://www.equalityhumanrights. com/our-work/our-human-rights-work/monitoring-and- promoting-un-treaties/un-convention-rights-persons*

Fulford, K. W. M. (2008). *Values-based practice: a new partner to evidence-based practice and a first for psychiatry? Mens Sana Monographs 6(1), 10–21.*

Fulford, K. W. M. (2011). *The value of evidence and evidence of values. Journal of Evaluation in Clinical Practice 17(5), 976–987.*

Fulford, K. W. M. (2013). *Values-based practice: Fulford's dangerous idea. Journal of Evaluation in Clinical Practice 19(3), 537–546.*

Fulford, K. W. M. and Woodbridge, K. (2008). *Practicing ethically: values-based practice and ethics—working together to support person-centred and multidisciplinary mental health care. In: T. Stickley and T. Basset, Eds., Learning About Mental Health Practice, pp. 79–103. Chichester: Wiley.*

Higher Education England (2020). *Mental Health Nursing Competence and Career Framework. London: Higher Education England.*

MacIntyre, A. (1985). *After Virtue, 2nd ed. London: Gerald Duckworth & Co., Ltd.*

Marzorati, C. and Pravettoni, G. (2017). *Value as the key concept in the health care system: how it has influenced medical practice and clinical decision-making processes. Journal of Multidisciplinary Healthcare 10, 101–106.*

Mental Health Taskforce (2016). *Five-Year Forward View for Mental Health. NHS England. Available at: https://www.england.nhs.uk/wp-content/uploads/ 2016/02/Mental-Health-Taskforce-FYFV-final.pdf*

Morgan, A., Felton, A., Fulford, K. W. M., Kalathil, J., and Stacey, G. (2016). *Values and Ethics in Mental Health: An Exploration for Practice. London: Palgrave.*

National Institute for Mental Health in England, Sainsbury Centre for Mental Health, and the National Health Service University (2004). *The national framework of values for mental health. In: The Ten Essential Shared Capabilities: A Framework for the Whole of the Mental Health Workforce, Appendix B. London: Department of Health.*

Newham, R. (2015). *Virtue ethics and nursing: on what grounds? Nursing Philosophy 16(1), 126–141.*

NHS Health Education England (2022). *Commitment and Growth: Advancing Mental Health Nursing Now and for the Future: Baroness Watkins of Tavistock Review of Mental Health Nursing in England. London: Health Education England.*

Nursing and Midwifery Council (2018). *The Code: Professional Standards of Practice and*

Behaviour for Nurses, Midwives and Nursing Associates. London: Nursing and Midwifery Council.

Oxford Learner's Dictionaries (2022a). *Principle. Oxford University Press. Available at: https://www.oxfordlearn ersdictionaries.com/definition/english/principle?q=Pri nciples*

Oxford Learner's Dictionaries (2022b). *Standard. Oxford University Press. Available at: https://www.oxfordlearn ersdictionaries.com/definition/english/standard_1?q= standard*

Raphael, D. D. (1981). *Moral Philosophy. Oxford: Oxford University Press.*

Rogers, C. R. (1979). *The foundations of the person-centered approach. Education 100(2) 98–107.*

Varkey, B. (2019). *Principles of clinical ethics and their application to practice. Medical Principles and Practice 30(1), 17–28.*

Woodbridge, K. and Fulford, K. W. M. (2004). *Whose Values? A Workbook for Values-Based Practice in Mental Health Care. London: Sainsbury Centre for Mental Health.*

3 Evidence-based mental health nursing practice

Patrick Callaghan   Paul Crawford

Learning outcomes

By the end of this chapter, you should be able to:

1 Describe the contested issues about evidence-based practice

2 Evaluate published evidence

3 Demonstrate your critiquing skills in academic work

4 Use evidence in practice.

▼ Introduction

The use of informed, up-to-date, high-quality evidence underlies every nursing interaction. Mental health nurses are increasingly called to account for their own practice in terms of evidence, and students need to master the skills of evaluating published evidence and guidelines, understanding the research process, and utilizing these to deliver best practice. The concept of the individual as a self-governing entity responsible for his or her own education, development, and evidence-based practice (EBP) is central to several initiatives that promote quality of care and service delivery (e.g. B. Brown and Crawford, 2003; S. Brown, 2018; Jolley, 2020). EBP has been embraced by health services as the antidote to ritualistic and 'outdated' practice, inappropriate variations in care delivery, and ineffective and wasteful service provision.

In this chapter we will describe the origins of EBP, examine contested issues about EBP, and show you how to evaluate published evidence.

▼ What is evidence-based practice?

In beginning to identify criteria against which to evaluate published evidence, you need to appreciate that there are two main models (or paradigms) for gaining knowledge of the world: positivism or quantitative research, and interpretivism or quantifiable research. Positivism seeks to establish universal laws and views knowledge as reducible to observable positive facts and numbers and the relations between them—it goes forth and quantifies (numbers-based research). Interpretivism seeks to understand the social world as actively constructed by human beings who are continuously making sense of or interpreting our social environments—it goes forth and qualifies (words-based research) (B. Brown et al., 2003).

Adopting one or other of these approaches, or combining them, shapes how we go about gathering knowledge. The choice taken by researchers will say something about their values and beliefs about the nature and utility of evidence. Unfortunately, over many years there have been heated debates about which is the best kind of research and what constitutes valid 'evidence' (Crawford et al., 2002), and objections have been raised to hierarchies of evidence. Indeed, many practitioners have complained that EBP demotes the evidence of clinical experience, or what has been called practice-based evidence, or 'overrules' the preferences of clients and patients.

Research, then, is not a single, straightforward entity—it is a competitive field in which accounts of 'what is what', 'what causes what', or 'what relates to what' are contested and preferred. Furthermore, the continuum of confidence in research can run from the idea that we can build knowledge 'upon a set of firm, unquestionable … indisputable truths' (Hughes and Sharrock, 1997, pp. 4–5)—so-called foundationalism—to an emphasis of the provisional nature of knowledge or, indeed, the impossibility of arriving at any truths at all—so-called anti-foundationalism. In beginning to critique research, a key starting point is to identify the underlying paradigm of any given study and to be aware of the researcher's 'take' on, or 'framing' of, evidence. This requires 'philosophy' skills from the student, identifying the kinds of thinking and wisdom behind attempts to gain knowledge of the world.

Nevertheless, there is evidence that EBP produces better patient outcomes (Connor et al., 2023), and a key example of high-quality care (Lehane et al., 2019).

There is considerable variation in how the concept of EBP is defined and described (e.g. Coyler and Kamath, 1999;

Box 3.1 Definition of evidence-based nursing

The conscientious, explicit and judicious use of theory-derived, evidence-based information, such as published empirical research, informed, expert opinion, anecdotes, clinical case studies, service users' preferences and expert opinion in making decisions about care delivery to individual service users, or groups of service users and in consideration of their individual needs and preferences.

Callaghan and Carter (2022), modified from
Ingersoll (2000, p. 151)

Evidence-based practice is the process by which nurses make clinical decisions using the best available research evidence, their clinical expertise and patient preferences, in the context of available resources.

DiCenso et al. (1998, p. 38)

McKenna et al., 2000). However, a useful definition that captures the range of views of evidence-based (mental health) nursing is shown in Box 3.1. The pursuit of EBP comprises several components, which are shown in Box 3.2.

Gray (1997) argues that patient care decisions are based on evidence, values, and resources. He goes on to state that the

Box 3.2 The components of evidence-based practice

- Clinical guidelines
- Patient and public choice
- Information on epidemiology
- Success or failure of certain interventions
- Evidence-based purchasing, reflecting audit outcomes and performance measures
- Health service management

- Organizational audit
- Financial audit and guidelines
- Education and training
- Curricula based on best available evidence
- Translating evidence to practice
- Skills in assessing evidence quality.

Source: data from von Degenberg, K. (1996). Clinical guidelines: improving practice at the local level. *Nursing Standard* 10(19), 37–39; and Callaghan, P. and Carter, T. (2022). Knowledge translation and linking evidence to practice. In: A. Higgins, N. Kilkku, and G. Kort Kristofersson, Eds., *Advanced Practice in Mental Health Nursing: A European Perspective*, pp. 405–426. Cham: Springer.

Box 3.3 Skills required of an evidence-based decision-maker

- An ability to define criteria such as effectiveness, safety, and acceptability
- An ability to find articles on the effectiveness, safety, and acceptability of a new test or treatment
- An ability to assess the quality of evidence
- An ability to assess whether the results of research are generalizable to the whole population from which the sample was drawn

- An ability to assess whether the results of the research are applicable to a 'local' population.

Source: data from Gray, J. A. M. (1997). *Evidence-Based Health Care*. London: Churchill-Livingstone, p. 2, and Callaghan, P. and Carter, T. (2022). Knowledge translation and linking evidence to practice. In: A. Higgins, N. Kilkku, and G. Kort Kristofersson, Eds., *Advanced Practice in Mental Health Nursing: A European Perspective*, pp. 405–426. Cham: Springer.

optimum use of resources will be evidence based. According to Gray (1997), the evidence-based decision-maker requires several skills, as shown in Box 3.3.

In assessing the quality of any evidence, Gray suggests the following helpful questions:

1 Is this the best type of research method to address the question?

2 Is the research of adequate quality?

3 What is the size of the beneficial effect and of the adverse effect?

4 Is the research generalizable to the whole population from which the sample was drawn?

5 Are the results applicable to a 'local' population?

6 Are the results applicable to this patient?

However, answering these questions requires a sound understanding of how to evaluate published evidence. We will now move on to this issue. It is not possible here to review all the arguments and counterarguments about the philosophical 'seeding' of research or what stands as 'best' evidence (see B. Brown et al. (2003) for a wide-reaching analysis), but rather to adopt a mainstream position in presenting foundational skills in evaluating or 'critiquing' evidence. To do this we will indicate how to judge both the quantitative and qualitative evidence that is put before us or we seek out.

▼ Evaluating research

There are two main approaches to evaluating research: individual and collegial. Individual critiquing is when a student or practitioner independently reviews published research papers, whereas collegial critiquing is conducted by groups of reviewers working together. The latter has evolved in response to the daunting task of reviewing large amounts of research and the need to facilitate practitioners in using research findings as part of EBP. Collegial critiquing can be formal and programmatic, as with Cochrane (formerly the Cochrane Collaboration), the Centre for Reviews and Dissemination at York University, and through bodies such as the National Institute for Health and Care Excellence (NICE) which produce guidelines for practice based on best available evidence. But collegial evaluation can also be informal and involve groups of practitioners joining forces to review and evaluate research relevant to their own area of clinical practice.

The skills of evaluation can begin only when the student/ practitioner or group of students/practitioners have developed sufficient knowledge of the research process itself. Even then, such skills are generally developed over time and through regular practice. With sufficient background knowledge and comprehension, a series of questions can be applied to any piece of research, rather as evidence may be examined in a courtroom context. The correct questions should elicit the strengths and weaknesses of the research; assess how such research relates to professional or clinical practice; and discriminate or differentiate between quantitative and qualitative research as part of the 'philosophy' skills outlined above previously.

Evaluation is concerned with examining each of the key components to research papers and 'making a value judgement on what is reported' or 'weighing what was done against accepted practice by researchers' (Parahoo, 2006, p. 401). The components that need to be 'weighed' are as follows: abstract, research question, literature review, methodology, sample, data collection, data analysis, results, discussion, and recommendations for practice or further research.

Good practice in reporting evidence is also key to evidence-based mental health nursing. Callaghan and Carter (2022) present detailed guidance on tools that nurses can use to report evidence that journals increasingly require in published papers.

In Box 3.4 we now consider the kinds of questions that we may skilfully deploy for each of these categories in making a general critique of any research paper, before going on to look specifically at quantitative and qualitative research.

Evaluating quantitative research

You are likely to be quite new to the process of evaluating published research-based evidence. To help you in this challenging task, and because there are several different

Box 3.4 General tips on evaluating published research-based evidence

Abstract

- Does the abstract provide a clear summary of the research paper, including the research question and methods applied?
- Are the key findings and the conclusions stated?

Research question

- Does the research paper identify a question or hypothesis?
- Is the question or hypothesis followed through into the conclusion?
- Were the chosen methods appropriate to the question at hand?

Literature review

- Is the literature comprehensive and up to date?
- Are gaps in the literature identified?
- Does the literature review support the case for further research?

Methodology

- Does the research paper indicate the research approach it is taking?
- How relevant is the methodological framing of the research?

- Are the best methods applied to answer the research question?

Sample

- Is the sample size included?
- Is the sample size appropriate to the aims of the research?
- Are the characteristics of the sample described?
- Is the response rate stated?

Data collection

- What method was used to collect data?
- What is the validity and reliability of the method?

Data analysis

- Does the research paper state how the data were analysed?
- Were these methods appropriate?

Discussion/conclusion

- Does the paper provide a balanced account or discussion of the findings?
- Were the limitations of the research indicated?
- Do the conclusions match the findings?
- Were recommendations reasonable or credible?

designs within quantitative research, we recommend that you use a checklist to help you conduct your evaluation. Checklists to help you evaluate different types of quantitative research design are widely available. In Table 3.1 we summarize many different checklists and signpost you to websites where you should find these to save and print off. In addition to the resources listed in Table 3.1, the *British Medical Journal* (BMJ) published a series of 'How to read a paper' articles between 19 July and 20 September 1997 (BMJ, Volume 315), written by Professor Trisha Greenhalgh, who is widely respected in the EBP field. This series provides excellent advice on how to read and understand papers reporting various types of research. We also recommend

that you look at these articles. In addition, the EQUATOR network (https://www.equator-network.org/) contains an extensive list of checklists for evaluating and reporting different types of studies.

Evaluating qualitative research

There are multiple approaches to qualitative research, and the skilled practitioner will need to build up knowledge of these to assist in the critiquing process. All such approaches share a focus on the meaning making of humans through texts and symbols without which it

Table 3.1 Checklists for reporting quantitative research papers

Research design	Checklist	Source of checklist
Randomized controlled trial (RCT)	Revised CONSORT statement (Moher et al., 2001)	www.consort-statement.org/ Statement/revisedstatement.org
Clustered RCT	CONSORT-PLUS (Campbell et al., 2004)	www.consort-statement.org
Non-randomized evaluations	TREND (Des Jarlais et al., 2004)	www.consort-statement.org
Observational studies in epidemiology	STROBE	www.strobe-statement.org
Studies testing diagnostic accuracy	STARD initiative (Bossuyt et al., 2003)	www.consort-statement.org/ Initiatives/newstard
Meta-analysis and systematic reviews of literature	QUOROM	www.consort-statement.org/ Evidence/evidence.html#quorom
Evaluating ethical probity of study	ASSERT	www.assert-statement.org
Cohort study	12 questions to help you make sense of a cohort study	Critical Appraisal Skills Programme: http://www.phru.nhs. uk/Pages/PHD/CASP.htm
Case–control study	12 questions to help you make sense of a case–control study	Critical Appraisal Skills Programme: http://www.phru.nhs. uk/Pages/PHD/CASP.htm
Economic evaluations	10 questions to help you make sense of economic evaluations	Critical Appraisal Skills Programme: http://www.phru.nhs. uk/Pages/PHD/CASP.htm

Box 3.5 Indicative questions for assessing qualitative research

- Were the aims of the research clearly stated?
- Is a qualitative methodology appropriate and justified in this case?
- Were theory and methods sound?
- Did the researchers include the context of the study?
- Were details of sampling provided?
- Was the sample sufficiently diverse to promote transferability?
- Is it clear how the data were collected?
- Was there a clear description of analysis?
- Were multiple methods used (triangulation) to test the validity of data and analysis?

- Did a second researcher conduct a separate analysis to test the reliability of both data and analysis?
- Did the researchers critically evaluate their own influence on the research process?
- Did the researchers 'return to the field' and check out their interpretation of the data with participants?
- Do the findings clearly relate to the research question?
- Can the findings be applied in other kinds of setting?
- Is the study relevant or important?
- Does it have implications for practice?

would be impossible to share an understanding of the world. This extends to interpreting the social and cultural construction of the world, making sense of the environments, traditions, activities of people, and their lived experiences. Broadly, qualitative research analyses aspects of human life rather as a literary critic might closely interpret a book.

Qualitative research tends to involve interviews, observation, action research, or documentary analysis. Box 3.5 outlines questions that can help you make sense of published qualitative research.

Whittemore et al. (2001) and Jorgensen (2006) advocate the following as primary criteria for evaluating qualitative research:

- Credibility
- Authenticity
- Criticality
- Integrity.

Credibility (Lincoln and Guba, 2000) relates to whether the results of the research reflect the experience of the participants in a believable way. Confidence in the themes derived by researchers from interviews or focus groups is strengthened when findings are discussed subsequently with participants. This enables refinements and corrections in the light of feedback, thus addressing the challenge 'of preserving participants' definitions of reality' (Daly, 1997, p. 350) through a process of participant validation. **Authenticity** is evident when researchers retain a reflective awareness of their preconceptions and the possibility of being surprised by findings. The criteria of **criticality** and **integrity** relate to the potential for many different interpretations to be made, dependent on the assumptions and knowledge background of the investigators. This calls for researchers to review emerging themes and to establish their credibility, plausibility, and resonance with experiences beyond the confines of the original study (Horsburgh, 2003).

✖ Tips on how to demonstrate skills in evaluation when writing assignments

As a student mental health nurse, you will be required to write assignments where you are asked to evaluate ideas, arguments, or positions people take in written work. Here are some tips on how you can demonstrate skills in evaluation:

1 Compare and contrast arguments using set criteria.
2 Look for evidence supporting arguments that authors make.
3 Think of some alternatives to these arguments.
4 Cite the source of your alternatives.

5 Justify your arguments (e.g. from clinical observations, your reading of other research).
6 Judge the position being taken, not the person taking it.
7 Separate facts from opinions—your own and others'.
8 Think about what you believe, and why you believe this.
9 Identify all possible sources of material that you can draw upon in forming your argument.
10 State the criteria against which you have made your judgement.

▼ Opportunities and obstacles in the pursuit of evidence-based practice

We know that multiple factors can conspire to inhibit the appearance of EBP (Crawford et al., 2002; Ray, 1999). It is important that the student and practising mental health nurse appreciate that EBP is not a step-by-step un-problematic process of reviewing or evaluating journal research papers and then applying the evidence in practice. Alongside the kind of stepwise process of judging the quality of a piece of research discussed previously, both student and practitioner will need to utilize skills, not least those around creating partnerships, in achieving the necessary conditions for accessing and evaluating evidence in the first place and then for making good use of this evidence in practice. S. Brown (2018) draws our attention to the 'research–practice connection' that should never be taken for granted but instead developed and exploited. Research evidence is only ever as useful as its application in building new knowledge or inspiring and informing practice. In other words, there needs to be a strategy for sustainable EBP. In Table 3.2 we outline some of the opportunities and obstacles in the pursuit of EBP.

You will need to work flexibly and creatively to promote EBP in the face of such obstacles. Box 3.6 gives four tips on how to overcome these obstacles.

Table 3.2 Opportunities and obstacles in the pursuit of evidence-based health care

Opportunities	Obstacles
Improved care	'Top-down' driven
Directing resources cost-effectively	Conflicting evidence
Advancing care	Disseminating and implementing evidence
Improved research	Lack of available evidence
Increased professionalism	Cross-cultural validity
Development of clinical guidelines	Inadequate managerial support
Partnerships in care	Reliance on types of evidence
'Doing the right things and doing things right'	Lack of time to retrieve and read evidence
Drawing upon expert knowledge	Research literacy of clinician
	Lack of time
	Poor access to information
	Conflicting ideologies

Sources: data from Miles, A., Hampton, J. R., and Hurwitz, B. (Eds.) (2000). *NICE, CHI and the NHS Reforms: Enabling Excellence or Imposing Control.* London: Aesculapius Medical Press; and Renfrew, M. (1997). The development of evidence-based practice. *British Journal of Midwifery* 5(2), 100–104.

Box 3.6 How to overcome the obstacles to evidence-based practice

1 Education and skills development: in searching and judging the literature (see text), utilizing or providing clinical supervision, and promoting EBP as a multidisciplinary activity.

2 Promoting access to evidence: requesting computer access in the workplace to evidence-based information packages and guidelines on key clinical practices or interventions.

3 Negotiating time: requesting that EBP is viewed as a core, formal activity in clinical practice that requires dedicated time.

4 Networking and sharing: using 'partnership' skills in setting up or joining journal clubs or groups discussing EBP; conducting informal, collegial critiquing; networking across institutions and between trusts and higher education providers; and sharing literature reviews and empirical research conducted as part of higher education course with colleagues.

Lomas (1993) identifies four factors that are central, in his view, to getting research into practice:

1 Quality of evidence (see Table 3.1 for checklists that help you to judge the quality of evidence)

2 Credible dissemination body (see Table 3.3 and Box 3.7 for factors that inhibit and enhance dissemination)

3 Overall practice environments (see Table 3.2 for a list of opportunities)

4 Obstacles to implementing EBP and external factors (e.g. how society views the evidence and its relationship to their lives; how the media report the evidence).

A good example of the last point is the report by Kirsch et al. (2008) into the effectiveness of antidepressant drugs. This paper was published and was the main news item in national news bulletins in the UK. Most of the media summarized the report to state bluntly that antidepressants in widespread use such as fluoxetine (e.g. Prozac®) did not work according to unpublished studies. This, however, is not the key message of the study, which reports the conditions under which the drugs work (but this was not how the media reported it). An important message from this paper and its reporting in the media is the difference in outcomes from reviews of research when you include published and unpublished studies. Unpublished studies are often hard to find and subsequently are excluded from reviews, but they often report negative findings. In many respects, what Lomas (1993) is suggesting makes sense. Table 3.3 shows how to introduce change effectively and the impediments to the change (Davies, 1999; Granados et al., 1997; Joyce, 1999).

Systematic reviews of literature are useful sources to a clinician with little time for reading as they often summarize a lot of literature in one paper. Based on a review of systematic reviews, we are better informed as to effective methods of getting evidence into practice. See Box 3.7.

▲ Conclusion

The premise that mental health nursing care should be based on the best available evidence is sound, but it is unclear at what point enough evidence is gathered to justify a clinical decision. Although integrating clinical acumen with current best evidence is our best hope of improving mental health nurses' competence and care, health problems are not neatly resolved by recourse to research trials and hierarchies of evidence. Questions relating to the care of patients are not all answered by science; health care is at the interface of many disciplines, and to understand fully the experience of health and ill health we need to draw from many types of evidence. In terms of getting evidence into practice, diffusion is the most common, but

least effective, approach. Methods to disseminate and implement evidence need to be (inter)active processes; dissemination and implementation involve change, and this takes time, resources, pragmatism, and flexibility. Furthermore, the sheer busyness of health care and its complexity does not lend itself to easy application of research evidence to practice. On this basis, Jolley (2020) argues that we need more so-called implementation-ready evidence that meets the standard of scientific criteria, and which takes us further than non-research or anecdotal forms of evidence alone, such as peer review, clinical audit, benchmarking, established clinical expertise, tradition, experience, policy, and guidelines.

Table 3.3 Enabling and inhibiting change

Introducing effective change	Impediments to effective change
Opinion leaders	Unclear objectives
Audit	Inappropriate means, messages, communicators, populations, incentives, timescales, and resources
Feedback	Top-down approaches
Informal education	Hierarchical and autocratic initiatives
Clinical guidelines	Advantage of introducing change is not clear
Financial incentives	Proposed change is incompatible with current beliefs and working practices
Role modelling	Proposed change increases complexity of clinical practice
Reflection on action	Perverse incentives
Action learning groups	Distortions of perception of risk
Research awareness groups	Lobbying by special interest groups
Timing	Bureaucratic manoeuvring
Direct contact with staff	Poor reward systems
Concise policy documents	Uncertainty of science—policymakers want certainty
Clear and compelling presentation style	Timing
Mass media	Peer pressure
	Lack of self-efficacy
	Information overload
	Opinion leaders with opposing views

Box 3.7 What works? Evidence-based methods of effective dissemination and implementation

Consistently effective interventions

- Educational outreach visits
- Reminders
- Multifaceted interventions, such as two or more of audit and feedback, reminders, local consensus processes, marketing (e.g. 'Closing the gap between research and practice: an overview of …')
- Interactive educational meetings.

Interventions of variable effectiveness

- Audit and feedback
- Local opinion leaders
- Local consensus processes
- Patient-mediated interventions.

Interventions that have little or no effect

- Simply providing educational materials
- Didactic educational meetings.

Sources: data from Bero, L. A., Grilli, R., Grimshaw, J. M., Harvey, E., Oxman, A. D., and Thomson, M. A. (1997). Closing the gap between research and practice: an overview of systematic reviews of interventions to promote the implementation of research findings. *British Medical Journal* 317(7156), 465–468; Cheung, A., Weir, M., Mayhew, A. Kozloff, N., Brown, K., and Grimshaw, J. (2012). Overview of systematic reviews of the effectiveness of reminders in improving healthcare professional behavior. *Systematic Reviews* 1, 36; Grimshaw, J. M., Eccles, M. P., Lavis, J. N., Hill, S. J., and Squires, J. E. (2012). Knowledge translation of research findings. *Implementation Science* 7, 50.

✖ Tips from service users

1 Ensure you understand the issue before your research begins. Is the issue for one patient or are other patients experiencing the same problem?
2 Manage any change in your practice with your patient(s) both on an individual basis and/or as a community. It may be that research shows things must change for both you as a clinician and for your patients as well.
3 Make sure they know you will be there for them in this journey.
4 Be honest with your patient(s). If you cannot solve a clinical issue, let them know you need to seek out further relevant learning from research, which may mean you also talk more with your colleagues for some additional research areas to look at.

W   Companion website

For extra resources on the topics covered in this chapter, visit the companion website at: www.oup.com/mhns

✚   References

Bero, L. A., Grilli, R., Grimshaw, J. M., Harvey, E., Oxman, A. D., and Thomson, M. A. (1997). *Closing the gap between research and practice: an overview of systematic reviews of interventions to promote the* *implementation of research findings. British Medical Journal 317(7156), 465–468.*

Bossuyt, P. M., Reitsma, J. B., Bruns, D. E., Gatsonis, C. A., Glasziou, P. P., Irwig, L. M., Lijmer, J. G., Moher, D.,

Rennie, D., de Vet, H. C., and Standards for Reporting of Diagnostic Accuracy (2003). *Towards complete and accurate reporting of studies of diagnostic accuracy: the STARD initiative. Clinical Chemistry 49(1), 1–6.*

Brown, B. and Crawford, P. (2003). *The clinical governance of the soul: 'deep management' and the self-regulating subject in integrated community mental health teams. Social Science and Medicine 56(1), 67–81.*

Brown, B., Crawford, P., and Hicks, C. (2003). *Evidence-Based Research: Dilemmas and Debates in Health Care. Milton Keynes: Open University Press.*

Brown, S. (2018). *Evidence-Based Nursing: The Research-Practice Connection, 4th ed. Burlington, MA: Jones & Bartlett Learning.*

Callaghan, P. and Carter, T. (2022). *Knowledge translation and linking evidence to practice. In: A. Higgins, N. Kilkku, and G. Kort Kristofersson, Eds., Advanced Practice in Mental Health Nursing: A European Perspective, pp. 405–426. Cham: Springer.*

Campbell, M. K., Elbourne, D. R., and Altman, D. G. (2004). *CONSORT statement: extension to cluster randomised controlled trials. British Medical Journal 328(7441), 702–708.*

Connor, L., Dean, J., McNett, M., Tydings, D. M., Shrout, A., Gorsuch, P. F., Hole, A., Moore, L., Brown, R., Melnyk, B. M., and Gallagher-Ford, L. (2023). *Evidence-based practice improves patient outcomes and healthcare system return on investment: findings from a scoping review. Worldviews on Evidence-Based Nursing 20(1), 6–15.*

Coyler, H. and Kamath, P. (1999). *Evidence-based practice. A philosophical and political analysis: some matters for consideration by professional practitioners. Journal of Advanced Nursing 29(1), 188–193.*

Crawford, P., Brown, B., Anthony, P., and Hicks, C. (2002). *Reluctant empiricists: community mental health nurses and the art of evidence-based praxis. Health and Social Care in the Community 10(4), 287–298.*

Daly, K. (1997). *Re-placing theory in ethnography: a postmodern view. Qualitative Inquiry 3(3), 343–365.*

Davies, P. (1999). *Introducing change. In: M. Dawes, Ed., Evidence-Based Practice: A Primer for Health Care Professionals, pp. 203–218. London: Churchill Livingstone.*

Des Jarlais, D., Lyles, C., Crepaz, N., and TREND Group (2004). *Improving the reporting of the quality of nonrandomized evaluations of behavioural and public health interventions. American Journal of Public Health 94(3), 361–366.*

DiCenso, A., Cullum, N., and Ciliska, D. (1998). *Implementing evidence-based nursing: some misconceptions. Evidence-Based Nursing 1(2), 38–39.*

Granados, A., Jonsson, E., Banta, H. D., Bero, L., Bonair, A., Cochet, C., Freemantle, N., Grilli, R., Grimshaw, J., Harvey, E., Levi, R., Marshall, D., Oxman, A., Pasart, L., Räisänen, V., Rius, E., and Espinas, J. A. (1997). *EUR-ASSESS project subgroup report on dissemination and impact. International Journal of Technology Assessment in Health Care 13(2), 220–286.*

Gray, J. A. M. (1997). *Evidence-Based Health Care. London: Churchill-Livingstone.*

Horsburgh, D. (2003). *Evaluation of qualitative research. Journal of Clinical Nursing 12(2), 307–312.*

Hughes, J. A. and Sharrock, W. W. (1997). *The Philosophy of Social Research, 3rd rev ed. London: Longman.*

Ingersoll, G. I. (2000). *Evidence-based nursing: what it is and what it isn't. Nursing Outlook, 48(4), 151–152.*

Jolley, J. (2020). *Introducing Research and Evidence-Based Practice for Nursing and Healthcare Professionals, 3rd ed. Abingdon: Routledge.*

Jorgensen, R. (2006). *A phenomenological study of fatigue in patients with primary biliary cirrhosis. Journal of Advanced Nursing 55(6), 689–697.*

Joyce, L. (1999). *Development of practice. In: S. Hamer and G. Collinson, Eds., Achieving Evidence-Based Practice: A Handbook for Practitioners, pp 109–127. Edinburgh: Baillière Tindall.*

Kirsch, I., Deacon, B. J., Huedo-Medina, T. B., Scoboria, A., Moore, T. J., and Johnson, B. T. (2008). *Initial severity and antidepressant benefits: a meta-analysis of data submitted to the food and drug administration. Public Library of Science Medicine 5(2), 260–268.*

Lehane, E., Leahy-Warren, P., O'Riordan, C., Savage, E., Drennan, J., O'Tuathaigh, C., O'Connor, M., Corrigan, M., Burke, F., Hayes, M., Lynch, H., Sahm, L., Heffernan, E., O'Keeffe, E., Blake, C., Horgan, F., and Hegarty, J. (2019). *Evidence-based practice education for healthcare professions: an expert view. BMJ Evidence-Based Medicine 24(3), 103–108.*

Lincoln, Y. S. and Guba, E. G. (2000). *Paradigmatic controversies, contradictions, and emerging confluences. In: N. K. Denzin, and Y. S. Lincoln, Eds., Handbook of Qualitative Research, 2nd ed., pp. 163–188. Thousand Oaks, CA: Sage Publications.*

Lomas, J. (1993). *Retailing research: increasing the role of evidence in clinical services for childbirth. The Millbank Quarterly 71, 439–475.*

McKenna, H., Cutcliffe, J., and McKenna, P. (2000). *Evidence-based practice: demolishing some myths. Nursing Standard 14(16), 39–42.*

Moher, D., Schultz, K. F., and Altman, D. (2001). *The CONSORT statement: revised recommendations for improving the reporting of parallel group randomised controlled trials. Lancet 357(9263), 1191–1194.*

Parahoo, K. (2006). *Nursing Research: Principles, Process and Issues, 2nd ed. London: Macmillan.*

Ray, L. (1999). *Evidence and outcomes: agendas, pre-suppositions and power. Journal of Advanced Nursing 30(5), 1017–1026.*

von Degenberg, K. (1996). *Clinical guidelines: improving practice at the local level. Nursing Standard 10(19), 37–39.*

Whittemore, R., Chase, S. K., and Mandle, C. L. (2001). *Validity in qualitative research. Qualitative Health Research 11(4), 522–537.*

4 Caring: The essence of mental health nursing

Carmel Bond
Theo Stickley

Gemma Stacey

Learning outcomes

By the end of this chapter, you should be able to:

1 Consider the concept of caring in terms of the language of caring and its ethical underpinnings

2 Demonstrate an awareness of the relevance of caring to contemporary mental health nursing practice when working with people in a recovery-focused way

3 Display the interpersonal and intrapersonal skills required to adopt a caring approach to practice

4 Transfer these skills into your nursing practice.

▼ Introduction

The chapter is divided into two parts. The first part examines the language of 'caring' in healthcare settings and identifies the core ethical principles and values that underpin the concept of care. The origins of mental health nursing will be considered by locating emotional and psychological caring in a historical context. The relationship between caring and treatment is examined, considering contemporary policy and models of practice.

The second part describes the skills associated with a caring approach to mental health practice. The skills are underpinned by acknowledging that human relationships are intrinsically complicated, and caring cannot be separated from the quality of both interpersonal and intrapersonal communication. In this part, we also provide an outline of basic interpersonal skills which will help you to learn how to listen attentively while caring. This aims to ensure caring remains the essence of mental health nursing practice.

▼ The concept of caring in mental health nursing practice

Evidence supports the healing power of caring and argues that nurses develop this healing approach by mobilizing hope, confidence, and trust between themselves and the person they are working with (Benner, 1984). The following section will provide the historical and theoretical justification for caring to remain the essence of mental health nursing practice while helping people towards recovery.

The ethics of caring

A caring practitioner will acknowledge the need to be physically present and demonstrate compassion, and offer consolation and support (Bond et al., 2022; Prince-Paul and Kelley, 2017). Such practical expressions of care are at the heart of mental health nursing practice. Caring for another can be seen as the nurse making informed, altruistic decisions which empower the person with whom they are working (Santangelo et al., 2018).

A caring approach requires the mental health nurse to make moral choices and justify their actions in the context of wider questions such as: 'How does the action taken agree or conflict with my own moral values?' 'How has the action taken enhanced the choice and well-being of the person I am working with?' What are considered reasonable actions will vary by person or situation. Caring must be underpinned by common principles, supported by the Nursing and Midwifery Council's (2018) Code of Practice:

1 Non-maleficence: to do no harm physically or psychologically.

2 Benevolence or beneficence, and compassion: to give positive help to people wherever necessary.

3 Justice: to treat people fairly or equally.

4 Autonomy: accepting that everyone has the right to make their own decision based on their own values (Haddad and Geiger, 2021).

These principles encourage you to base your actions on duty and obligation. Such obligations need to be understood, interpreted, and applied by you. They are inseparable from your character and the moral qualities and values you possess. Considering caring as a moral quality or individual value allows you to recognize caring towards another as a complex situation in which the moral character, the role of emotion, and the significance of the relationship between you and the person with whom you are working are fully acknowledged.

The language of care: 'caretakers' or caring nurses?

The word 'care' is perhaps one of the most overused words in mental health practice:

- 'Care plans'
- 'Care coordinator'
- 'Care programme approach'
- 'Care managers'
- 'Healthcare assistant'.

Not only does the word show up in health settings but it appears in other contexts too; for example, we tell people to 'take care' when we leave them; we sometimes ask, 'Would you care for a cup of tea?' The building where you work or study may have a 'caretaker', someone who takes care of the premises. As with any word, when it is used so much in so many contexts, it can easily lose its meaning. For example, is there much difference between caring for a building and caring for a person? We would argue that there is a huge difference and unless we understand the meaning of 'care' and put that meaning into practice, we may as well become caretakers of buildings rather than people.

The good caretaker takes pride in the building and protects it from harm. However, the personal needs of vulnerable people are much greater than the physical demands of the caretaker of buildings. As a mental health nurse (the 'caretaker' of vulnerable people), you are inevitably caught up in the tricky business of human relationships. We discuss the complexities of this kind of work in practice later in the chapter. We also argue that you need skills to implement care to complement your moral values and character.

Historical context

In 1952, psychiatric nurse Hildegard Peplau wrote *Interpersonal Relations in Nursing* in which she identified a relational model for mental health nursing, placing emphasis upon the nurse-client relationship. As psychologist, Carl Rogers (1951, 1963), did much to introduce a 'scientific' approach to the realm of 'client-centred therapy', thus, Peplau gave mental health nursing a theoretical base from which mental health nurses could give a meaningful rationale for caring. Mental health nursing subsequently developed as a profession with a theoretical cornerstone of caring through interpersonal relating and caring by way of the therapeutic relationship, and the deliberate use of self 'within' this relationship became core to the mental health nursing role. The idea that caring occurs 'within' the therapeutic relationship has generally been maintained throughout the mental health nursing literature, notably through Peplau (1952), Altschul (1985), Watkins (2001), and Barker (2003).

Contemporary context of caring

The current context of caring is one of transformation, reflecting a movement towards understanding mental health as occurring on a continuum (Johnstone, 2019). This directs thinking towards a 'recovery-focused' approach. The recovery approach is centred around several principles that emphasize the importance of working in partnership with patients and carers to identify realistic life goals and enable their achievement. Recovery is an individual journey, accepting that the person is the 'expert' in their life. Care should, therefore, be guided by the person. Those you work with might not always make decisions you agree with, or you might not necessarily approve of people's preferred recovery strategies. Co-creating care **with** people and deciding together what works best for **them** is where you need to stop and think carefully about how your own values might influence care. It is this inherently relational nature of caring which makes mental health nursing complex.

The principles of recovery are crucial for maximizing choice and autonomy in the care people receive. These principles have been reflected in policy reforms (Department of Health and Social Care, 2019; NHS England, 2019), changes to the Mental Health Code of Practice (Legislation.gov.uk, 2007; Sustere and Tarpey, 2019), and the Mental Health Nursing Competency Framework (Health Education England, 2020). We also recommended that you familiarize yourself with the following models: the Tidal Model (Barker and Buchanan-Barker 2004), the Wellness Recovery Action Plan (WRAP®; Copeland, 1997), and the Strengths Perspective (Ibrahim et al., 2014). These models form the basis of recovery principles. A caring approach, therefore, represents the foundation for the therapeutic relationship which can act as a vehicle towards recovery.

However, you may be frequently faced with dilemmas which involve striking a balance between promoting recovery through adopting a caring approach, and the necessity to protect individuals and communities from harm. Mental health nurses are expected to be able to predict and develop measures to manage the behaviour of individuals experiencing mental health difficulties. In some environments, managing risk can often dominate the decision-making process (Felton et al., 2018), hence a more controlling than caring line of practice is justified.

Studies have shown that patients feel that professionals prioritize medication management and symptom monitoring to manage risk (Eldal et al., 2019). This is at the expense of providing space and time for individual work, where the person can raise issues that are important to them and in which they feel heard and cared for. It is suggested that this dissonance of priorities can be explained by the continued dominance of a medicalized understanding of mental distress within mental health services. The consequence of this is a conflict of values and understandings which ultimately prevents shared decision-making and the promotion of autonomy, which are essential to recovery (Waldemar et al., 2016). The primary objective of mental health nursing should always be to form therapeutic human relationships.

▼ Skills for caring in mental health nursing practice

Caring in the context of mental health nursing is complicated. It is far easier on human skills and emotions to be a caretaker of buildings than it is to become a caregiver of vulnerable people. There are, however, skills that can be developed to enable 'care in action'. The historical and theoretical foundations of mental health nursing emphasize the importance of interpersonal and intrapersonal skills which are essential for building therapeutic relationships. At the heart of these relationships is a caring approach, which can be communicated to the people you work with using basic interpersonal and intrapersonal communication skills.

Interpersonal skills for caring

The basic interpersonal skills which communicate a caring approach are listed below. Each of these skills will be described and explained. Exercises are given for you to practise each of these skills. We suggest that you conduct these practical tasks with your fellow students and take turns to adopt the various roles outlined in the tasks. This will give you an opportunity to

experience the skill in a safe environment where it is okay to make mistakes before practising in your placements. We also suggest you take the opportunity to reflect upon adopting each of the roles as a way of enhancing your understanding of how it feels to be placed in the varied positions within the interaction.

- Non-verbal communication
- Asking open questions
- Clarifying
- Reflecting content
- Reflecting feeling
- Using silence

When all the skills are being used together, the proper, respectful conditions for personal growth to take place are provided. The kind of environment and space that is created is caring and therapeutic. By employing these skills in your individual work you may be able to provide an effective way of truly listening, and in doing so communicate genuine care. Not only does the person benefit from being offered these

Box 4.1 Interpersonal skills practice scenarios

Scenario A

Client: you are Amanda, aged 28. Having experienced many abusive relationships, you went into prostitution and began to use drugs and alcohol regularly. You were admitted to an acute ward after getting drunk one night. You have been detained under the Mental Health Act and you do not know why you are there and feel very angry that your freedom has been curtailed.

Nurse: you have been asked to talk with Amanda who is 28. She has been detained under Section 2 of the Mental Health Act. You know nothing about her past, other than she has a history of drink and drugs. She was admitted to an acute ward after claiming to be the 'Virgin Mary' and running around a local park with few clothes on.

Scenario B

Client: you are Bev, aged 22. You have been admitted to the acute ward after a serious attempt on your life. You have now been an inpatient for 6 weeks. It is totally impractical for you to go back to your parents as you have a very destructive relationship with them. You have got no ideas for your future. Everything seems hopeless.

Nurse: you have been asked to spend time with Bev who is 22. She was admitted to the acute ward after a serious attempt on her life. She has now been an inpatient for 6 weeks. You are under a great deal of pressure to discharge her into a women's hostel.

To practise skills for caring using these scenarios it is useful for three people to work together: a client, a helper, and an observer. The observer's role is to sit to one side and silently make notes about the skills the worker is using. The observer should give the worker feedback at the end of the session. Usually when these scenarios are being used, 10 minutes should be allowed for practising.

---

conditions, but the nurse can also learn to develop empathic understanding in the process of exercising the skills.

We cannot emphasize enough the need to practise these skills and one of the best ways to do this is to create role play scenarios. In Box 4.1 we have included several scenarios that might be useful.

The six skills for listening and communicating care

1 Non-verbal communication

In establishing a caring relationship, non-verbal communication is of the upmost importance. Much of all the communication that takes place between people is non-verbal. When we meet someone for the first time, we automatically make judgements about people, and this is invariably communicated non-verbally. It is important that we are always aware of our non-verbal communication.

Sadly, there are many stories of people being admitted to hospital for the first time and are then left alone. At this critical moment, it is imperative that a person is warmly greeted and a member of staff is dedicated to sitting with the person. These action will create a therapeutic space from the outset.

We have developed an acronym (SURETY) to help facilitate this therapeutic space:

S Sit at an angle to the client

U Uncross legs and arms

R Relax

E Eye contact

T Touch

Y Your intuition

Compare the photographs in Figure 4.1. Assuming this sort of positioning may seem common sense, but it is not. You need to practise awareness of body language when working therapeutically.

- Sit at an angle to the client. If we sit directly opposite somebody who is feeling in any way vulnerable, this may be interpreted as confrontational. Sitting exactly next to a person (as in a waiting room), is impersonal. If, however, we sit at a slight angle, it creates a non-confrontational, comfortable seating arrangement, ideal for one-to-one work.

- Uncross legs and arms. Research into non-verbal communication (Lee et al., 2019) has shown that crossed arms and legs communicate defensiveness. Depending on the

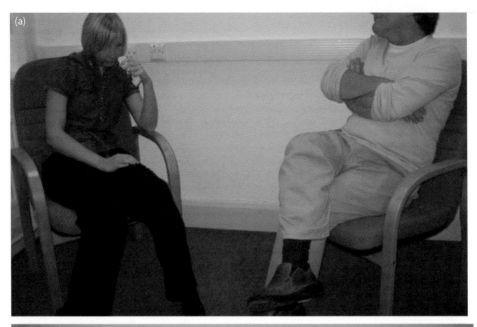

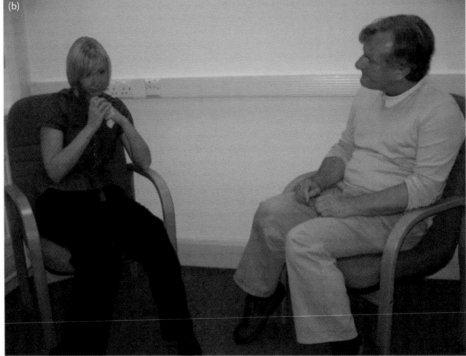

Figure 4.1 Comparisons of (a) ineffective and (b) effective non-verbal communication

whole-body position, crossed arms and legs may also communicate that we are not interested. Purposefully uncrossing arms and legs communicates openness and that we are receptive to the person.

- Relax. Despite the prescriptive nature of this method of deliberate non-verbal communication, it is most important that the listener learns to relax in the assumed position. It

may feel awkward at first, but it is worth it, and furthermore, it works!

- Eye contact. Maintaining appropriate eye contact is a powerful way of communicating respect and that you are paying attention. Eyes that wander to windows or the clock are sure to be read as lack of interest or attention.

'Appropriate' eye contact is different to staring. Appropriate eye contact breaks on occasions. It is always important to have eye contact at the ready if a client is distressed and perhaps looking down. If they momentarily look up and your eyes are not waiting for them, they may lose trust.

- Touch. The appropriate use of touch is not universal and cultural sensitivity is essential. Hugs or kisses are not appropriate in mental health care although respectful use of touch can communicate compassion, empathy, and understanding. Always seek informed consent from the person first.

- Your intuition. Our final point here is the need for workers to trust their intuition. There are no set guidelines for every situation, but as the practitioner grows in confidence, so they should learn to trust their intuition.

2 Asking open questions

A closed question is a question that elicits a yes or no answer. An open question invites the client to think, explore, and talk freely.

Examples of open and closed questions are shown in Table 4.1

Look again at Table 4.1 and you will see that closed questions usually begin with do, did, or are. Open questions usually begin with how, when, what, and tell. Can you think of more?

We advise against using the word 'why'. Often, when people are in distress, being asked 'why' can be infuriating. People often do not know 'why'.

3 Clarifying

When clarifying factual information, it is fine to ask closed questions: 'Did you say your husband was George?'

Table 4.1 Examples of open and closed questions

A woman has been admitted to a word having taken a large overdose. The worker is conducting an assessment.

Closed	Open
Did you really want to die?	How were you feeling when you overdosed?
Do you live alone?	Tell me about your home life?
Do you work?	
Are you feeling suicidal?	What do you do for a living?
	How are you feeling now?

Box 4.2 Examples of reflecting content

Example 1

Service user: I don't know why I've been sent here to talk to you.
Student nurse: You don't know why you are here.

Example 2

Client: I don't know what's the matter with me, the doctor says one thing, my son says something else, and I don't know what to do.
Nurse: You're getting conflicting advice and you are unsure what to do.

Unfortunately, however, assessments often sound like a tick list of information giving and receiving, and little time is given to open exploration.

Clarifying is essential if we are muddled about factual information. People are generally happy to clarify if we have misheard or made a wrong assumption.

4 Reflecting content

Reflecting to the person the content what they are saying:
- Demonstrates you are listening
- Ensures accuracy
- Communicates empathetic understanding
- Creates dialogue

Two examples of reflecting are provided in Box 4.2 and Box 4.3.

These responses may not be perfect and there is no absolute right or wrong. Here you are attempting to avoid judgement and to focus on being reflective.

5 Reflecting feeling

Reflecting feelings is the same as reflecting content but instead there is a focus on the person's feelings (Box 4.3). These may be communicated verbally or non-verbally.

Once again, we stress the need to practise these skills. They are quite straightforward in principle but take a long time to develop. Do not underestimate the effectiveness of using skills of reflection. As people feel listened to and empathically understood, trust will inevitably develop, and the person may feel able to engage.

Box 4.3 Examples of reflecting feelings

'You had tears in your eyes when you said that.'

'You sounded angry when you said that.'

'You sound sad.'

'You look very tense.'

'I can see your fists clenched.'

'You look afraid.'

'You look pleased about that.'

Examples of reflecting feelings communicated verbally

For this, use the same expressions as before but this time we add the reflection of feelings:

'…and you sound confused.'

'…and you sound sad.'

'…and you sound worried.'

'…and you look angry.'

'…and you look frightened.'

Box 4.4 Pause for thought

How often do you experience silence?

How do you feel?

Why not sit in silence now for 10 minutes?

This is often very difficult to achieve, have you noticed?

The world was a much quieter place years ago. Before technology brought us recorded music and mobile phones!

6 Using silence

The use of silence in attentive listening and communicating care is essential. While silence is common between people who are intimate, it is often considered uncomfortable in regular conversation. We have provided some questions for you to consider in Box 4.4. Working therapeutically needs to be more than typical, everyday, conversation and the use of silence has to be practised (Box 4.5).

In using attentive listening skills for individual work, it is necessary to allow adequate pauses between the client speaking and your next response/intervention.

Box 4.5 Using silence

Example without a pause:

Client: I don't know why I've been sent to talk to you.
Nurse: You don't know why you are here?

Now with a pause the dialogue changes:

Client: I don't know why I've been sent to talk to you.
[Pause]
Client: Maybe it's for my own good.
[Pause]
Nurse: You don't know why you are here but maybe it's for your own good.

The first pause allows the client to think for themselves. The second pause allows you to reflect. We recommend a pause of 5 seconds.

Now when you practise your skills, count to five in your mind before making your next intervention. If you can introduce this very simple skill into your work, it will have an immediate impact on the style and tone of the interaction. From the outset we have argued for the significance of respect in the caring relationship. The use of silence is a way of communicating that respect. Silence conveys several messages:

- The person is important to you
- You have time for them
- This is more than a normal conversation
- Interventions are considered
- It is okay to be with someone without feeling the need to **do** something

Using the skills in practice

Whenever you are given the opportunity to work with someone, we believe that it is necessary to employ interpersonal skills such as those presented in this chapter. It is not enough to just rely on personality or charm. The work of building, sustaining, and ending therapeutic relationships is complex and if it is to be 'therapeutic' then relationship building takes time, patience, and skill (see also Chapter 6). Our critics may accuse us of oversimplifying the skills needed for working in caring relationships. What we assert is that if the practitioner masters the skills in this chapter their work will be greatly enhanced. It may be helpful to access the 'transferring skills into your practice' self-assessment provided on the companion website to help you to prepare, plan, implement, and evaluate the use of these skills in your placement.

Intrapersonal skills for caring

There is much emotional and psychological distress all around us and we are not immune to mental health difficulties. At times, we all need somebody who will offer us the human qualities to provide a caring relationship. In clinical practice, this support should come from your supervisor, who themselves has experience in mental health work and supervisory training. On occasions, it may be necessary for mental health nurses to receive counselling or psychotherapy. It is perfectly understandable that people who are regularly exposed to the distress of others may be affected in some way.

▲ Conclusion

Communicating care towards another is part of a wider human experience. It requires both emotional and thoughtful responses, but often leads to tension. The values of the nurse are not always in line with those of the patient or those of the healthcare institution or system they are working within. Therefore, caring often requires making decisions which are justified by conveying a compassionate response to the person with whom you work (Straughair, 2019). Caring is more than a principle or ingredient of mental health nursing practice, but part of the core which underpins every therapeutic interaction.

✖ Tips from service users

1 Show me that you are listening to me and at least 'trying' to understand me as a person (not just a diagnosis).
2 Think about 'What is right for this person?', knowing that this might alter as things change as my condition fluctuates.

3 Validating my feelings and experiences is a huge thing for me and a very important aspect of my care.

W   Companion website

For extra resources on the topics covered in this chapter, visit the companion website at: www.oup.com/mhns

✚   Further reading

Recovery-informed approach

National Empowerment Centre: http://www.power2u. org/index.html

Recovery and the Conspiracy of Hope: http://www. patdeegan.com/

Research into Recovery: www.researchintorecov ery.com

Slade, M. (2009). *The contribution of mental health services to recovery. Journal of Mental Health 18(5), 367–371.*

Strengths-based approach

Ibrahim, N., Michail, M., and Callaghan, P. (2014). *The strengths based approach as a service delivery model for severe mental illness: a meta-analysis of clinical trials. BMC Psychiatry 14, 243.*

Tidal model

Barker, P. (2001). *The tidal model: developing an empowering, person-centred approach to recovery within psychiatric and mental health nursing. Journal of Psychiatric and Mental Health Nursing 8(3) 233–240.*

Barker, P. and Buchanan-Barker, P. (2004). *The Tidal Model: A Guide for Mental Health Professionals. London: Brunner-Routledge. Available at: http://www.tidal-model.co.uk/*

WRAP[®]

Wellness and Recovery Action Planning (WRAP[®]): http://www.*mentalhealthrecovery.com/*

✚   References

Altschul, A. (1985). *Psychiatric Nursing: A Concise Nursing Text, 6th ed. London: Baillière Tindall.*

Barker, P., Ed. (2003). *Psychiatric and Mental Health Nursing: The Craft of Caring. London: Arnold.*

Barker, P. and Buchanan-Barker, P. (2004). *The Tidal Model: A Guide for Mental Health Professionals. London: Brunner-Routledge.*

Benner, P. (1984). *From Novice to Expert: Excellence and Power in Clinical Nursing Practice. Menlo Park, CA: Addison-Wesley Publishing Company.*

Bond, C., Hui, A., Timmons, S., Wildbore, E., and Sinclair, S. (2022). *Discourses of compassion from the margins of health care: the perspectives and experiences of people with a mental health condition. Journal of Mental Health 1–9.*

Copeland, M. E. (1997). *WRAP: Wellness Recovery Action Plan™. West Dummerston, VT: Peach Press.*

Department of Health and Social Care (2019). *Modernising the Mental Health Act: Increasing Choice, Reducing Compulsion. Available at: https://www.gov.uk/government/publications/modernising-the-mental-health-act-final-report-from-the-independent-review*

Eldal, K., Natvik, E., Veseth, M., Davidson, L., Skjølberg, Å., Gytri, D., and Moltu, C. (2019). *Being recognised as a whole person: a qualitative study of inpatient experience in mental health. Issues in Mental Health Nursing 40(2), 88–96.*

Felton, A., Repper, J., and Avis, M. (2018). *Therapeutic relationships, risk, and mental health practice. International Journal of Mental Health Nursing 27(3), 1137–1148.*

Haddad, L. M. and Geiger, R. A. (2021). *Nursing Ethical Considerations. StatPearls Publishing. Available at: https://www.ncbi.nlm.nih.gov/books/NBK526054/*

Heath Education England (2020). *Mental Health Nursing Competence and Career Framework. Available at: https://www.hee.nhs.uk/sites/default/files/documents/HEE%20Mental%20Health%20Nursing%20Career%20and%20Competence%20Framework.pdf*

Ibrahim, N., Michail, M., and Callaghan, P. (2014). *The strengths based approach as a service delivery model for severe mental illness: a meta-analysis of clinical trials. BMC Psychiatry 14, 243.*

Johnstone, L. (2019). *Do you still need your psychiatric diagnosis? Critiques and alternatives. In J. Watson, Ed., Drop the Disorder!: Challenging the Culture of Psychiatric Diagnoses, pp. 8–23. Monmouth: PCCS Books Ltd.*

Lee, S. W. H., Thomas, D., Zachariah, S., and Cooper, J. C. (2019). *Communication skills and patient history interview. In: D. Thomas, Ed., Clinical Pharmacy Education, Practice and Research, pp. 79–89. Amsterdam: Elsevier.*

Legislation.gov.uk (2007). *Mental Health Act 2007. Available at: http://www.opsi.gov.uk/acts/acts2007/ ukpga_20070012_en_1*

NHS England (2019). *Mental Health Implementation Plan 2019/20–2023/24. Available at: https://www.longtermp lan.nhs.uk/wp-content/uploads/2019/07/nhs-mental-health-implementation-plan-2019-20-2023-24.pdf*

Nursing and Midwifery Council (2018). *Future Nurse: Standards of Proficiency for Registered Nurses. Available at: https://www.nmc.org.uk/globalassets/ sitedocuments/standards-of-proficiency/nurses/future-nurse-proficiencies.pdf*

Peplau, H. E. (1952). *Interpersonal Relations in Nursing. New York: G. P. Putnam and Sons.*

Prince-Paul, M. and Kelley, C. (2017). *Mindful communication: being present. Seminars in Oncology Nursing 33(5), 475–482.*

Rogers, C. R. (1951). *Client-Centred Therapy. Boston, MA: Houghton & Mifflin.*

Rogers, C. R. (1963). *Toward a science of the person. Journal of Humanistic Psychology 3(2), 72–92.*

Santangelo, P., Procter, N., and Fassett, D. (2018). *Mental health nursing: daring to be different, special and leading recovery-focused care? International Journal of Mental Health Nursing 27(1), 258–266.*

Straughair, C. (2019). *Cultivating compassion in nursing: a grounded theory study to explore the perceptions of individuals who have experienced nursing care as patients. Nurse Education in Practice 35, 98–103.*

Sustere, E. and Tarpey, E. (2019). *Least restrictive practice: its role in patient independence and recovery. Journal of Forensic Psychiatry & Psychology 30(4), 614–629.*

Waldemar, A. K., Arnfred, S. M., Petersen, L., and Korsbek, L. (2016). *Recovery-oriented practice in mental health inpatient settings: a literature review. Psychiatric Services 67(6), 596–602.*

Watkins, P. (2001). *Mental Health Nursing: The Art of Compassionate Care. Oxford: Butterworth-Heinemann.*

5 Interpersonal communication: Heron's Six Category Intervention Analysis

Jean Morrissey

Learning outcomes

By the end of this chapter, you should be able to:

1 Describe Heron's Six Category Intervention communication framework

2 Demonstrate an understanding of how Heron's Six Category Intervention framework can be used in clinical practice

3 Identify factors that may influence the application of Heron's Six Category Intervention

4 Use Heron's Six Categories in practice.

▼ Introduction

Communication underlies everything we do daily, as well as in our professional practice. In mental health nursing, communication has been recognized as a fundamental component of all therapeutic interventions and essential for the delivery of quality nursing care since the work of Peplau in 1952 (Peplau, 1988). The knowledge and interpersonal skills that a mental health nurse conveys are important aspects of helping the person who is experiencing mental health problems as well as facilitating the development of a positive nurse–service user relationship. The therapeutic relationship underpins all interactions provided to service users and is a powerful intervention (Morrissey and Callaghan, 2011). Hence, in the therapeutic relationship, the therapeutic use of communicating is an interpersonal and interactive process that aims to involve the service user in decision-making about their care and to improve both nurses' and service users' experiences of care (Farrelly et al., 2014; Moreno-Poyato et al., 2018; Wykes et al., 2018). This chapter outlines Heron's (2001) Six Category Intervention Analysis model of communication and its application in mental health nursing.

Traditionally, the views of mental health service users have received minimal attention; however, more recently it has been acknowledged that service users are the experts, with an invaluable experience of how mental illness can impact their lives (Barker and Buchanan-Barker, 2004; Deegan, 1995). Involving service users and carers in the planning and delivery of mental health care is therefore an essential component of high-quality mental health services. Government policy and patient advocacy groups, both in the UK and other countries, have emphasized the importance of engagement within mental health settings and promoted the concept of patient-centred communication and service user involvement as central to the delivery of quality health care and service delivery (Department of Health, 2006; Mind, 2011, 2017). Despite this, research over the years has failed to demonstrate engagement in practice (Bee et al., 2006; McAllister et al., 2019; Stomski et al., 2017). Mental health charities report that both service users and their carers have complained about the lack of therapeutic engagement in mental health services (Mind, 2011,

2017). Given the evidence that shows the effectiveness of mental health nursing is dependent on engagement between nurses and service users (Browne et al., 2012), the need to formulate a holistic understanding of the essential components of engagement with service users is urgent. Evidence suggests that, in practice, therapeutic contact time between nurses and service users is minimal, and that when interactions do occur, 'they are neither purposely therapeutic nor theoretically informed' (Cameron et al.,

2005, p. 65). Acquiring new skills and learning how to use them effectively can facilitate an improvement in mental health nurses' knowledge and skill base so that they can deliver best practice in a variety of clinical situations. This chapter describes Heron's (2001) model of communication, Six Category Intervention Analysis; illustrates how each category can be used in clinical practice; and examines some of the factors that may influence the therapeutic outcome of each category.

▼ What is Six Category Intervention Analysis?

Six Category Intervention Analysis is a communication/counselling framework developed by John Heron in 1975 at the Human Potential Research Project, University of Surrey (Heron, 1975). It is a way of classifying a large range of skills under six types of interventions that include six different purposes or intentions. As a therapeutic framework it provides a very useful and practical tool for mental health nurses to select, monitor, and reflect on their communication skills and interactions with service users, carers, and other key people involved in their care. All six categories can be used in a wide range of communication encounters whereby one person (the mental health nurse) is the **listener** and the facilitator, and the other person (the service user) is the **talker**—the one who is dealing with some issue that needs the time, attention, and service of another human being. The aim of this helping relationship is to offer a helping service and skill that is grounded fundamentally in a person/service user-centred attitude.

As a communication/counselling framework, each of the six categories and the respective interventions that fall under each category are **theoretically neutral**, that is, they are not aligned with any theoretical perspective of psychology or psychotherapy, for example, a humanistic approach, cognitive behavioural therapy, and others (Heron, 2001). Nevertheless, the Six Category system can be used as a tool to compare the therapeutic practice of different theoretical approaches. Like other psychotherapeutic approaches, the quality of the nurse–service user relationship is central to the therapeutic use and effectiveness of each of the six categories. Sensitive and skilled use of verbal and non-verbal communication can offer the necessary core conditions of all therapeutic relationships with service users and their carers, including genuineness, respect, empathetic understanding, and openness (Rogers, 1957).

Authoritative and facilitative interventions

The Six Categories and their designations are classified into two main groups: authoritative and facilitative. **Authoritative or directive** interventions are so called because in each case the practitioner is taking a more overtly assertive or directive role. When using authoritative interventions, the emphasis is more on what the mental health nurse is **doing** to or with the service user; they include prescriptive, informative, and confronting interventions.

Facilitative interventions are less obtrusive, and the role of the practitioner is more discreet. The emphasis is on the **effect** of the intervention on the service user, and interventions may be cathartic, catalytic, or supportive.

What is an intervention?

An intervention is an identifiable piece of verbal and/or non-verbal behaviour that is part of the nurse's clinical work or role with the service user (Heron, 2001). There is no set way of defining an intervention; it can have many verbal forms. Although the six interventions refer mostly to the nurse's verbal skills, components of non-verbal behaviour, such as eye contact, gestures, and body language, are equally important in determining how the verbal interventions come across to the service user. Therefore, you should be mindful not only about what you say, but also about how it is expressed. Furthermore, it is important that verbal and non-verbal messages are congruent, that is, they match the core message being conveyed at the time. For a more detailed coverage of verbal and non-verbal skills in clinical practice, see Morrissey and Callaghan (2011).

Intention

All six categories comprise a specific intention that determines the ultimate choice of intervention. Each intervention can be defined in terms of its intention or purpose: what it is that you want to achieve by your intervention. Table 5.1 outlines the Six Categories and their intentions.

It is important to remember that the authoritative categories are not more or less valuable or effective than the facilitative interventions; it all depends on:

- the nature of the nurse's role
- the needs of the service user at the time
- the content or focus of the intervention.

In practice, authoritative interventions have traditionally tended to be overused. Burnard and Morrison's seminal (1988, 1989, 1991) studies of qualified nurses' perceptions of their own interpersonal skills using Six Category Intervention Analysis found that nurses generally perceived themselves to be more skilful in the authoritative than in the facilitative categories. Although authoritative interventions are not **bad**

Table 5.1 The Six Categories and their intentions

	Aim	Example
Authoritative interventions		
Prescriptive	To direct the behaviour of the service user by demonstration, advice, suggestion, command	'I think you might feel less anxious if you talk about some of the reasons why you do not want to be discharged.'
Informative	To impart new knowledge or information to the service user by telling, informing	'Your medication may cause you to feel drowsy.'
Confronting	To raise the consciousness (awareness) of the service user about some limiting attitude, belief, or behaviour that he or she is unaware of by challenging, giving direct feedback in a supportive manner	'Are you aware that your Mum feels frightened when you shout at her?'
Facilitative interventions		
Cathartic	To enable the service user to share, express, or discharge painful emotions (primarily grief, fear, and anger) by encouraging and supporting the person to express his or her feelings	'It's okay to feel angry about the abuse you experienced as a child.'
Catalytic	To enable the service user to learn and develop by self-direction, problem-solving, and self-discovery within the context of nurse–service user encounter, but also beyond it	'What have you done in the past that helps you regulate your feelings of wanting to self-harm?'
Supportive	To affirm the worth and value of the service user's person, qualities, attitudes, or actions by enhancing the self-esteem of the person by giving encouraging, validating feedback.	'I know it was not easy for you to talk about your experience of voice hearing in the group; but you made a great effort, and the group members appreciated it.'

Source: data from Heron, J. (2001). *Helping the Client: A Creative Practical Guide*, 5th ed. London: Sage.

or **incorrect** per se, they can become ineffective and therefore non-therapeutic when they are used to the exclusion of facilitative interventions. Equally, the sole use of a facilitative approach can also lead to ineffective interventions and outcomes because it excludes the use of the nurse's professional authority in an appropriate way. For example, in practice there may be occasions when it is part of your role and responsibility to guide or direct the service user's behaviour, provide information, and challenge them to meet the service user's needs at that time. However, as Heron (2001) points out, balancing authoritative and facilitative interventions is all about the appropriate use of power in clinical practice, that is:

1   Your power over the service user

2   The power the practitioner and the service user share with each other

3   The autonomous power within the service user.

All three forms of power need one another, and always in the right amount and according to the changing needs of the service user throughout the therapeutic encounter.

▼ Applying Six Category Intervention Analysis in practice

Each of the six interventions is **value neutral**, that is, each intervention is neither more nor less significant and important than any other when used in an appropriate context. All six categories embrace patient-centred communication—'communication which invites and encourages the patient to participate and negotiate in decision making regarding their own care' (Langewitz et al., 1998, p. 230)—and, most importantly, are of any real value only if they are rooted in care and concern for the service user. Although the Six Categories are independent of one another and have a specific intention or purpose, there are also significant areas of overlap between them. Where such overlap occurs, the intervention is classified under the category that covers its primary purpose, as illustrated in the practice example in Box 5.1. The practice example illustrates the use of all six interventions, although this interaction reflects a more facilitative approach (see also Box 5.2).

In learning how to use the Six Categories, the nurse is acquiring a set of analytical and behavioural tools to select, monitor, and evaluate his or her own therapeutic interactions in terms of their therapeutic outcome. Each intervention can be evaluated only by testing it against the evidence in a practical context to determine whether the selected interventions elicited the desired result. In principle, each intervention can be checked, rechecked, amended, and modified by personal inquiry and in clinical supervision. For many nurses, it is not a question of starting from scratch with a whole new system. Many of the listed interventions identify and describe interventions that nurses will realize they have already been using, whereas other interventions will be new and enable nurses to extend their knowledge and skill base. Learning to use the Six Categories in practice can increase your confidence and efficacy. In practice, the skilled nurse aims to:

- be equally proficient in a wide range of interventions in each of the categories

- be able to move skilfully from one type of intervention to any other as the developing situation and purpose of the interaction require

- know what category they are using, and why, at any given time

- know when to lead and when to follow the service user

- know that the value of an intervention is a function of the total situation at the time and the purpose of the nurse's role in relation to the service user.

Factors that may influence the application of Six Category Intervention Analysis in practice

Given the uniqueness of each therapeutic relationship, every interaction with a service user will require different skills and interventions, based on the aim of the therapeutic communication, the context of the therapeutic encounter, the nurse's stage of professional development and level of competence, as well as the nature of the therapeutic relationship. As such, each interaction presents different learning opportunities and challenges that are often interchangeable and context dependent. However, to recognize the learning to be gained and the implications for practice, the nurse needs to reflect on the above and other potential factors, for example, the timing of the interaction, the service user's well-being, the nurse's cognitive and affective state, and many more that may affect the therapeutic outcome and quality of the therapeutic alliance.

The questions in Box 5.2 are intended to be used as an aide-memoire rather than a definitive checklist to assist you in monitoring, reviewing, and evaluating your use of the six

Box 5.1 Practice example

Service user: 'I feel really fed up; it's getting worse every day.'

Nurse: 'I am sorry to hear that you are feeling fed up, would you like to tell me more about what it is that might be making you feel this way?' [Supportive and Catalytic]

Service user: 'It's the voices, they are getting louder and louder. I just can't cope anymore with them, they never stop.'

Nurse: 'Constantly hearing loud voices must be very challenging for you. What are the voices saying to you? [Supportive and Catalytic]

Service user: 'They say my family don't care about me anymore.'

Nurse: 'You have told me that your family, especially you parents are very important to you so I can imagine that must be very difficult for you.' [Supportive]

Service user: 'I feel sad, angry at the voices … my family try so hard to help me … I am afraid that they will think I have let them down.'

Nurse: 'It's okay to have all these feelings—sadness, anger, fear.' [Cathartic]

Service user: [Begins to cry] 'I don't know what to do.'

Nurse: 'I notice that you have stopped doing your distraction techniques.' [Confronting]

Service user: 'I want to do them, but I sometimes forget, and I find it difficult doing them on my own.'

Nurse: 'Okay, would it help if I reminded you to do them?' [Supportive]

Service user: 'Yes, that might help.'

Nurse: 'Do you remember I gave you information about voice hearing and the use of distraction techniques. Would it help for us to discuss that again?' [Catalytic]

Service user: 'Yes, it would. I don't always hear things.'

Nurse: 'Okay, I will explain it again and I would like you to tell me to stop if you don't hear me or if I am explaining it too quickly or you don't understand what I am saying.' [Prescriptive]

Box 5.2 A guide to using Heron's six interventions in practice

Consider the following reflective questions:

- What was my primary intention or purpose during this interaction?
- Was my intention appropriate for this interaction and service user? If not, why not?
- What interventions did I use during this interaction?
- What was my intention in using these interventions?
- How did I use each category (intervention) in terms of the timing of the intervention; amount—too much or too little; tone; and body language?
- How competent did I feel using these interventions?
- Which interventions did I think were effective for the service user and how do I know they were effective?
- What factors enhanced my use of the chosen categories?
- What components of the interaction were less effective and for what reasons?
- What factors hindered my use of the chosen categories?
- What would I do differently in the future and why?
- What have I learned from reflecting on this interaction?
- What am I aware of about my interpersonal communication that I was unaware of before reflecting on this interaction?
- What intervention do I need to develop/improve in the future?
- What interventions do I tend to overuse?
- What interventions do I tend to underuse?

interventions in practice. These questions may also be useful when using a model of reflection, such as the Gibbs reflective cycle (Gibbs, 1988).

▲ Conclusion

In this chapter I have outlined the principles and practice of Heron's Six Category Intervention Analysis. For the developing practitioner, this communication framework provides a flexible and user-friendly tool to learn, acquire, and develop a range of interpersonal skills that can be used in various clinical encounters. However, it is not enough simply to learn the specific interventions; they must be applied in practice, whereby real learning takes place. As with all new learning, this will require time, practice, and a willingness to be open to inquiry, reflection, and feedback from service users, carers, and colleagues about the usefulness of your therapeutic communication in clinical practice. While I hope that this chapter is useful to you in developing your repertoire of communication skills and style of engaging with service users, it is not intended to be the only source for your ongoing learning and development as a mental health nurse. Notwithstanding, this chapter provides a useful framework to identify and clarify what you are doing, when, how you are doing it, and, more importantly, how you know your communication/interventions are useful and therapeutic for the service user.

✖ Tips from service users

1 When using any of the interventions make sure the language you use is understandable to your service user or carer.
2 If one intervention is not working, do not put the blame on the service user. It is worth exploring whether it is only the case with that client or if there are similar issues with other service users and/or carers.
3 Use self-reflection regularly on how you move through the interventions. Do not be afraid to use your supervision to explore the reasons why something may not be working and how to move forward.

✚ References

Barker, P. and Buchanan-Barker, P. (2004). *The Tidal Model: A Guide for Mental Health.* London: Brunner-Routledge.

Bee, P., Richards, D., Loftus, S., Baker, J., Bailey, L., Lovell, K., Woods, P., and Cox, D. (2006). *Mapping nursing activity in acute inpatient mental healthcare settings. Journal of Mental Health 15(2), 217–226.*

Browne, G., Cashin, A., and Graham, I. (2012). *The therapeutic relationship and mental health nursing: it is time to articulate what we do! Journal of Psychiatric & Mental Health Nursing 19(9), 839–843.*

Burnard, P. and Morrison, P. (1988). *Nurses' perceptions of their interpersonal skills: a descriptive study using Six Category Intervention Analysis. Nurse Education Today 8(5), 266–272.*

Burnard, P. and Morrison, P. (1989). *What is an interpersonally skilled person? A repertory grid account of professional nurse's views. Nurse Education Today 9(6), 384–391.*

Burnard, P. and Morrison, P. (1991). *Nurses' interpersonal skills: a study of nurses' perceptions. Nurse Education Today 11(1), 24–29.*

Cameron, D., Kapur, R., and Campbell, P. (2005). *Releasing the therapeutic potential of the psychiatric nurses: a human relations perspective of the nurse-patient relationship. Journal of Psychiatric and Mental Health Nursing 12(1), 64–74.*

Deegan, P. (1995). *Coping with recovery as a journey of the heart. Psychiatric Rehabilitation Journal 19(3), 91–97.*

Department of Health (2006). *Best Practice Competencies and Capabilities for Pre-Registration Mental Health Nurses in England: The Chief Nursing Officer's Review of Mental Health Nursing. London: Department of Health.*

Farrelly, S., Brown, G., Smukler, G., Rose, D., Birchwood, M., Marshall, M., Waheed, W., and Thornicroft, G. (2014). *Can the therapeutic relationship predict 18-month outcomes for individuals with psychosis? Psychiatry Research 220(1–2), 585–591.*

Gibbs, G. (1988). *Learning by Doing: A Guide to Teaching and Learning Methods. Oxford: Further Education Unit, Oxford Polytechnic.*

Heron, J. (1975). *Six Category Intervention Analysis. Guildford: University of Surrey.*

Heron, J. (2001). *Helping the Client: A Creative Practical Guide, 5th ed. London: Sage.*

Langewitz, W. A., Eich, P., Kiss, A., and Wossmer, B. (1998). *Improving communication skills—a randomized controlled behaviourally oriented intervention study for residents in internal medicine. Psychosomatic Medicine 60(3), 268–276.*

McAllister, S., Robert, G., Tsianakas, V. and McCrae, N. (2019). *Conceptualizing nurse-patient therapeutic engagement on acute mental health wards: an integrative review. International Journal of Nursing Studies 93, 106–118.*

Mind (2011). *Listening to Experience: An Independent Inquiry into Acute and Crisis Mental Healthcare. London: Mind.*

Mind (2017). *Ward Watch: Mind's Campaign to Improve Hospital Conditions for Mental Health Patients. London: Mind.*

Moreno-Poyato, A., Delgado-Hito, P., Suarez-Perez, R., Lluch-Canut, T., Roldan-Merino, J. F., and Monteso-Curto, P. (2018). *Improving the therapeutic relationship in inpatient psychiatric care: assessment of the therapeutic alliance and empathy after implementing evidence-based practices resulting from participatory action research. Perspectives Psychiatric Care 54(2), 300–308.*

Morrissey, J. and Callaghan, P. (2011). *Communication Skills for Mental Health Nurses. Maidenhead: McGraw-Hill/Open University Press.*

Peplau, H. (1988). *Interpersonal Relations in Nursing. Basingstoke: Macmillan Education.*

Rogers, C. (1957). *The necessary and sufficient conditions of therapeutic personality change. Journal of Consulting Psychology 21(2), 95–103.*

Stomski, N., Morrison, P., Whitely, M., and Brennan, P. (2017). *Advocacy processes in mental health: a qualitative study. Qualitative Research in Psychology 14(2), 200–215.*

Wykes, T., Csipke, E., Williams, P., Koeser, I., Nash, S., Rose, D., Craig, T., and McCrone, P. (2018). *Improving patient experiences of mental health inpatient care: a randomised controlled trial. Psychological Medicine 48(3), 488–497.*

6 Understanding therapeutic relationships in mental health nursing

Greg Rooney
Stephen McKenna Lawson

Michael Coffey

Learning outcomes

By the end of this chapter, you should be able to:

1 Appreciate the policy and context related to therapeutic relationships for mental health nursing

2 Understand some of the research and evidence related to therapeutic relationships in mental health nursing

3 Identify approaches, tools, and strategies required for recovery-focused therapeutic relationships skills.

Introduction

The therapeutic relationship is central to mental health nursing. There is evidence (Coffey et al., 2019; Horgan et al., 2021; Simpson et al., 2016) that service users have better experiences and outcomes where their mental health nurses are skilful in therapeutic relationships. Poorer experiences and outcomes result where service users do not perceive their care to be characterized by good therapeutic relationships (McAllister et al., 2021). The nature of therapeutic relationships in mental health nursing has changed over time. Our goal is to gain a therapeutic alliance, facilitating maximum involvement of service users in decisions made. Therapeutic relationships are complex. We hope that this chapter will help you understand that complexity. Whether you are beginning your journey as a mental health nurse, or you are building your existing skills, this chapter will help you understand and think actively about skills in therapeutic relationships.

Policy context

The last decade of UK policymaking has seen strategic plans implemented in each of the four nations (Department of Health, 2021; Scottish Government, 2017; Welsh Government, 2012). There has also been a push to either supplement or reform the most fundamental legislation, with an independent review (Department of Health and Social Care, 2018) of the Mental Health Act (1983) leading to the White Paper on *Reforming the Mental Health Act* (Department of Health and Social Care, 2021).

Beyond the statute book, two reports take mental health nursing as their specific focus: *Laying Foundations* (Palmer et al., 2020), and the broader *Commitment and Growth* review (Watkins, 2022).

This latter review identifies aspects of mental health nursing work as indispensable. The introduction makes this plain: 'Service users and their families have highlighted that mental health nurses possess empathy, communication skills and the ability to build strong therapeutic relationships' (Watkins, 2022, p. 5).

The report explicitly identifies how therapeutic skills deserve attention and fortification across the domains of clinical practice, research, education, and training.

Education and training have also undergone substantial change with the implementation of *Future Nurse: Standards of Proficiency for Registered Nurses* by the Nursing and Midwifery Council (2018). The standards make clear that nursing is a complex profession requiring high levels of skill, in which mental health knowledge and interpersonal therapeutic skills are featured alongside competencies in physical health, assessment, health promotion, safety, leadership, and care coordination.

▼ Therapeutic traditions within mental health nursing

UK mental health nurses when describing their work indicate that their identity, therapeutic self, skills, and relationships are critical (McKenna Lawson, 2022). Although contemporary literature captures the sense that the mental health nurse as a psychotherapeutic practitioner is a fading phenomenon (Hurley et al., 2020), traces of two distinct but often conflated historical psychotherapeutic traditions can be identified in self-descriptions: Hildegard Peplau's theory of interpersonal relations (Peplau, 1988) and Carl Rogers' model of client-centred therapy (Rogers, 1951).

It is not the presence of Peplau and Rogers' legacy per se that is noteworthy. Rather, it is their fusion and presentation as a de facto philosophy of nursing that deserves comment, for there are fundamental differences between these approaches, not least that Peplau's work emerges from within nursing and Rogers' without. Each describes conflicting formulations of how to engage with people in distress. Their combination arguably represents a therapeutic incoherence within the profession.

Peplau stressed the importance of interpersonal relations, insisting that positive outcomes are **necessarily** the product of a respectful but pragmatic discrepancy in knowledge and function between the nurse and patient (D'Antonio et al., 2014). In contrast, Rogerian counselling rests on the rejection of any hierarchy between the persons involved in therapy (Clarke, 1999). The words, thoughts, and experiences of the person are centred in a non-directed fashion, as opposed to a particular process being followed. Through the adoption of absolute presence, empathy, and acceptance, the counsellor enables a therapeutic relationship to develop (Rogers, 1951).

In short, where Peplau outlines stages and functions for the professional, Rogers emphasizes the embodiment of attitudes that do not require professional knowledge. Where Peplau emphasizes the nurse as the agent of change, Rogers de-emphasizes the professional and privileges the relationship itself. Where Peplau seeks direction, Rogers throws away the map.

▼ Evidence base

Our knowledge of what works in therapeutic relationships is partly derived from the psychotherapeutic field. Mental health nurses, however, operate in contexts that are markedly different to usual arrangements for psychotherapy. These include working with people in acute wards and psychiatric intensive care, community settings, and in specialist services such as dementia care. This range of contexts requires that we consider what works, for whom, and when. For example, Hewitt and Coffey (2005) noted that people who experience relationships as therapeutic had better outcomes but also that while these relationships were necessary, they were not sufficient alone when helping people with severe mental illness. Hartley et al. (2020) concluded that the evidence base for therapeutic relationships was poor despite being fundamental to the nursing role and a major contributor to positive outcomes. This conclusion, however, says as much about the quality and relative absence of research as it does about therapeutic relationships. Farrelly and Lester (2014) found that what works for people diagnosed with psychosis is a relationship based on mutual trust, demonstration of mutual respect, and shared decision-making, qualities that appeared difficult to achieve in routine practice. Felton et al. (2018) showed that the more significant the decision, the more distant from the service user it is made. It is therefore possible that shared decisions are reserved for more mundane issues. Ahmed et al. (2021), for example, concluded that there was little evidence of collaboration in decisions about risk and safety. They identified barriers including power issues and professional responsibility, but also that a key enabler is therapeutic relationships. In other words, therapeutic relationships provide the means for deeper and more meaningful work to keep people safe.

We know, too, that people using services value the relationships they have with nurses as care coordinators in community services (Simpson et al., 2016), associating this with better recovery, and that nurses and service users in acute settings rate relationships highly (Coffey et al., 2019). A recurring issue for mental health care is delivery of interventions that fail to acknowledge the experience of people using services. McAllister et al. (2021) developed a theory-informed intervention to improve nurse–patient therapeutic relationships. The resulting intervention addressed four joint priorities of service users and clinicians. These were to improve communication with withdrawn people, nurses to help service users help themselves, nurses to feel confident when engaging with service users, and improving team and ward culture.

The evidence is growing on the value of establishing good-quality therapeutic relationships. These relationships are associated with satisfaction, quality of life, and ultimately can help the person achieve recovery.

▼ The context for practice

Therapeutic relationships are based on reciprocal engagement in the process. Each person in the interaction is ordinarily there by choice, usually they have made autonomous decisions to engage with each other. One person is assumed to be seeking help and the other person is there to provide that help. If everything goes to plan then a relationship is formed that is confiding, supportive, and facilitative, creating the basis for help to be provided. In mental health settings, however, people using services are sometimes coerced into care. They can be required to see the nurse when on community treatment orders, or sometimes they are detained in hospital. The nurse, too, is somewhat compelled; it is their professional duty, their reason for being there. They may also be anxious, frightened, and uncertain. This context may fundamentally alter the basis for the relationship. One party's autonomous decision to participate is in doubt. There is ambivalence at play in the interaction. And yet, the interaction is still required, and somehow both parties must find a way, a middle ground on which to discuss difficult issues. Part of the work required here is to reflect and acknowledge this context. These are not situations we would ordinarily choose for building relationships. These are situations that require skilful attempts at creating a connection.

Good-quality therapeutic relationships involve person centredness. This is the intent for active participation of individuals in decisions about their own care so that their needs, circumstances, preferences, and values are placed at the centre of the help they receive (Health Foundation, 2016). The focus is on the person first and not the illness or condition. The Health Foundation suggests four principles of person-centred care:

1 Affording people dignity, compassion, and respect

2 Offering coordinated care, support, or treatment

3 Offering personalized care, support, or treatment

4 Supporting people to recognize and develop their own strengths and abilities to enable them to live an independent and fulfilling life.

Therapeutic relationships based on person-centredness can help nurses keep people safe (Felton et al., 2018). Deploying therapeutic skills to create meaningful relationships facilitates service user knowledge contributions to shared plans for care.

▼ Relationships skills for mental health nurses

Interpersonal skills are the foundation of therapeutic relationships, the bedrock of mental health nursing (Felton et al., 2018). Many of these relationship skills are the same as those used in social communication and so all mental health nurses, even the most inexperienced student, will have some communication and relationship skills. Therapeutic relationships are more specialized; they are a conscious and deliberate use of specific skills designed to create a safe environment, to foster service user engagement, and to facilitate their recovery (Wright, 2021). It is through these relationships that we can better understand the service user's experiences. In this section, we discuss what is required to develop effective therapeutic relationships and so foster an enabling alliance between the mental health nurse and the service user. We address the role of self-awareness as well as the specific communication skills required, including the phases of the relationship. McAllister et al. (2021) suggest that negative service user experience such as self-harm and aggression are substantially correlated with a low-quality emphasis on therapeutic relationships within mental health settings.

In mental health nursing, we include the personal as well as the professional. The mental health nurse's self is an inevitable aspect of the therapeutic alliance. To address this, we must consider self-awareness. The ability to reflect and become more self-aware is critical in the development of therapeutic relationships (Barker and Williams, 2018). Self-awareness enables us to reflect on what shapes us, our values, and emotions. Self-awareness can help us identify attributes that help in therapeutic relationships. For example, we may reflect that our own life experiences help us empathize with someone who is frightened. But self-awareness also enables us to explore what, within ourselves, may be an impediment to therapeutic relationships. It may be

that you noticed that you feel frustrated when working with a particular service user. Therapeutic relationships require the mental health nurse to adopt a non-judgemental attitude. This can be challenging especially when, for example, working with service users whose beliefs, behaviours, or life choices contradict your own values. Reflection is the process where you try to understand why this may be so. Access to clinical supervision is one way to strengthen the positive elements that enable therapeutic relationship skills and discuss concerns identified through reflection.

✖ Exercise

Conduct an internet search on 'self-awareness'. Try to find resources that can help you build your self-awareness. Take time to practise some techniques to help you grow your

self-awareness. Think about how this might help you in therapeutic relationships. Spend time with a trusted friend, colleague, tutor, or family member and discuss your experiences.

Ellis and Day (2018) suggested that, in therapeutic relationships, the mental health nurse has several roles. They must be clear and **purposeful** so that both parties understand the aims and purpose of the relationship. The mental health nurse needs to be **connected**; this is to be able to demonstrate their understanding of the person's experience by listening and showing empathy. Throughout the relationship, the mental health nurse must be **facilitative** and be able to forge a therapeutic alliance where both service user and nurse can play a meaningful part. This requires the mental health nurse to be **supportive** and encouraging. Finally, the mental health nurse needs to be **influential** and be able to inspire confidence so that the person can feel able to make positive changes.

There are four distinct but overlapping stages of the therapeutic relationship (Figure 6.1). These are **exploration**, **understanding**, **action**, and **resolution**. The therapeutic relationship can last from hours, such as in a liaison team, to months or even years, for example, when working with people with persistent mental health needs. Regardless of these variations, these stages will help the mental health nurse consider what skills and approaches to use to achieve desired aims.

The therapeutic relationship begins with the exploration stage. To make a success of this phase, you need to carefully consider the environment and the context. Is the environment safe? Is it comfortable? Is it free from distraction and other factors that might impede communication? Adjustments to the environment may be needed to facilitate the important exploration stage.

Exploration

Aim is to establish rapport and build therapeutic relationship

Understanding

Aim is to understand the service user experience and to identify key issues

Action

Aim is to collaborate in recovery-focused problem-solving

Resolution

Aim is to encourage service user autonomy and resilience

Figure 6.1 Four stages of the therapeutic relationship

The exploration stage is about 'getting to know you'—but remember, the service user will want to get to know you too. Consequently, your first impression is vital. Non-verbal communication skills help you foster a helpful, trusting, and meaningful relationship. Think about your tone of voice and how you might come across to, for example, someone who is scared or confused. Is your voice too loud or too soft? Do you speak too fast? Your facial expression and body language are also important. Think about your posture and about the use of touch. Again, depending on the needs and concerns of the service user, you might need to modulate elements of your non-verbal communication. This is because non-verbal communication, especially eye contact, may be easily misinterpreted.

During the exploration stage, encourage the service user to share their thoughts, feelings, and experiences. Thinking about modern, recovery-focused mental health care, you will want to explore not just their difficulties and problems, but get to know the person, their hopes, ambitions, and strengths. Listening skills are used during this phase. **Active** listening is more than just listening; it includes non-verbal skills such as leaning forward and using your posture and gestures—for example, nodding at responses. Active listening is an intentional form of listening and demonstrates attentiveness. Active listening contributes to fewer incidents of misunderstanding, more accurate assessments and care planning, and stronger therapeutic relationships (Arnold and Boggs, 2020).

Open questions feature prominently in the exploration phase. These are questions that cannot usually be answered in one word or short replies. They are also known as process questions as they invite the person to think through answers. Open questions give the person the opportunity to describe and discuss their perspective in their own words. By asking open questions such as 'Tell me about your family', the mental health nurse may gain rich, detailed replies. This will be helpful in aiding your understanding of the service user's perspective. Being able to speak freely is likely to be appreciated by service users, many of whom may not have felt that their voice was previously heard. However, some service users may have trouble in processing open questions or articulating their reply. Consider a person who is confused: they may not be able to manage the demands of a complex open question. The person may be experiencing features of severe depression and may not be able to respond to such questions. In these circumstances, it might be useful to use **closed questions**. These are questions that invite one-word or short replies, such as 'When did you start feeling this way?' or 'How old is your daughter?' Closed questions can be used by the mental health nurse to clinch specific detail. In most circumstances, the mental health nurse will use both open and closed questions. Typically, they use open questions to gain insights ('Tell me about your experience') and follow these with closed questions to clinch detail ('When did this begin?').

The exploration phase allows the nurse to communicate empathy, acceptance, and genuineness and so establish rapport. Using **affirming statements** enables the mental health nurse to accentuate service user positives and strengths. These demonstrate empathy and illustrate positive recovery values. Examples include 'Despite feeling discouraged, it's great that you aren't giving up'. **Paraphrasing** is when you use your own words to convey that you have understood what has been said. These skills are used in the next stage of the process—the understanding stage.

While the focus of the exploration stage is to gain insights and establish rapport, in the **understanding phase** it is to add understanding to what the service user is saying and how they come across. Skills used in the first stage are developed and there is a greater emphasis on gaining a detailed understanding of the service user experience. Questions are now used to gain clarity and elaboration. The mental health nurse will, at this stage, be listening for themes, patterns, and gaps. They will be using their observation of the person to consider factors such as congruence. An example of this is when a person has limited eye contact, looks glum, and talks slowly, yet they say that they are not depressed. The mental health nurse will want to better understand the situation, perhaps by sharing their observations with the service user. The greater focus in this phase might be driven by the mental health nurse's knowledge. For example, in the exploration phase, the service user has talked about how distressed they are by medication-induced weight gain. The mental health nurse may draw upon their knowledge of medicines and medicines management to formulate specific questions. However, it is important that this process does not begin too early in the therapeutic relationship as it may prevent the service user from talking fully about their experiences and give the sense that it is the nurse's agenda and not theirs which is important.

Demonstrating empathy, acceptance, and genuineness is vital throughout the therapeutic relationship (Horgan et al., 2021). This maintains and builds rapport. Recovery values drive us to consider the person as an active partner in the therapeutic alliance. In the understanding phase, the mental health nurse will identify the service user's readiness for this partnership and reflect on their own. Relationship skills can be used to foster hope and develop the person's sense of empowerment, by focusing on strengths and using affirmative statements. These are vital in the next stage, the action stage.

In modern mental health services, we strive to engage service users at every stage of their care. This is known as co-production and involves collaboration and agreement on the problems and concerns, what the goals are, and how these might be achieved—together. Skills required by the mental health nurse include those used in previous stages. There is a greater focus on steps to alleviate problems and concerns.

Using relationship skills, the mental health nurse can facilitate service user problem-solving tools and techniques. These can be used in managing the different life events and stressors that they experience. This would include identifying the main concerns and problems and then generating solutions and ideas that could be useful. For example, a service user may discuss their self-harming. The mental health nurse will use their interpersonal skills of questioning, listening, paraphrasing, and conveying empathy to elicit from the person any strategies that could be helpful. It is important that ideas and possible strategies emanate from the service user; simply telling them of the strategies (even if you know them) is likely to be counterproductive in terms of autonomy. It is important that problem-solving adopts an optimistic outlook, with a view that problems can be solved.

▲ Conclusion

The descriptions of interpersonal skills offered here, and their philosophical origins, rest on the assumption that the therapeutic relationship will be established and maintained in physical space. The impact of COVID-19 upon ways of working in healthcare have been profound, and those professions engaging with the mentally distressed are no exception. It is possible, if not probable, that over time therapeutic relationships will be increasingly mediated through multiple technological entities including screens, smartphone apps, online platforms, and virtual assistants. One of the many questions this poses is whether productive therapeutic relationships enabling healing can occur between people and objects, programmes, or systems, as opposed to other people.

Neither Peplau nor Rogers could have envisioned this development, so it will be up to the practitioners and theorists of the twenty-first century to adapt and reforge the foundational interpersonal principles and skills sufficiently for nurses and service users to be included in the inevitable redesign of healthcare delivery.

✖ Tips from service users

1 Treat every interaction, no matter how short, as a therapeutic interaction. Service users appreciate the demands on the mental health nurse's time, but don't want this busyness to prevent therapeutic interaction.
2 **All** interactions should be about conveying empathy, compassion, and understanding. Service users feel that too many are merely about information exchange.
3 Always think about different perspectives and how this guides your therapeutic relationship. Each service user is unique. Their uniqueness, including gender, ethnicity, and age, all matter.

W   Companion website

For extra resources on the topics covered in this chapter, visit the companion website at: www.oup.com/mhns

➕   References

Ahmed, N., Barlow, S., Reynolds, L., Drey, N., Begum, F., Tuudah, E., and Simpson, A. (2021). *Mental health professionals' perceived barriers and enablers to* *shared decision-making in risk assessment and risk management: a qualitative systematic review. BMC Psychiatry, 21(1), 594.*

Arnold, E. and Boggs, K. U. (2020). *Interpersonal Relationships: Professional Communication Skills for Nurses, 8th ed. St. Louis, MO: Elsevier.*

Barker, S. and Williams, S. (2018). *Compassionate communication in mental health care. In K. Wright and M. McKeown, Eds., Essentials in Mental Health Nursing, pp. 297–313. London: Sage Publications.*

Clarke, L. (1999). *Carl's world. In: Challenging Ideas in Psychiatric Nursing, pp. 32–45. London: Routledge.*

Coffey, M., Hannigan, B., Barlow, S., Cartwright, M., Cohen, R., Faulkner, A., Jones, A., and Simpson, A. (2019). *Recovery-focused mental health care planning and co-ordination in acute inpatient mental health settings: a cross national comparative mixed methods study. BMC Psychiatry 19(1), 115.*

D'Antonio, P., Beeber, L., Sills, G., and Naegle, M. (2014). *The future in the past: Hildegard Peplau and interpersonal relations in nursing. Nursing Inquiry 21(4), 311–317.*

Department of Health (2021). *Mental Health Strategy: 2021–2031. Belfast: Department of Health.*

Department of Health and Social Care (2018). *Modernising the Mental Health Act: Increasing Choice, Reducing Compulsion. London: Department of Health and Social Care.*

Department of Health and Social Care (2021). *Reforming the Mental Health Act: Government Response. London: Department of Health and Social Care.*

Ellis, M. and Day, C. (2018). *The therapeutic relationship: engaging clients in their care and treatment. In: I. J. Norman and I. Ryrie, Eds., The Art and Science of Mental Health Nursing: Principles and Practice, 4th ed., pp. 125–139. London: McGraw Hill/Open University Press.*

Farrelly, S. and Lester, H. (2014). *Therapeutic relationships between mental health service users with psychotic disorders and their clinicians: a critical interpretive synthesis. Health & Social Care in the Community 22(5), 449–460.*

Felton, A., Repper, J., and Avis, M. (2018). *Therapeutic relationships, risk, and mental health practice. International Journal of Mental Health Nursing 27(3), 1137–1148.*

Hartley, S., Raphael, J., Lovell, K., and Berry, K. (2020). *Effective nurse–patient relationships in mental health care: a systematic review of interventions to improve the therapeutic alliance. International Journal of Nursing Studies 102, 103490.*

Health Foundation (2016). *Person-Centred Care Made Simple: What Everyone Should Know About Person-Centred Care. London: The Health Foundation.*

Hewitt, J. and Coffey, M. (2005). *Therapeutic working relationships with people with schizophrenia: literature review. Journal of Advanced Nursing 52(5), 561–570.*

Horgan, A., O'Donovan, M., Manning, F., Doody, R., Savage, E., Dorrity, C., O'Sullivan, H., Goodwin, J., Greaney, S., Biering, P., Bjornsson, E., Bocking, J., Russell, S., Griffin, M., MacGabhann, L., van der Vaart, K. J., Allon, J., Granerud, A., Hals, E., Pulli, J., Vatula, A., Ellilä, H., Lahti, M., and Happell, B. (2021). *'Meet me where I am': mental health service users' perspectives on the desirable qualities of a mental health nurse. International Journal of Mental Health Nursing 30(1), 136–147.*

Hurley, J., Lakeman, R., Cashin, A., and Ryan, T. (2020). *The remarkable (disappearing act of the) mental health nurse psychotherapist. International Journal of Mental Health Nursing 29(4), 652–660.*

McAllister, S., Simpson, A., Tsianakas, V., and Robert, G. (2021). *'What matters to me': a multi-method qualitative study exploring service users', carers and clinicians' needs and experiences of therapeutic engagement on acute mental health wards. International Journal of Mental Health Nursing 30(3), 703–714.*

McKenna Lawson, S. (2022). *How we say what we do and why it is important: an idiosyncratic analysis of mental health nursing identity on social media. International Journal of Mental Health Nursing 31(3), 708–721.*

Nursing and Midwifery Council (2018). *Future Nurse: Standards of Proficiency for Registered Nurses. Available at: https://www.nmc.org.uk/globalassets/sitedocuments/standards-of-proficiency/nurses/future-nurse-proficiencies.pdf*

Palmer, W., Hutchings, R., and Leone, C. (2020). *Laying Foundations: Attitudes and Access to Mental Health Nurse Education. Nuffield Trust. Available at: https://www.nuffieldtrust.org.uk/research/laying-foundations-attitudes-and-access-to-mental-health-nurse-education*

Peplau, H. E. (1988). *Interpersonal Relations in Nursing: A Conceptual Frame of Reference for Psychodynamic Nursing, 1988 ed. Houndmills: Palgrave.*

Rogers, C. R. (1951). *Client-Centered Therapy: Its Current Practice, Implications and Theory. London: Constable.*

Scottish Government (2017). *Mental Health Strategy: 2017–2027. Available at: https://www.gov.scot/ publications/mental-health-strategy-2017-2027/*

Simpson, A., Hannigan, B., Coffey, M., Barlow, S., Cohen, R., Jones, A., Všetečková, J., Faulkner, A., Thornton, A., and Cartwright, M. (2016). *Recovery-focused care planning and coordination in England and Wales: a cross-national mixed methods comparative case study. BMC Psychiatry 16(1), 147.*

Watkins, B. (2022). *Commitment and Growth: Advancing Mental Health Nursing Now and for the Future. London: Health Education England.*

Welsh Government (2012). *Together for Mental Health. Available at https://www.gov.wales/sites/default/files/ publications/2019-04/together-for-mental-health-summ ary.pdf*

Wright, K. M. (2021). *Exploring the therapeutic relationship in nursing theory and practice. Mental Health Practice. https://doi.org/10.7748/mhp.2021.e1561*

7 Assessment in mental health nursing

Helen Rees
Adam Chillman

Zaynab Yasin Sohawon

Learning outcomes

By the end of this chapter, you should be able to:

1 Understand the purpose of mental health assessment

2 Describe the components of a mental health assessment and the reason for their inclusion

3 Demonstrate how the patient's voice can be heard throughout assessment

4 Be mindful and respectful of patient experience.

▼ Introduction

Nurses are frequently required to complete mental health assessments, which are used to determine access to appropriate services, current mental state, the formulation of a patient's experiences, and the use of legislation/restrictive practices. Since nursing assessments are highly influential over the care an individual receives, it is essential that the patient's preferences, values, and personalized formulations of their experiences are represented throughout the assessment process.

The value of mental health nursing assessment is recognized by Health Education England's *Mental Health*

Nursing: Competence and Career Framework (2020) and changes to the Mental Health Act in 2008, which made nursing reports for First-Tier Tribunals a statutory duty (Patyal, 2010). However, while this chapter will focus primarily on mental health nursing assessment, the core skills involved with this are relevant for anyone working in health and social care. Indeed, the relevance of mental health assessment to all fields of nursing is highlighted in the Nursing and Midwifery Council *Future Nurse* standards (2018).

▼ Evidence base and background

Historically, mental health assessment was aligned to the diagnostic criteria included within medical classification manuals. While these criteria still exist, modern mental health assessment also has the flexibility to engage patients who do not understand their symptoms within a diagnostic narrative. This stems primarily from activism from the survivor and critical psychiatry movements, who influenced a move towards the recovery model of mental illness and a

biopsychosocial-spiritual approach to mental health assessments (Trenoweth, 2016).

Early access to mental health support reduces mental health crises and improves health outcomes (World Health Organization, 2013). Supporting universal access to timely mental health support is therefore a key area of public health policy (Mental Health Taskforce, 2016); comprehensive and timely assessment is key to achieving these aims.

✖ Patient perspective: case study

Zaynab, a young person and mental health advocate, recounts her experiences being assessed in mental health settings. She states:

> I was sectioned five times under the Mental Health Act over a period of 4 years. I was in psychiatric intensive care units and psychiatric secure settings. My diagnoses were psychosis, autism, and complex trauma.
>
> I was assessed numerous times under the Mental Health Act for a Section 2, Section 3, and a Community Treatment Order. What I think is incredibly important about Mental Health Act assessment is relationship-based practice. For me to be open about what I was struggling with, I would need a basis to connect with the assessor. If the assessor was asking me questions about my difficulties and symptoms, without getting to know me properly, I would be likely to disengage and become hostile. The best Mental Health Act assessments I had begun with a clinician trying to find common ground. Easy ways to do this include asking about what the patient likes to be identified as, e.g. the pronouns they prefer to use for themselves, or any nicknames they like to use that they prefer. Often simple ways to encourage connection include asking what a patient likes to do for fun or what their hobbies are, followed by sharing of one's own. This relieves patient anxiety, reducing the 'me versus clinicians' power dynamic, allowing room to build and sustain trust. In turn, this will encourage the patient to engage more meaningfully and feel safer to do so. In mainstream statutory services, there is a power dynamic of having 'helper–helpee' relationships where the assessor is the 'helper' and the patient is the 'helpee'. This can lead to non-conducive power imbalances in assessment and so the approach of 'learning together' while displaying an attempt towards 'collaboration' is usually favoured by the patient. A little mutuality goes a long way.
>
> A patient having to repeat their story repeatedly feels like having to relive the trauma all over again. It is as if having to endure all the same emotions attached to their story. For me, I would keep having to tell each clinician about my self-harm and childhood trauma, which was distressing. Sometimes I would feel like I was reliving the experiences by having to tell this to each professional. It became emotionally draining and fatiguing. What can help is acknowledging this temporary distress with the patient, explaining that the only purpose of telling their story is for the best interests of the patient, to assess their needs to enable them to access the best care pathway.

▼ Preparation

Situativity theory (Durning and Artino, 2011) states that who we are, who the patient is, and the assessment itself are complex products of time, place, culture, context, and environment; according to this theory, different words will have different meanings depending on the context of the person saying it and the person hearing it.

Preparing a respectful mental health assessment begins before a health care professional has direct contact with a patient, that is, it is at this stage that decisions are made about the assessing environment, when the assessment will happen, who will be involved in the assessment, and what sources of information are important to consider.

Consider who the patient is to you

Before beginning an assessment, health care professionals should consider both their personal safety (since the assessment process may trigger violence/aggression) and the safety of the patient (since mental health patients are more likely to have experienced trauma, including trauma because of their involvement with mental health services). They should also ask themselves whether they have met the patient before, what previous contact the patient has had with mental health services, and what the purpose is of the assessment. When doing this the assessor should consider what information is clinically relevant and what sources of information are available. When using lots of different sources of information, it is pivotal that the patient's own voice remains central. Remember that local patient information systems may not give a complete or up-to-date picture; there is no national database for mental health services, so confidential communication with colleagues from across provider boundaries may be important to consider.

Consider where the assessment is taking place

Mental health assessments take place in a variety of settings. Assessors should therefore be mindful that there may be different guidelines for assessing patients in different places, such as the *Quality Standards for Liaison Psychiatry Services* (Baugh et al, 2020).

Consideration of environmental risks is an important part of the assessment process. This should entail scanning the environment for potential weapons, evidence of alcohol/substance use, and items blocking an exit (most lone working guidelines recommend that assessors situate themselves near to a clear exit). If an assessor is worried that the environment poses safety risks, then they should consider ways of mitigating this, such as completing the assessment with another practitioner and/or making other practitioners aware of where you will be and what time you expect to be finished. It may also be important to consider the timing of the assessment and whether this needs to be changed to minimize any identified risks.

The Equality Act 2010 (Legislation.gov.uk, 2010) places a legal duty upon public sector organizations to ensure that people with protected characteristics are not disadvantaged in accessing their services. It is therefore essential that health care professionals make reasonable adjustments to the assessing environment to promote patient safety and take any safety concerns seriously. Taking a universal approach to tailoring the assessment environment to the individual ensures best practice.

✖ Patient perspective

Be aware of diversity. Is the patient neurodiverse? How can you adapt your approach to suit the needs of their neurodiversity? For example, for an autistic person, allowing sensory toys or having the assessment take place in a quiet room with minimal people can often help. Having an informal option of telling the patient that they could leave to go to another quiet room if they wished also helps with a patient feeling more comfortable with sharing their difficulties.

Consider who else may be involved in the assessment

If the patient gives permission, supporters can be a useful source of information for a mental health assessment. Sometimes it may be appropriate to approach a patient's support network without patient permission; this decision needs to be clinically justified and clearly documented. It is always best practice to ensure that if involving a patient's support network, the patient is also given the opportunity to speak to the assessor alone. This should be applied universally but particularly if there are safeguarding concerns.

▼ Meeting the patient

When completing assessments for the purposes of determining care provision, the process should be explained to the patient at the outset. Patients have a right to understand what is involved in health care procedures and to be given the information required to do this. Outlining how the Data Protection Act 2018 (Legislation.gov.uk, 2018) applies to the mental health assessment is also an important part of informed consent.

All assessments should begin with introductions; this provides an opportunity for the patient and assessor to know who everyone is, their roles, and their preferred names and pronouns—it is important that this information is requested universally, and not assumed based on appearance and stereotypes. According to the Armed Forces Covenant and NHS Constitution, health care professionals also have a responsibility to ensure that people in the armed forces, reservists, their families, and veterans are not disadvantaged in accessing health services (Ministry of Defence, 2021). It can therefore be useful to ask patients if they, or a member of their family, serve or have served in the Armed Forces (and if so, what was their experience of discharge?).

✖ Patient perspective

The best assessments I had was when the clinician had read my notes beforehand and when they showed empathy. Sometimes going the extra mile can make a dramatic difference to a patient's day. I was first sectioned a few days before my 14th birthday. The assessing nurse went out of her way to request the ward to buy me a smoothie book as she had remembered that my parents were getting me a smoothie blender for my birthday. It was a touching gesture since I was hopelessly suicidal and believing I was better off dead.

What helped me to engage more meaningfully with the assessor was when I felt the assessor cared. If I was shown compassion, empathy, respect, and understanding, I would establish a greater sense of trust in the assessor and would comply.

▼ Presenting complaint and history of presenting complaint

When taking a clinical history, it is standard practice to start with understanding the problem, or problems, that the patient is presenting with. This is an opportunity to understand what has led to the mental health assessment and develop a critical awareness and person-centred understanding of the patient's experiences. Building a timeline is a useful way of helping the assessor to conceptualize how the patient perceives their problems, how their symptoms have evolved over time, and any identifiable precipitating/relieving factors. Identifying the onset of symptoms can also be a useful way of determining whether further investigations are required to rule out organic causes; it is therefore important to spend sufficient time talking to the patient about their symptoms and raising any concerns with the wider team.

✖ Patient perspective: being trauma-informed

Be considerate and mindful as to if there is pre-existing trauma and adapt a trauma-informed approach, where you are not assuming severe abuse but acknowledging there may be sensitivities or triggers for a patient. Often it helps to shift your thinking or style of questioning from 'What is wrong with you?' to 'What has happened to you?' Further information about this approach can be found at The British Psychological Society website (www.bps.org.uk/PTM-main). This is an overall more compassionate approach to mental health assessment and expresses empathy. It is good to be respectfully curious about what is going on for the patient and to visualize yourself in the patient's shoes to understand their presentation.

▼ Past psychiatric, medical, and surgical history

The next stage of the assessment involves taking a wider view of the patient's involvement in health services, including their medical/surgical history. Diagnostic overshadowing is a phenomenon where people with a mental health diagnosis are less likely to be referred, screened, or treated for physical health conditions because their symptoms are assumed to be related to their mental disorder (Public Health England, 2019). This is particularly problematic given that people experiencing

mental illness are more likely to have long-term physical health problems. Mental health nurses are therefore in a key position to advocate for patients and ensure that their physical health needs are met. Assessing a patient's medical/surgical history is also a way of identifying predictors of poor outcomes and developing a differential diagnosis. This is particularly relevant when mental and physical health conditions can present in similar ways.

▼ Family history and medication history

During an assessment it is important to identify whether other members of the patient's family experience mental distress. Growing up in a family where other people have serious and enduring mental illness can increase the risk of exposure to adverse childhood experiences (Isobel and Delgado, 2018). There is also evidence that there may be a genetic predisposition to some mental disorders (Sandstrom et al., 2020), and that childhood trauma and/or adverse childhood events may have an intergenerational impact (Narayan et al., 2021).

It is also important to ask about any medication the patient is taking or has taken in the past. This supports effective treatment planning by identifying medications that have been ineffective or associated with intolerable side effects. Assessors should also ask patients about non-prescribed medications since some of these may have psychotropic properties and/or interact with commonly prescribed psychiatric drugs.

▼ Alcohol and recreational drug use

To avoid making assumptions, it is important that all patients are routinely asked about alcohol and recreational drug use. Knowing about this is important for assessment because alcohol and recreational drug use can be implicated in precipitating and perpetuating mental distress (e.g. abrupt alcohol withdrawal can be life-threatening for people with alcohol dependence). Alcohol use can be quantified by asking patients how much they drink (either in units, strength, or volume) and how often, but assessors should bear in mind that excessive alcohol consumption is not always a predictor of dependence. In terms of brief screening, the Alcohol Use Disorders Identification Test (AUDIT) is recommended by the World Health Organization and can be a supportive tool in identifying problematic alcohol use (Barbor et al., 2001).

Recreational drug use can be quantified in a similar way to alcohol (by asking about frequency, cost, and drug weight); remember to qualify any terms used that you are unsure about the meaning of.

Every clinical interaction is a potential opportunity for health promotion; if a patient presents with excessive alcohol/recreational drug use then mental health assessments should also include an assessment of the patient's motivation to change. As assessment of motivation to change can be supported with the Readiness to Change Questionnaire (Heather and Rollnick, 1993). People with problematic alcohol/recreational drug use are frequently exposed to negative judgements/stigma so careful communication is required to demonstrate unconditional positive regard.

▼ Personal and social history

Taking a personal and social history from a patient involves starting at pregnancy/childbirth and asking about developmental milestones (this often requires collateral history

from other family members). Asking the patient about their school experience, qualifications, and employment history may also provide insight into the duration of their symptoms and/or any adverse experiences/trauma (e.g. bullying). Understanding the patient's social network is also an important way of identifying their coping style and may give an indication of who should be included in their recovery plan. When taking a patient's personal history, the assessor will also need to ask questions about historically taboo topics (e.g. abuse). It is important these topics are discussed sensitively and universally: people experiencing severe and enduring mental disorders are more likely to have experienced abuse then the general population and asking about this is in line with a trauma-informed approach to mental health care (Khalifeh et al., 2014). It is also an important time to consider any additional safeguarding/risk planning.

This part of the assessment provides an important opportunity to build up a picture of protective factors and sources of resilience for the patient.

▼ Forensic history and premorbid personality

During a mental health assessment, it is important to ask patients universally if they have had involvement with the criminal justice system. This is important for accurate risk assessment and may give an indication of the patient's mental health status in the past.

Understanding what someone was like before the presenting issue started is important and is often referred to as premorbid personality. This helps identify any changes to the individual's personality and behaviour as well as providing structure for discussions around what recovery may look like for that individual.

✖ Patient perspective

Often in my journey, I would feel that I would not receive good care due to being a young South Asian female and would be conscious that I did not look like any of the assessors. In assessment, it is key to understand that sometimes mental illness can look different in marginalized and ethnically diverse communities.

▼ Mental state examination

Mental state examination is a standardized component of all mental health assessments and provides a useful way of documenting how patients present, even if they are unable to answer questions or unwilling to engage in the assessment process. Under these circumstances, mental state examination is essential in deciding whether immediate action is required to alleviate the patient's distress and/or reduce their risks. The components of the mental state examination are as follows.

Appearance

Health care professionals should only comment on a patient's appearance if it is relevant to the assessment and/or there is a clear justification for its inclusion (e.g. self-harm scars, bruising, and self-care). Noting extremes of weight may also be useful for patients with disordered eating and/or as part of an overall assessment of the patient's health (eating disorders require a specialist assessment and it is important referrals contain as much information as possible to allow for appropriate triaging). Ill-fitting clothes may also cue questions about possible recent acute weight gain or loss, or potential financial concerns. Tattoos and body art may be meaningful to the patient so they should be given an opportunity to discuss these, if necessary/appropriate.

Behaviour

Many mental disorders have a behavioural component, so it is useful to document any unusual findings during an assessment. Is the patient demonstrating signs of anxiety, such as hand wringing, pacing, or foot tapping (be aware that the assessment itself may be responsible for some of this anxiety). Is the patient able to concentrate during the assessment and answer questions appropriately? Is the patient avoiding eye contact or staring? Is the patient presenting with signs of hostility or paranoia? Remember that if the patient is demonstrating aggressive behaviour and the assessor is unable to mitigate environmental risks, the assessor should leave the assessment immediately and follow this up appropriately with support from the multidisciplinary team.

Speech

Is the patient's speech normal in rate, tone, and content? Rate refers to the speed at which the patient is talking, for example, rapid speech may suggest that the patient is anxious or manic in some circumstances. Tone refers to the ability to speak with varied tonality, for example, monotone speech may suggest that the patient is low in mood. Content refers to the variety of speech offered by the patient, for example, severe depression can reduce the ability to generate spontaneous thought, leading to short, closed loops of sentences.

Mood

Mood should be assessed either subjectively or objectively. Subjective mood involves trying to understand the patient's own perception of their mood (e.g. by asking the patient directly or using rating scales). Objective mood is estimated by considering any signs or cues that the patient presents with.

Affect refers to the outward presentation of someone's mood. Incongruent affect occurs when the patient's presentation does not match the mood, they describe (e.g. they are smiling/laughing but describing their mood as low). Blunted affect refers to a reduction or absence of expressive mood (e.g. reduced facial expressions). This may occur as part of many mental health conditions, including depression, psychosis, and trauma.

Thoughts and perceptions

Is the patient expressing unusual or bizarre ideas that they may not be able to support with evidence? Thoughts of unevidenced persecution and paranoia may also suggest an underlying mental disorder. However, cultural literacy demands that we listen to patients and understand what is normal for them. It is therefore essential that unusual ideas are not dismissed as evidence of mental illness.

Switching topics quickly with no obvious links or stopping mid-sentence with no obvious cause may indicate that the patient is having difficulty with their thought processes. Thought blocking occurs when patients experience obstructions to their thought processes that they are unable to move past. In some psychotic disorders, patients also describe thoughts being inserted or withdrawn from their consciousness by an external agent.

All assessors should routinely enquire about thoughts of self-harm, suicidal ideation, and thoughts of anger or aggressions towards others. If the patient indicates that they are experiencing these thoughts, this may prompt a specialist assessment. If there is any doubt with regard to risk in these areas, it is important that this is discussed with the multidisciplinary team and a clear plan is made, documented, and shared with the patient and their supporters.

Hallucinations can occur in any sensory modality, but auditory and visual hallucinations are linked to several mental health conditions. Physical health screening should be considered for new and/or rapidly occurring hallucinations. Olfactory (smell) and gustatory (taste) hallucinations also suggest a possible underlying organic pathology.

Disassociation occurs when patients believe they are not in control of their actions or are experiencing them as though observing another person.

▼ Cognition and insight

A very simple test of a patient's cognition is to determine whether they are orientated to time, date, and place. Assessors can also use bedside tests to assess the patient's attention, concentration, and memory. Insight refers to the patient's ability to recognize the nature of their symptoms and assessing this gives an indication to the assessor of whether the patient is likely to accept input from mental health services. It is important to respect patients' views and symptoms attributions; having an alternative explanation does not always mean that the patient lacks insight.

▼ Documentation

Following assessment, documentation in a timely way that is in line with local and national policy is important to reduce the risk of patients needing to repeat information and to ensure continuity of care.

✖ Patient perspective

It was good practice, from my experience as a patient, when an assessor would ask me after the assessment how I felt about their practice. This also gives the patient a voice and a choice, both of which is relatively rare for a patient to have, especially when undergoing mental health act assessment.

▲ Conclusion

This chapter introduces the history of mental health assessment, the nursing role in mental health assessment, and how the patient's voice can be heard throughout the mental health assessment process. The nursing process highlights that assessment underpins all clinical interactions. As such, this skill should be continually revisited, developed, and reflected upon and practitioners should consider including assessment in any revalidation and feedback opportunities.

✖ Patient perspective: hope-based collaboration

Don't lose hope in your patient. Many clinicians thought I would be in receipt of mental health services until late in my adult life. Upon assessment, many clinicians would see me at my absolute-worst state of mental illness. Offering hope, even at the stage of assessment, can lead to a patient feeling significantly more empowered and in control of their journey.

✖ Tips from service users

1. Mental health assessments may be routine for health care professionals, but not for patients. Assessments should involve learning together through a collaborative discussion. This will help keep the focus on the patient and reduce the risk of a tick-box approach.
2. Ensure patients are prepared for assessments and make any necessary adaptations beforehand. This will increase the chance of the patient feeling able to engage with the assessment. Consider what triggers may be present for the patient, without making judgements, and ensure appropriate support is provided.
3. Trust in health care professionals cannot, and should not, be assumed. Showing compassion, empathy, respect, and understanding throughout the assessment process is important to help work towards building this trust.
4. Addressing the power imbalance in the assessment is vital to offer a voice to the patient and facilitate shared decision-making. Ask patients at the end of the assessment how they found your practice, respect this feedback, and be open to continual professional development.

✚ References

Barbor, T. F., Higgins-Biddle, J. C., Saunders, J. D., and Monteiro, M. G. (2001). *AUDIT. The Alcohol Use Disorders Identification Test. Guidelines for Use in Primary Care.* *Department of Mental Health and Substance Dependence, World Health Organization. Available at: https://www.who. int/publications/i/item/WHO-MSD-MSB-01.6a*

Baugh, C., Blanchard, E., and Hopkins, I. (2020). *Quality Standard for Liaison Psychiatry Services. Royal College of Psychiatrists. Available at: https://www.rcpsych.ac.uk/docs/default-source/improving-care/ccqi/quality-networks/psychiatric-liaison-services-plan/quality-standards-for-liaison-psychiatry-services---sixth-edition-2020.pdf?sfvrsn=389bb253_0*

Durning, S. J. and Artino, A. R. (2011). *Situativity theory: a perspective on how participants and the environment can interact: AMEE Guide no. 52. Medical Teacher 33(3), 188–199.*

Health Education England (2020). *Mental Health Nursing: Competence and Career Framework. Available at: https://www.hee.nhs.uk/sites/default/files/documents/HEE Mental Health Nursing Career and Competence Framework.pdf*

Heather, N. and Rollnick, S. (1993). *Readiness to Change Questionnaire: User's Manual (Revised Version). National Drug and Alcohol Research Centre. Available at: https://ndarc.med.unsw.edu.au/resource/readiness-change-questionnaire-users-manual-revised-version*

Isobel, S. and Delgado, C. (2018). *Safe and collaborative communication skills: a step towards mental health nurses implementing trauma informed care. Archives of Psychiatric Nursing 32(2), 291–296.*

Khalifeh, H. (2014). *Domestic and sexual violence against patients with severe mental illness. Psychological Medicine 45(4), 875–886.*

Legislation.gov.uk (2010). *Equality Act 2010. Available at: https://www.legislation.gov.uk/ukpga/2010/15*

Legislation.gov.uk (2018). *Data Protection Act 2018. Available at: https://www.legislation.gov.uk/ukpga/2018/12/enacted*

Mental Health Taskforce (2016). *The Five Year Forward View for Mental Health. NHS England. Available at: https://www.england.nhs.uk/publication/the-five-year-forward-view-for-mental-health/*

Ministry of Defence (2021). *The Armed Forces Covenant and Veterans Annual Report. Available at: https://ass ets.publishing.service.gov.uk/government/uploads/system/uploads/attachment_data/file/1040571/Armed_Forces_Covenant_annual_report_2021.pdf*

Narayan, A. J., Lieberman, A. F., and Masten, A. S. (2021). *Intergenerational transmission and prevention of adverse childhood experiences (ACEs). Clinical Psychology Review 85, 101997.*

National Institute for Health and Care Excellence (2023). *How should I screen for problem drinking? Available at: https://cks.nice.org.uk/topics/alcohol-problem-drinking/diagnosis/how-to-screen/*

Nursing and Midwifery Council (2018). *Future Nurse: Standards of Proficiency for Registered Nurses. Available at: https://www.nmc.org.uk/globalassets/sitedocuments/standards-of-proficiency/nurses/future-nurse-proficiencies.pdf*

Patyal, A. (2010). *What to expect when giving nursing evidence at a first-tier tribunal. Mental Health Practice 13(5), 32–34.*

Public Health England (2019). *NHS RightCare Toolkit: Physical Ill-Health and CVD Prevention in People with Severe Mental Illness (SMI). Available at: https://www.england.nhs.uk/rightcare/wp-content/uploads/sites/40/2019/03/nhs-rightcare-toolkit-cvd-prevention.pdf*

Sandstrom, A., MacKenzie, L., Pizzo, A., Fine, A., Rempel, S., Howard, C., Stephens, M., Patterson, V. C., Drobinin, V., Van Gestel, H., Howes Vallis, E., Zwicker, A., Propper, L., Abidi, S., Bagnell, A., Lovas, D., Cumby, J., Alda, M., Uher, R., and Pavlova, B. (2020). *Observed psychopathology in offspring of parents with major depressive disorder, bipolar disorder and schizophrenia. Psychological Medicine 50(6), 1050–1056.*

Trenoweth, S. (2016). *Promoting Recovery in Mental Health Nursing. London: Learning Matters.*

World Health Organization (2018). *Comprehensive Mental Health Action Plan 2013–2030. Geneva: World Health Organization. Available at: https://www.who.int/publications/i/item/9789240031029*

8 Working in partnership

Alan Simpson   **Geoff Brennan**

Learning outcomes

By the end of this chapter, you should be able to:

1 Demonstrate an understanding of skills required to work in partnership with service users

2 Describe the potential areas of conflict in working collaboratively and how to resolve them

3 Identify some of the theories and approaches that underpin these skills

4 Use the partnership working skills in practice.

▼ Introduction

Developing and sustaining a positive therapeutic relationship with the service user, their family, and other carers is central to the role of the mental health nurse and is recognized as a core competency for nurses in policies across the UK's four nations.

It also offers the solid foundation for collaborative working, which is a key feature of the recovery approach (Box 8.1) and an empowering way of helping the service user. To work in partnership requires the relationship between the mental health nurse and service user to be positive, meaningful, and based on trust.

The key principles of the recovery approach inform mental health nursing practice in all areas of care and underpin service structures, individual practice, and educational preparation (Department of Health, 2006). Nurses need to:

- value the aims of service users
- work in partnership and offer meaningful choice
- be optimistic and offer hope about the possibilities of positive change
- value the social inclusion of people with mental health problems.

Working collaboratively as a nurse is to recognize the unique knowledge and expertise the service user has about their own life and experiences. We all tend to carry age-old ideas about nurses caring for the patient, and doing things for the patient (and sometimes this is still what is required in the short term), so working in partnership is not necessarily easy for either party.

In this model of working, the nurse uses the opportunities within a positive therapeutic relationship to enable the service user to find their own ways forward. The nurse draws on their expertise and knowledge to help the person recognize the choices they have and to resolve problems in beneficial and acceptable ways that help them to regain control over their health and life.

The pursuit of jointly agreed strategies is more empowering for the service user as the nurse is not taking over and making decisions for them. The nurse helps the person develop and draw on their own interests and skills to deal with challenges on their personal journey to recovery.

In this chapter, we outline some of the skills and approaches that mental health nurses need to work in partnership and will consider these across the various life stages the nurse is likely to encounter in their work. We also identify some of the challenges that may be encountered when trying to implement these skills in the 'real world' of mental health services, where staff often face huge demands and insufficient resources (Brennan et al., 2006; Coffey et al., 2019).

Box 8.1 Recovery approach and mental health nursing

Recovery can be defined as a personal process of tackling the adverse impacts of experiencing mental health problems, despite their continuing or long-term presence. It involves personal development and change, including acceptance there are problems to face, a sense of involvement and control over one's life, the cultivation of hope and using the support from others, including direct collaboration in joint problem solving between people using services, workers, and professionals. Recovery starts with the individual and works from the inside out. For this reason, it is personalised and challenges traditional service approaches.

Frak (2005, p. 1)

▼ Why form a partnership?

Why do nurses form partnerships with service users? The simple answer is that partnerships are forged to help the person to get better. But then we must ask, what does 'better' mean? Well, 'better' means helping a person create a healthier future, with more quality of life, and better mental and physical health, combined with opportunities for meaningful relationships, accommodation, employment, and education. All these are aspects of the recovery approach. In essence, then, we form partnerships with service users to facilitate recovery.

We are still left with questions, however, as recovery has different meaning for people with different issues. Many aspects of 'recovery' are dependent on individual characteristics, cultural norms, and stage of life. Look at Table 8.1 and ask yourself if you agree with the broad statements about recovery as applied to different user groups.

Table 8.1 Approaches to recovery

For people who are dealing with . . .	Recovery allows . . .	Recovery should not include . . .
Dementia	• Recognition of personhood (personality, life history, choices, preferences) • Realignment of key relationships • Comfort and dignity as condition progresses • Dignity in end of life	• Denial of the progressive worsening of the condition • False hope for user and carer • Dismissal of previous biography and life choices
Psychosis	• Remission or control of psychotic symptoms • Access to same life choices as people without psychotic symptoms • Active and visual confrontation of stigma	• False hope for user and carer • Denial of the disabling effects of psychosis for many • Denial of social needs such as housing and employment
Personality disorder	• Acknowledgement of the right to access care • Supportive relationships which set boundaries and allow growth • Recognition of the difficulties in processing emotion	• Denial of right to treatment • User being blamed for difficulties • Iatrogenic problems through inappropriate treatments
Depression and suicidal urges	• Protection from self-destructive impulses • Hope for a better future	• Freedom to take their life • Inability to take therapeutic risks

Therefore, recovery needs to be defined for any given client with any given problem. This makes it impossible to discuss recovery in any more than general terms unless related to an individual. It should also be remembered that recovery came from the service user movement and that nurses 'borrow' the term when they use it (Davidson, 2005). In addition, within specific services such as those for people with dementia, there is debate about the appropriateness of the word 'recovery', with concern that the word reads as 'cure' or a return of full function (Adams, 2007). In general, therefore, while we may all agree with the principles of the personal focus and respect for personhood in the concept of recovery, we may have to find careful ways to communicate these ideals within specific services.

▼ Policy and evidence base

Best practice in mental health nursing is underpinned by several frameworks that shape and inform the outcomes of mental health education and training. Working in partnership is included in the Nursing and Midwifery Council (2014) *Standards for Competence for Registered Nurses* and as a core competency of Health Education England's (2020) *Mental Health Nursing: Competence and Career Framework*. Partnership working is now an essential aspect in:

- respecting the person's diversity
- providing care and treatment
- challenging inequality, stigma, and discrimination
- promoting recovery
- identifying people's needs and strengths
- providing person-centred care and in promoting safety and positive risk-taking.

In other words, partnership working is at the heart of good mental health nursing.

In community mental health services, care is delivered within a framework of **case management** where service users' needs are assessed and addressed by a **care coordinator** working as part of a **multidisciplinary team**. This role is most often carried out by mental health nurses.

The care coordinator is required to work in partnership with the service user to understand their strengths and abilities, to identify their health, social care, and safety needs, to write a care plan in collaboration with the user, and then ensure the care plan is implemented and reviewed by members of the multidisciplinary team and other agencies. Members of the person's family and other informal carers should also be consulted when appropriate and should be provided with a copy of the plan.

There has long been concern that the care planning **processes** are overly bureaucratic, and the 'form filling' can dominate the work of nurses and others at the expense of partnership working and providing therapeutic interventions (Simpson, 2005). A systematic review of the literature on service users' and carers' views on mental health nursing suggested that mental health nurses too often fail to ensure that partnership working takes place (Department of Health, 2006, p. 56). While service users tend to place a positive value on mental health nurses and hold their listening skills in high regard, nurses do not provide them with sufficient information to make informed choices and tend not to provide suitable opportunities for collaborating in their own care.

More recent studies of the care planning and coordinating processes in community and inpatient settings reported similar findings (Coffey et al., 2019; Simpson et al., 2016) and contributed to the publication of *The Community Mental Health Framework* (NHS England et al., 2019). This amplified the need for partnership working by calling for: 'High-quality co-produced, holistic, personalised care and support planning for people with severe mental health problems living in the community … with service users actively co-producing brief and relevant care plans with staff' (NHS England, 2022, p. 3).

While there has been analysis of partnership working, the 'gold standards' of research are difficult to apply in such complex contexts of this approach (Repper and Brooker, 1997). This is because partnership working tends to grow out of a therapeutic relationship built on empathic understanding, warmth or positive regard, and genuineness or congruence. These are the three conditions that Carl Rogers identified through research and practice as 'necessary and sufficient' in any person trying to help another achieve personal growth or therapeutic change (Rogers, 1961). Consequently, it is difficult and arguably futile to tease out or unpack those aspects of such a relationship most associated with 'partnership working' and subject them to a randomized controlled trial.

It is also difficult to measure and regulate components of a partnership relationship which necessarily involves participants' personalities, personal styles, and culture. Similarly, it would be difficult to control for the influences of personal histories, experiences, and contextual factors such as age, gender, and ethnicity. It would also be unethical to measure good partnership working by deliberately allocating people to a group where abusive or no-partnership working was taking place to measure against where good practice was the norm.

Despite these challenges, we can identify specific skills associated with partnership working and provide evidence through methods like individual reflective analysis, case studies, and learning through experience. Often, useful sources are key texts which deal directly with the formulation of partnership working and what that is like for the worker. These often come from practitioners with counselling and psychotherapeutic skills, as well as mental health nursing, and tend to be derived from many years of experience in working with service users and supervising workers. We can also draw on studies that have collated and analysed the accounts and perspectives of service users, especially studies designed and conducted by or co-produced with service user researchers (Sweeney et al., 2014; Trevillion et al., 2022).

There is a growing body of research into the effectiveness of various interpersonal, psychotherapeutic, or conversational approaches for various conditions (Barth et al., 2016; Huhn et al., 2014; Orfanos et al., 2015; Roth and Fonagy, 1996). Many of these are being adapted and employed in mainstream mental health and psychiatric settings (Cahill et al., 2010; Jacobsen et al., 2018; Parry, 1996). **Cognitive behavioural therapy (CBT)** is considered effective for a range of conditions (Mendez-Bustos et al., 2019; Newell and Gournay, 2000) with variable evidence available as to effectiveness in routine practice (Currid et al., 2011; Durham et al., 2000, Wood et al., 2020).

CBT helps people talk about how they think about themselves and the people around them and how what they do affects their thoughts and feelings. It can help people change how they think (cognitive) and what they do (behaviour), which can help them feel better and in more control. CBT focuses on 'here and now' problems and difficulties, rather than searching for the causes of distress or symptoms in the past and can help to make sense of overwhelming problems by breaking them down into smaller parts. **Psychosocial interventions** have been developed for people with psychosis which take many of the principles and techniques of CBT and use them alongside family work and case management to assist the person with psychotic experiences (Healy et al., 2006). Within substance misuse services, **motivational interviewing** techniques serve a similar function in assisting the service user to understand their motivation to change and take them through the difficulties of change (Rollnick and Miller, 1995).

Understandably, service users may initially feel overwhelmed and powerless in the face of mental distress and experiences that are frightening, and disorientating. This can be reinforced by stigmatized and discriminatory attitudes frequently shown in society towards people with mental illness—even among mental health professionals (Henderson et al., 2014). Where such beliefs are reinforced by staff, perhaps influenced by a limiting, medicalized view of mental distress, nurses and others can wrongly act **for** service users and reduce their autonomy—sometimes when it is not necessary.

Another approach that provides an empowering framework for partnership working with users is Egan's (1994) **skilled helper model**. Developed in psychological counselling, this person-centred, problem-solving approach has been adapted by many people working in psychiatric settings. Egan argued that people are often poor at solving problems and mental distress develops when people try to ignore or deny problems. Alternatively, they get stuck repeatedly attempting the same unsuccessful solutions. The nurse's task within this approach is to help the service user become more able to manage the problems they are faced with. To achieve this, Egan identifies three stages:

1. Help the person identify and clarify their difficulties, needs and problems, but also the things that are going well.

2. Help the person identify what they would like to do and achieve—to help them construct a better future.

3. Help the person create strategies to move towards those goals.

The nurse aims to engage the person in a process that moves through the three stages, while acknowledging the person brings a unique knowledge and understanding of their life story and situation. The nurse shares knowledge of the helping processes for people to become more resourceful and self-supporting (Watkins, 2001). We shall look at these approaches in more detail later.

In helping the person develop better problem-solving we should recognize that many people already use strategies that are helpful. Seminal research studies conducted with people diagnosed with schizophrenia (Barrowclough and Tarrier, 1997) and bipolar disorder (Lam et al., 1999) found that most people employed various coping techniques with varying success. Today, it us widely acknowledged that such strategies are useful and effective (Longden et al., 2018).

By acknowledging the service user's own attempts to manage situations, the nurse actively demonstrates a commitment to partnership working and reinforces the person's determination to self-manage. Nurses then draw on their knowledge and experience to suggest additional coping mechanisms to help the user broaden and strengthen their repertoire. Watkins (2001) suggests that several interventions drawn from solution-focused therapy are effective in helping people find strategies to move forward in their recovery. The nurse asks solution-focused questions that help the person identify strategies they employ and to encourage them to develop new ones.

However, it is also important that nurses adapt and integrate such skills within a conversational, collaborative style of working that recognizes nurses' unique role (Gamble and Brennan, 2023; Repper and Perkins, 1996). This helps normalize the application of these complex skills (Brandon 1996), making their use more acceptable.

Finally, we must consider that partnership working sometimes involves an element of risk: 'The possibility of risk is an inevitable consequence of empowered people taking decisions about their own lives' (Department of Health, 2007, p. 8).

Research into recovery-focused ways of working found that mental health nurses and colleagues address issues of risk and safety within the multidisciplinary team but too often fail to involve the service user or their family (Coffey et al., 2016; Simpson et al., 2016). There is insufficient space in this chapter to detail these issues, but it is worth readers noting guidance that supports the principle of empowerment through managing choice and risk in a responsible, considered way. This guidance encourages multidisciplinary teams and services to foster a common, agreed approach to risk and to share responsibility for risk in a transparent and constructive way (Department of Health, 2007).

▼ Step-by-step guide to partnership working

How do we form a partnership?

There are basic behaviours that any nurse should adhere to in interactions. These include:

- being respectful
- keeping promises
- being honest (e.g. about availability)
- paying attention to privacy and dignity.

While these have been covered in previous chapters, it is worth remembering that partnerships are based on mutual respect. Nurses show this respect in the first instance by paying attention to the basic courtesies. This may include welcoming people, making eye contact, smiling, showing interest in the person, and being sensitive to the situation that may be very anxiety provoking for the individual. Once a respectful relationship has been established (and there are service users—and indeed some nurses—who find it very difficult to build a respectful relationship), partnership working can be defined by two basic features. These two features are engagement and problem-solving.

Engagement

Astute readers may be asking: 'What is the difference between a respectful relationship and engagement?' The difference is that you enter a respectful relationship, but you then engage with each other towards a specific goal. Engagement, therefore, 'can be defined as the act of beginning and carrying on of an activity with a sense of emotional involvement or commitment and the deliberate application of effort' by both parties (Lequerica and Kortte, 2010, p. 416).

Problem-solving

Problem-solving is the vehicle that allows the partnership to achieve set goals. Problem-solving can be broken down into distinct steps (Box 8.2) and builds on Egan's (1994) model identified earlier.

Difficulties

In many ways the practice example in Box 8.3 is an ideal position in that two capable people put their expertise together and aim to problem-solve a difficulty. There can, however, be factors which negatively impact the formation of a partnership between the user and the nurse (Table 8.2).

Working in partnership and agreeing on a plan can be extremely difficult and challenging for some people and trusting another person and working with them closely can be frightening. In good partnership working, the nurse will encourage sensitive discussion of the challenging emotions this arouses. Sometimes you will need to temporarily stop the

Box 8.2 Steps in problem-solving

Helping users identify and clarify needs and problems

- Helping them tell their story ('Why are you here?').

- Helping them unload.

- Avoiding assumptions, interpretations, our solutions.

- Establishing shared understanding of what the situation is and what needs to change.

- Measure the need or problem and how it affects the user.

- Identifying how we can help them.

Develop an intervention or set of interventions designed to satisfy the need or alleviate the problem

- Bring in prior knowledge or find knowledge about the evidence base for that problem or need.

- Negotiate areas of responsibility in carrying out the intervention.

- Describe, in terms the user can understand, who will do what within a time frame.

- Record this, again in ways understood by the user of the service. This is the basis of good care planning.

Evaluate the intervention

- We do this simply by measuring the outcome against our previous measurement (e.g. a recognized measurement of anxiety or depression (quantitative) and asking the user 'Did it work?!' (qualitative)).

- If it didn't achieve the required outcome, change. It is important in this that nurses avoid blaming the user or themselves. If the attempt was honest, we have learnt a valuable lesson. It is important to know what does not work at a given time. It gets us nearer to what will work.

- Few interventions are completely successful in all departments right away. We learn what we can from each attempt.

Box 8.3 Practice example: problem-solving erratic sleep

Jane is on an acute ward recovering from an acute psychotic relapse. She is well enough to undertake a mental state examination with Jack, the nurse. In this she has no ongoing psychotic symptoms but an erratic and distressing sleep pattern. Jane and Jack agree to work on this. They use a sleep diary and an anxiety scale to measure the problem.

Jane believes in the power of crystals and meditation. Jack gets some information on sleep hygiene. After looking at Jane's night routine they agree to changes, including Jane's ideas (using crystals and practising yoga in the evening) and ideas from Jack (reduction in caffeine and use of digital devices before trying to sleep). Although there is limited success at first in terms of increased hours sleep, Jane feels less anxious. The intervention is changed to include listening to soothing music at night. Over time the intervention is felt to be working by Jane. There is a reduction in her anxiety score, and she states she is less anxious. Hours slept does not improve.

problem-solving to reassure, renegotiate, and re-establish the partnership.

The nurse's good intentions to work respectfully and collaboratively can also be frustrated as we repeatedly encounter people that are weary, suspicious, mistrustful, ambivalent, and angry—or who appear to undermine or mistrust genuine attempts at partnership. Recent research provides greater understanding of the factors that may be involved in developing and sustaining partnerships with people with such complex emotional needs (Foye et al., 2022; Trevillion et al., 2022).

Compassion and emotional energy are not inexhaustible commodities and continually stressful encounters can cause intense anxiety leading nurses to withdraw psychologically

Table 8.2 Circumstances and considerations affecting partnership working

Circumstance	Considerations
An absence of capacity in the service user. Can be due to many reasons, e.g.: • confusion (as in dementia) • acute psychosis	Be aware of the Mental Capacity Act and guidance. Work with wider network but still including and informing the user. Do not make decisions in isolation but discuss with other colleagues and carers and take consideration of previous life choices such as advanced directives
Service user does not identify nurse as someone who can help them. Can be due to: • difficulties in accepting condition • perceptions of nurse by the service user	Accept where the person is rather than force the issue. Maintain a position of open and honest working. Allow the user to choose other workers (including those outside services such as advocates or peer workers) and support this partnership
External factors which influence partnership: • partnership working within the criminal justice system, or • partnership working within forensic services • partnership working within the mental health act	Be totally honest regarding what will happen to shared information. Accept that there may be conflicts of interest and be honest about any external demands for information outside of the partnership. Allow the user to judge how much to collaborate in the partnership. Share any written or verbal feedback to others if possible and appropriate
The nurse lacks competence or knowledge	Be honest about your weaknesses and lack of knowledge. Allow yourself to learn. Seek information and supervision. Actively seek out role models from whom you can learn. Ask service users how other nurses have helped them

and physically from the service user (Bray, 1999; Menzies, 1960). We often hear complaints of nurses spending too much time in the office, rather than engaging with patients. To be consistently present, to apply interactive skills, and to work collaboratively with enthusiasm and empathy, mental health nurses need to be enabled and encouraged to use personal reflection, supportive colleagues, teamwork, and clinical supervision.

Endings

Partnership between a service user and a nurse will inevitably end. It is important for both nurse and client to recognize that ending is important. Given that partnership working involves the investment of emotional energy, the ending of the partnership should be as healthy as possible for both parties. Nurses will, inevitably, form many partnerships during their career. Some of these partnerships will adhere to the positive

principles outlined in this chapter. Some will be stymied by the difficulties outlined. To remain optimistic and giving of oneself, all partnerships need to be reflected upon, as indicated above. In our experience, many nurses remain optimistic and giving because they experience both positive partnerships with clients and positive support from colleagues when difficulties arise.

If it is possible to end the partnership in a healthy manner, it is important for nurses and clients to meet and evaluate. In this, both parties can learn valuable lessons as to what helped and what hindered the partnership. This meeting should be structured to allow the exchange of experiences and, if appropriate, a reflection on difficulties. If it is not possible to meet the client, nurses should use supervision to reflect on the partnership and any feelings they are left with. While it is sometimes appropriate to communicate these reflections to the client via a letter or phone call, the nurse should always be clear that the client is able to receive these communications in the spirit they are given. In other words, nurses should ensure that their motives for communicating are not to lecture, blame, or punish, but a genuine attempt at reconciliation of the partnership. It is important to remember that many clients will continue to use services and form other partnerships and the nurse has a responsibility beyond their own interaction with clients in allowing them to believe that the services are aimed at truly assisting them despite any difficulties.

▲ Conclusion

All services are now signed up to the **principles** of recovery, even if it is difficult to use the word 'recovery' for all service areas. This commitment is enshrined in many of the policy documents of the last decade. At the core of recovery is a new focus for the relationship between clients and mental health professionals, including nurses. In this there has been an active shift towards collaborative work aimed at assisting clients to solve the effects of mental health problems rather than prescriptive interventions that fail to account for personal preferences. This collaborative work is what partnership working is all about. Nurses need to actively attend to the principles of partnership working, despite the many difficulties.

✖ Tips from service users

1 Ask me what has been happening and what matters to me.
2 Find out who is important to me (e.g. family members, friends, neighbours, and members of faith community) and how much I would like them involved.
3 Check out what my priorities are and try hard to respect that—and be honest with me if you are not able to do that.

W   Companion website

For extra resources on the topics covered in this chapter, visit the companion website at: www.oup.com/mhns

✚   References

Adams, T. (2007). *Dementia Care Nursing: Promoting Well-being in People with Dementia and their Families.* London: Palgrave.

Barrowclough, C. and Tarrier, N. (1997). *Families of Schizophrenic Patients: Cognitive Behavioural Interventions.* London: Thornes.

Barth, J., Munder, T., Gerger, H., Nuesch, E., Trelle, S., Znoj, H., Juni, P., and Cuijpers, P. (2013). *Comparative efficacy of seven psychotherapeutic interventions for patients with depression: a network meta-analysis. Plos Medicine. https://doi.org/10.1371/journal. pmed.1001454*

Brandon, D. (1996). *Normalising professional skills. In: T. Heller, J. Reynolds, R. Gomm, R. Muston, and S. Pattison, Eds., Mental Health Matters, pp. 297–303. Basingstoke: Macmillan/Open University Press.*

Bray, J. (1999). *An ethnographic study of psychiatric nursing. Journal of Psychiatric & Mental Health Nursing 6(4), 297–305.*

Brennan, G., Flood, C., and Bowers, L. (2006). *Constraints and blocks to change and improvement on acute psychiatric wards—lessons from the City Nurses project. Journal of Psychiatric and Mental Health Nursing 13(5), 475–482.*

Cahill, J., Barkham, M., and Stiles, W. B. (2010). *Systematic review of practice-based research on psychological therapies in routine clinic settings. British Journal of Clinical Psychology 49, 421–453. https://doi. org/10.1348/014466509X470789*

Coffey, M., Cohen, R., Faulkner, A., Hannigan, B., Simpson, A., and Barlow, S. (2016). *Ordinary risks and accepted fictions: how contrasting and competing priorities work in risk assessment and mental health care planning. Health Expectations 20(3), 471–483.*

Coffey, M., Hannigan, B., Barlow, S., Cartwright, M., Cohen, R., Faulkner, A., Jones, A., and Simpson, A. (2019). *Recovery-focused mental health care planning and co-ordination in acute inpatient mental health settings: a cross national comparative mixed methods study. BMC Psychiatry 19(1), 115.*

Currid, T., Nikcevic, A., and Spada, M. (2011). *Cognitive behavioural therapy and its relevance to nursing. British Journal of Nursing 20(22), 1443–1447.*

Davidson, L. (2005). *Recovery, self-management, and the expert patient—changing the culture of mental health from a UK perspective. Journal of Mental Health 14(1), 25–35.*

Department of Health (2006). *From Values to Action: The Chief Nursing Officer's Review of Mental Health Nursing. London: Department of Health.*

Department of Health (2007). *Independence, Choice, and Risk: A Guide to Best Practice in Supported Decision Making. London: Department of Health.*

Durham, R. C., Swan, J. S., and Fisher, P. L. (2000). *Complexity and collaboration in routine practice of CBT: what doesn't work with whom and how might it work better? Journal of Mental Health 9(4), 429–444.*

Egan, G. (1994). *The Skilled Helper: A Problem-Management Approach to Helping, 5th ed. Pacific Grove, CA: Brooks/Cole Publishing.*

Foye, U., Stuart, R., Trevillion, K., Oram, S., Allan, D., Broecklemann, E., Jeffreys, S., Jeynes, T., Crawford, M. J., Moran, P., McNicholas, S., Billings, J., Dale, O., Simpson, A., and Johnson, S. (2022). *Clinician views on best practice community care for people with complex emotional needs and how it can be achieved: a qualitative study. BMC Psychiatry 22(1), 72.*

Frak, D. (2005). *Recovery Learning: A Report on the Work of the Recovery Learning Sites and other Recovery-Orientated Activities and its Incorporation into The Rethink Plan 2004–08. London: Rethink.*

Gamble, C. and Brennan, G., Eds. (2023). *Working with Serious Mental Illness: A Manual for Clinical Practice, 3rd ed. London: Elsevier.*

Healy, H., Reader, D., and Midence, K. (2006). *An introduction to and rationale for psychosocial interventions. In: C. Gamble and G. Brennan, Eds., Working with Serious Mental Illness: A Manual for Clinical Practice, 2nd ed., pp. 55–70. London: Elsevier.*

Health Education England (2020). *Mental Health Nursing: Competence and Career Framework. Available at: https://www.hee.nhs.uk/sites/default/files/docume nts/HEE%20Mental%20Health%20Nursing%20Career%20 and%20Competence%20Framework.pdf*

Henderson, C., Noblett, J., Parke, H., Clement, S., Caffrey, A., Gale-Grant, O., Schulze, B., Druss, B., and Thornicroft, G. (2014). *Mental health-related stigma in health care and mental health-care settings. Lancet Psychiatry 1(6), 467–482.*

Huhn, M., Tardy, M., and Spineli, L. M. (2014). *Efficacy of pharmacotherapy and psychotherapy for adult psychiatric disorder: a systematic overview of meta-analyses. JAMA Psychiatry 71(6), 706–715. doi:10.1001/ jamapsychiatry.2014.112*

Jacobsen, P., Hodkinson, K., Peters, E., and Chadwick, P. (2018). *A systematic scoping review of psychological therapies for psychosis within acute psychiatric in-patient settings. The British Journal of Psychiatry 213(2), 490–497. doi:10.1192/bjp.2018.106*

Lam, D. H., Jones, S., Hayward, P., and Bright, J. (1999). *Cognitive Therapy for Bipolar Disorders: A Therapist's Guide to Concepts, Methods, and Practice. Chichester: Wiley and Sons.*

Lequerica, A. H. and Kortte, K. (2010). *Therapeutic engagement. American Journal of Physical Medicine & Rehabilitation 89(5), 415–422.*

Longden, E., Read, J., and Dillon, J. (2018). *Assessing the impact and effectiveness of hearing voices network self-help groups. Community Mental Health Journal 54(2), 184–188.*

Mendez-Bustos, P., Calati, R., Rubio-Ramirez, F., Olie, E., Cortet, P., and Lopez-Castroman, J. (2019). *Effectiveness of psychotherapy on suicidal risk: a* *systematic review of observational studies. Frontiers in Psychology 10. https://doi.org/10.3389/fpsyg.2019.00277*

Menzies, I. (1960). *Social systems as a structured defence against anxiety. Human Relations 13, 95–121.*

Newell, M. and Gournay, K. (2000). *Mental Health Nursing: An Evidence-Based Approach. Edinburgh: Churchill Livingstone.*

NHS England (2022). *Care Programme Approach: Position Statement. Available at: https://www.england.nhs.uk/publication/care-programme-approach-position-statement/*

NHS England, NHS Improvement, and the National Collaborating Central for Mental Health (2019). *The Community Mental Health Framework for Adults and Older Adults. Available at: https://www.england.nhs.uk/publication/the-community-mental-health-framework-for-adults-and-older-adults/*

Nursing and Midwifery Council (2014). *Standards for Competence for Registered Nurses. Available at: https://www.nmc.org.uk/globalassets/sitedocuments/standards/nmc-standards-for-competence-for-registered-nurses.pdf*

Orfanos, S., Banks, C., and Priebe, S. (2015). *Are group psychotherapeutic treatments effective for patients with schizophrenia? A systematic review and meta-analysis. Psychotherapy and Psychosomatics 84(4), 241–249. https://doi.org/10.1159/000377705*

Parry, G. (1996). *NHS Psychotherapy Services in England: Review of Strategic Policy. London: Department of Health.*

Repper, J. and Brooker, C. (1997). *Difficulties in the measurement of outcome in people who have serious mental health problems. Journal of Advanced Nursing 27(1), 75–82.*

Repper, J. and Perkins, R. (1996). *Working Alongside People with Long Term Mental Health Problems. London: Chapman & Hall.*

Rogers, C. (1961). *On Becoming a Person: A Therapist's View of Psychotherapy. London: Constable.*

Rollnick, S. and Miller, W. R. (1995). *What is motivational interviewing? Behavioural and Cognitive Psychotherapy 23(4), 325–334.*

Roth, A. and Fonagy, P. (1996). *What Works for Whom? A Critical Review of Psychotherapy Research. London: Guilford Press.*

Simpson, A. (2005). *Community psychiatric nurses and the care co-ordinator role: squeezed to provide 'limited nursing'. Journal of Advanced Nursing 52(6), 689–699.*

Simpson, A., Hannigan, B., Coffey, M., Barlow, S., Cohen, R., Jones, A., Všetečková, J., Faulkner, A., Thornton, A., and Cartwright, M. (2016). *Recovery-focused care planning and coordination in England and Wales: a cross-national mixed methods comparative case study. BMC Psychiatry 16, 147.*

Sweeney, A., Fahmy, S., Nolan, F., Morant, N., Fox, Z., Lloyd-Evans, B., Osborn, D., Burgess, E., Gilburt, H., McCabe, R., Slade, M., and Johnson, S. (2014). *The relationship between therapeutic alliance and service user satisfaction in mental health inpatient wards and crisis house alternatives: a cross-sectional study. PLoS One 9(7), e100153.*

Trevillion, K., Stuart, R., Ocloo, J., Broeckelmann, E., Jeffreys, S., Jeynes, T., Allen, D., Russell, J., Billings, J., Crawford, M. J., Dale, O., Haigh, R., Moran, P., McNicholas, S., Nicholls, V., Foye, U., Simpson, A., Lloyd-Evans, B., Johnson, S., and Oram, S. (2022). *Service user perspectives of community mental health services for people with complex emotional needs: a co-produced qualitative interview study. BMC Psychiatry 22(1), 55.*

Watkins, P. (2001). *Mental Health Nursing: The Art of Compassionate Care. London: Butterworth-Heinemann.*

Wood, L., Williams, C., Billings, J., and Johnson, S. (2020). *A systematic review and meta-analysis of cognitive behavioural informed psychological interventions for psychiatric inpatients with psychosis. Schizophrenia Research 222, 133–144. https://doi.org/10.1016/j.schres.2020.03.041*

9 Dementia: A person-centred perspective

Helen Pusey
Simon Burrow

John Keady

Learning outcomes

By the end of this chapter, you should be able to:

1

Describe the biopsychosocial factors that influence the well-being of those living with dementia

2 Recognize best practice approaches to person-centred dementia care and support.

▼ Introduction

We have titled this chapter 'Dementia: a person-centred perspective' because we believe that it is vital for mental health nurses to enact person-centred values and to see the **person** rather than just the 'dementia'. Mental health nurses will work alongside people living with dementia in several different settings. These are likely to be through inpatient assessment wards in mental health hospitals, community mental health teams, nursing homes, memory clinics, and liaison teams within acute general hospitals. Our ambition for this chapter is to encourage you to think about how to deliver best practice in all of these settings by drawing upon the principles of person-centred dementia care.

▼ What is dementia?

Dementia is not a specific illness but a syndrome, or collection of symptoms, leading to cognitive deterioration. Dementia is caused directly or indirectly by numerous diseases with the most common being Alzheimer's disease, vascular disease, Lewy body disease, and diseases of the frontal temporal areas of the brain, often referred to as frontal temporal dementia. Although many forms of dementia may share similar symptoms, for example, memory loss, disorientation, or difficulties with communication, the exact symptoms will vary depending not only on the cause, but also from person to person depending on the part of the brain affected. Have a look at Table 9.1 for a summary of the main changes. Not everyone will experience all these changes, but it highlights the common difficulties people might have. The key issue is that everyone's experience of dementia will be unique to them. Later in this chapter, we will explore the other factors that influence this experience, but the starting point is to recognize that dementia is only an umbrella term covering a wide range of different illnesses.

There are an estimated 944,000 people living with dementia in the UK and over 50 million people worldwide. Dementia is not an inevitable part of ageing and most older people do not have dementia. However, the biggest risk factor for dementia is ageing; around two in 100 people develop the condition between the ages of 65 and 69 and this rises to one in five for those aged between 85 and 89 (Alzheimer's Research UK, 2022). Dementia is much less common in younger age groups,

Table 9.1 Summary of the most common types of dementia and their main changes

Type of dementia	Main changes
Alzheimer's disease	Gradual decline in cognitive function
	Memory loss
	Word-finding difficulties
	Recognition and perceptual difficulties
	Disorientation
	Increasing problems with everyday tasks
Vascular dementia	Similar to Alzheimer's disease but onset can be abrupt with 'stepwise' progression
	Specific difficulties will depend on the part of the brain affected
Lewy body dementia	Hallucinations
	Fluctuations between lucidity and confusion
	Physical symptoms of Parkinson's disease
	Disturbed sleep
	Risk of falls
	Highly sensitive to neuroleptic medication
Frontal lobe dementia (number of variants including semantic dementia and primary progressive aphasia)	Reduced motivation
	Reduced empathy
	Personality change
	Disinhibition
	Obsessive–compulsive behaviours
	Difficulties with language and comprehension
	Change in eating habits (often drawn to sweet foods)

but in the UK, there are likely to be over 42,000 people under 65 with dementia, with Alzheimer's disease the most common diagnosis for both the younger and older population groups (Prince et al., 2014).

▼ Development of the person-centred approach

The person-centred approach to dementia care grew out of the pioneering work of the social psychologist Tom Kitwood (1997). He questioned the notion that the experience of dementia and that the behaviour of people living with dementia could be attributed solely to the damage caused to the brain. He found that some people with very little brain pathology appeared to have severe impairment, while others were found to have significant pathology but appeared to have much less difficulty in coping with everyday life. Following extensive experience and research he concluded that the attitude and behaviour of other people towards the person with dementia will significantly impact their well-being. Alongside the attitude and behaviour of others, he proposed that the experience of dementia is influenced by a range of other factors. He combined all these elements to develop what has since become known as the 'enriched model of dementia' (Figure

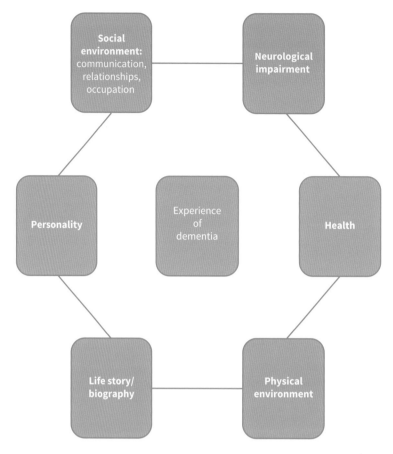

Figure 9.1 An adapted version of the 'enriched model of dementia'

Source: data from Kitwood, T. (1997). *Dementia Reconsidered: The Person Comes First*. Milton Keynes: Open University Press.

9.1). This model gives nurses the opportunity to make a substantial difference in well-being by being aware of these elements and addressing those factors where practice can be enhanced.

We will now work our way around this model to consider how people experience dementia and how we, as mental health nurses, can minimize impairment and maximize the well-being of people living with dementia.

Neurological impairment

As we saw in Table 9.1, dementia can impact across a range of different cognitive domains depending on where the damage to the brain is located. Although these impairments will vary from person to person, it is important to not see the person solely in terms of their deficits and to focus on their strengths.

Health

The next element in the model is health. If we can ensure optimum physical and mental health, we can make a significant contribution to enhancing well-being. However, in mental health settings, physical health has not always been sufficiently addressed and it has been argued that many biopsychosocial approaches to dementia do not adequately consider the physical dimensions of care (Keady et al., 2013). Furthermore, the physicality of nursing, such as attending to bodily fluids and eliminations, is often downplayed in mental health but considering how we approach these needs is a key feature of person-centred care. As Keady et al. (2013) point out: 'It is unglamorous work but arguably it is the very essence of nursing through the act of upholding (in another person) a sense of their dignity and worth as a human being' (p. 2773).

It is important to recognize that people living with dementia will experience the same range of health concerns as everyone else. However, unfortunately, sometimes health professionals are unable to see beyond a diagnosis, such as dementia. This can be referred to 'overshadowing' (Jones et al., 2008). This overshadowing can lead to the assumption that a symptom of a physical or mental health problem, or perhaps behaviour arising from a physical health problem, is due to a person's dementia rather than the actual cause. This can mean a delay in diagnosing serious diseases such as cancer or diabetes or addressing specific mental health problems such as depression. This overshadowing can also mean that everyday health concerns such as headaches or toothache are missed because staff are focusing on the dementia diagnosis. Finally, it can mean that attempts by the person to communicate their physical or emotional distress are labelled as 'challenging behaviour' and we will return to this issue later in the chapter.

People with dementia often experience difficulties with eating and drinking as their illness progresses. Some of the main issues are a reduction in appetite, a reduction in motor skills and sensory awareness, the impact of memory difficulties, and unhelpful physical and social environments. It is important to monitor the level of fluid intake as dementia can accelerate the decline in kidney function and the hormone that detects thirst. Common physical symptoms of dehydration are a dry mouth, lips, and tongue, dry skin, low blood pressure, drowsiness, **confusion**, dizziness, and **disorientation**. It can also affect **memory** and concentration. As you can see, some of these symptoms mirror dementia and may not be recognized by staff.

Similarly, malnutrition can occur when people with dementia forget to eat, have a reduced appetite, or difficulty in feeding themselves. As well as weight loss, malnutrition can lead to low mood, tiredness and dizziness, and an increased risk of infections.

People with dementia experience pain in the same way as everyone else. Unfortunately, this is not always recognized and acted upon quickly by health professionals. Furthermore, we all express our pain in different ways, and we have to be mindful of trying to know when someone with dementia may be experiencing pain in any practice setting. Appropriate and regular analgesia should always be considered.

Physical environment

Although Kitwood (1997) did not include the physical environment in his model, we have added it into our adapted version because the physical world in which we live can have a profound impact on our well-being. As mental health nurses,

we have an opportunity to adapt and change elements of physical environments and spaces, making them more accessible and enabling for people who are living with dementia. These key design principles are recommended in the *World Alzheimer Report* 2020 (Fleming et al., 2020).

- Ensure the internal and external environment is safe and easy for the person to move around in.

- Ensure the size of the environment and number of people doesn't overwhelm.

- Allow people to see and be seen by ensuring good visual access and appropriate signage.

- Reduce unhelpful stimulation such as unnecessary noise and visual clutter.

- Optimize helpful stimulation by using lighting, personal items, and signage to help the person know where they are and what they can do.

- Support movement with well-defined pathways and points of interest and the opportunity to engage.

- Create a familiar space with personalized objects.

- Provide opportunities to be alone or with others.

- To reduce stigma and improve connections, physically link the space to the wider community.

- Ensure the space fits the person-centred philosophy of care—even small changes can make a huge difference.

Personality/life story work/biography

These parts of the model highlight the importance of recognizing the individuality of each person with dementia and using that understanding to inform how we adapt our engagement, communication, and approach to best meet the needs of the individual.

If we have time to get to know someone, we can build our knowledge and understanding of them but sometimes using a tool can help. If we have less time, the leaflet 'This is Me' (https://www.alzheimers.org.uk/get-support/publications-factsheets/this-is-me) produced by the Alzheimer's Society provides useful prompts for recording cultural considerations, important people, and events, preferences, and routines.

People living with dementia will be affected in their own unique way. However, there are important issues to consider with respect to how people in minority or disadvantaged groups may experience dementia and access the services and supports that exist for people with dementia and their families. For example, to what extent is your service accessible and acceptable to people of ethnic heritage, the LGBTQI+ community, the Travelling community, and people who are deaf? This list is not exhaustive, but hopefully encourages you to think about meeting the needs of our diverse community.

Social environment

The final section of the 'enriched model' is the social environment or, as Tom Kitwood called it, 'social psychology'. This part of the model concerns factors such as relationships, care provision, and opportunities for meaningful activity. This is a particularly important element to consider because it can present the greatest opportunity for mental health nurses to enhance quality of life. The social world which people with dementia inhabit presents the opportunity to support and enhance well-being. However, where this is poor—and in care settings, where practice needs to be improved—this can cause feelings of ill-being in the person with dementia.

▼ Communication

Communication is at the heart of care and relationships and is a vital opportunity to influence well-being. Hamilton (2008) describes everyday conversation as a dance: communication is seen less as a **product** (that is correct or not) and more as a **moment-to-moment process**. Kindell et al. (2017) propose that good communication is about drawing on the resources and abilities the person with dementia retains and 'scaffolding' to support the person to engage in conversation. In a similar fashion to Hamilton (2008), Kindell et al. (2017) also argue that the **social function** of conversation is as important as the more conventional concept of communication as a 'transfer of information'.

We often think about verbal communication when we think about communication skills, but arguably our non-verbal communication is of even greater significance. Even if people can no longer understand verbal speech, they will understand your tone and the feelings you are conveying.

> As we become more emotional and less cognitive, it's the way you talk to us, not what you say, that we will remember … We know the feeling but do not know the plot. Your smile, your laugh, your touch is what we will connect with. We're still here in emotion and spirit—if only you could find us.
>
> (Bryden, 2005, p. 138)

As dementia progresses, receptive and expressive verbal communication can become more problematic for people, but non-verbal communication remains a strength. This means we need to focus on the non-verbal ways in which people with dementia communicate with us, and how we use our non-verbal skills to communicate with them. These hints and tips by the Alzheimer's Society (2020) on how best to communicate, may be helpful:

- Stand or sit where the person can see and hear you as clearly as possible.
- Try to be at eye level with the person.
- Be as close to the person as is comfortable for you both.
- Communicate clearly and calmly.
- Go at a slightly slower pace than usual if the person is struggling to follow you.
- Use short, simple sentences.
- Do not talk to the person as you would to a child.
- Allow time between sentences for the person to process the information and respond.
- Try to communicate with the person in a conversational way, rather than asking question after question, which may feel quite tiring or intimidating.
- Try to let the person complete their own sentences.
- Include the person in conversations with others.
- If the person becomes tired easily, then short, regular conversations may be better.
- Prompts can help, for instance, pointing at a photo of someone or encouraging the person to hold and interact with an object you are talking about.
- Try to make sure your body language is open and relaxed. Avoid speaking sharply or raising your voice.
- Listen to the person's intonation. This may be communicating more than the words themselves. Focus on the feeling behind the words.

▼ Truth and deception

A common ethical dilemma that faces nurses working in the field of dementia is how we respond to someone whose perception of reality differs from our own. For example, this might be an older person asking for their mother or worrying about their young children. Although lying in these types of scenarios is generally not talked about among staff (Turner et al., 2017), it is likely that many nurses have used some degree of deception in our communication (Mental Health Foundation, 2016) and this is sometimes referred to as 'therapeutic lying'. Truth telling is a complex topic and responses can be considered on an axis from whole truth telling, through to looking for alternative meaning, distracting, going along with, to lying.

The Mental Health Foundation (2016) has published useful guidance to ensure a person-centred approach:

- Nurses should find out the meaning for people of these different beliefs and realities using knowledge of people's life story, values, and experiences.
- Start as close as possible to whole truth telling but move along the axis if this will cause unnecessary distress.
- Avoid environment lies; spaces designed to deceive such as painted shop fronts; it is much better to have a real shop.
- Responses should be consistent across the team and fully documented.

▼ Meaningful occupation

Kitwood had a useful definition of occupation, he called it 'To be occupied means to be involved in the process of life in a way that is personally significant, and which draws on a person's abilities and powers' (Kitwood and Brooker, 2019, p. 94).

Engagement in a meaningful occupation can enhance well-being and as Brooker and Latham (2016) state: 'seeing somebody light up with delight when engaged in an activity that has meaning for them is evidence enough that it is a worthwhile endeavour' (2016, p. 100).

However, an absence of activity can be detrimental and can lead to boredom, apathy, loss of self-esteem, depression, social exclusion, and loneliness (Kolanowski et al., 2006).

Being meaningfully occupied is important for a person wherever they happen to be and however advanced their dementia may be. As people with dementia lose abilities, we need to find ever more creative ways to enable them to use their strengths to engage in activity that is meaningful to them. Care settings like hospitals pose additional challenges, but creative approaches that tailor to individual personalities and needs can be found.

▼ Creativity and the arts

For people living with dementia who may have difficulty with conventional modes of communication, the creative arts can provide a gateway for both them and for those who care for them.

Art can also provide valuable insight into the person with dementia for carers. Finding out that someone can express themselves in other ways provides not only information about who this unique person with dementia is, but also enables a whole wealth of new avenues to explore so that connections can be made.

The creative arts have always been seen as a means of communication for everyone. Music, poetry, and the visual arts can capture or enhance a mood, resonate a feeling, or provide a critical outlet of expression. None of this changes when we develop dementia and for some people it can remain a

vital mode of communication long after more conventional methods elude them and those who care for them. Indeed, some people find wholly new ways of expressing themselves through the creative arts.

Creative arts also provide an opportunity for people living with dementia to engage with and share an experience. Unlike much care delivery, participatory art is where the experience happens alongside others and where it is not something that is 'done to the person'.

Creative arts, in all their forms, provide an ideal vehicle for being 'in the moment' for people with dementia and for those who are supporting or caring for them. 'In the moment' is an expression of a feeling or a connection with others. It is not a test of cognitive ability, and it is impossible to fail at art. Being 'in the moment' is crucial for people living with dementia; they may not have memories of some aspects of the past and the future may seem uncertain. Celebrating and living 'in the moment' is free from judgement and has a worth that sits outside a person's diagnosis of dementia.

▼ Behaviours that challenge

When we pull the elements of the 'enriched model of dementia' together (Figure 9.1), it can help us to understand the concept of 'behaviours that challenge'. These are behaviours and actions of people with dementia that attract labels such as 'aggressive', wanderer', or 'sexually inappropriate'. These labels are unhelpful and even harmful for people with dementia; they lead to judgements and people being blamed. They emphasize the 'dementia' rather than the 'person' and they lead to a focus on 'behaviour'. The reasons behind the behaviour are not identified by such labels and underlying needs remain unmet. Humans do not only communicate through words, but we also communicate through our actions and our behaviours. This is certainly the case for people living with dementia.

James and Jackman (2017) describe how these behaviours we often view as 'challenging' may be the result of an unmet need. In essence, a person's actions are communicating to other people that they are experiencing an unmet need and/or the expression of a feeling or emotion. People with dementia may be communicating through more than just words; actions are also a means of communication. There is often a tendency to label actions as 'behaviours' or 'symptoms' of dementia, but in doing so, this has the potential to distract from what those actions are communicating about the person's physical, emotional, or social needs. Imagine it as an iceberg: the behaviour we see (e.g. pacing, shouting, resisting care) is only the tip of the iceberg, but underneath there could be a host of needs that we don't see: Feeling lost or misunderstood, the effects of medication, a differing perception of reality, fear, pain, delirium, a need for comfort or familiarity, visuo-spatial or cognitive difficulties, a need to be occupied, or physical needs such as hunger or thirst.

▼ Person-centred perspective in practice

The person-centred perspective was developed further by Dawn Brooker (Brooker and Latham, 2016) who wanted to provide a simple model for practice. The VIPS model (Table 9.2) involves all levels of an organization and provides a framework for person-centred dementia care.

Table 9.2 VIPS model

V	**Valuing** people with dementia and those who care for them
I	Treating people as **Individuals**
P	Looking at the world from the **Perspective** of the person with dementia
S	Providing a supportive **Social** environment

Source: data from Brooker, D. and Latham, I. (2016). *Person-Centred Dementia Care: Making Services Better*. London: Jessica Kingsley Publishers.

Brooker and Latham (2016) pose the following questions which can help you consider the extent to which your practice environment is 'person centred':

Inclusion: are people helped to feel part of what is going on around them and supported to participate in a way in which they are able?

Respect: does the support we provide show people that they are respected as individuals with unique identities, strengths, and needs?

Warmth: does the atmosphere we create help people to feel welcomed, wanted, and accepted?

Validation: are people's emotions and feelings recognized, taken seriously, and responded to?

Enabling: does the support we provide help people to be as active and involved in their lives as possible? Are people treated as equal partners in their care?

Part of the community: does our service do all it can to keep people connected with their local community and the community connected to the service?

Relationships: do we know about, welcome, and involve the people who are important to a person?

▲ Conclusion

This chapter has presented the enriched model of dementia as a framework for promoting a person-centred approach to practice. Mental health nurses can use this model to consider how they can actively enhance the well-being of those living with dementia.

✖ Tips from service users

These final thoughts come from our colleague, Dr Ann Johnson. Ann has lived with dementia for many years and campaigned nationally to raise awareness and challenge stigma.

1 You may have dementia, but you have a life to live, and you must live it the best way you can.

2 No two people with dementia are alike; if you've met one person with dementia, you've met one person with dementia.

3 Purpose and fulfilment are vital; support people to realize their potential no matter how far their dementia has progressed.

W Companion website

For extra resources on the topics covered in this chapter, visit the companion website at: www.oup.com/mhns

Acknowledgements

As a person living with dementia, we would like to acknowledge Dr Ann Johnson for her vital contribution over the years to teaching programmes on dementia at the University of Manchester and in particular for her wise words that we have incorporated into this chapter.

✚ References

Alzheimer's Research UK (2022). *Dementia Statistics Hub: Prevalence and Incidence. Available at: https://www.dementiastatistics.org/statistics-about-dementia/prevalence-2/*

Alzheimer's Society (2020). *How to Communicate with a Person with Dementia. Available at: https://www.alzheimers.org.uk/about-dementia/symptoms-and-diagnosis/symptoms/tips-for-communicating-dementia*

Brooker, D. and Latham, I. (2016). *Person-Centred Dementia Care: Making Services Better. London: Jessica Kingsley Publishers.*

Bryden, C. (2005). *Dancing with Dementia: My Story of Living Positively with Dementia. London: Jessica Kingsley.*

Fleming, R., Zeisel, J., and Bennett, K. (2020). *World Alzheimer Report 2020: Design, Dignity, Dementia: Dementia-Related Design and the Built Environment. Alzheimer's Disease International.*

Available at: https://www.alzint.org/resource/world-alzheimer-report-2020/

Hamilton, H. E. (2008). *Language and dementia: sociolinguistic aspects. Annual Review of Applied Linguistics 28, 91–110.*

James, I. and Jackman, L. (2017). *Understanding Behaviour that Challenges: A Guide to Assessment and Treatment. London: Jessica Kingsley.*

Jones, S., Howard, L., and Thornicroft, G. (2008). *'Diagnostic overshadowing': worse physical health care for people with mental illness. Acta Psychiatrica Scandinavia 118(3), 169–171.*

Keady, J., Jones, L., Ward, R., Koch, S., Swarbrick, C., Hellström, I., Davies-Quarrell, V., and Williams, S. (2013). *Introducing the bio-psycho-social-physical model of dementia through a collective case study design. Journal of Clinical Nursing 22(19–20), 2768–2777.*

Kindell, J., Keady, J., Sage, K., and Wilkinson, R. (2017). *Everyday conversation in dementia: a review of the literature to inform research and practice. International Journal of Language and Communication Disorders 52(4), 392–406.*

Kitwood, T. (1997). *Dementia Reconsidered: The Person Comes First. Milton Keynes: Open University Press.*

Kitwood, T. and Brooker, D., Eds. (2019). *Dementia Reconsidered Revisited: The Person Still Comes First. London: Open University Press.*

Kolanowski, A., Buettner, L., Litaker, M., and Yu, F. (2006). *Factors that relate to activity engagement in nursing home residents. American Journal of Alzheimer's Disease and Other Dementias 21(1), 15–22.*

Mental Health Foundation (2016). *What is Truth? An Inquiry About Truth and Lying in Dementia Care. London: Mental Health Foundation.*

Prince, M., Knapp, M., Guerchet, M., McCrone, P., Prina, M., Comas-Herrera, M., Wittenberg, A., Adelaja, R., Hu, B., King, B., Rehill, D., and Salimkumar, D. (2014). *Dementia UK: Update. London: Alzheimer's Society. Available at: https://www.alzheimers.org.uk/about-us/policy-and-influencing/dementia-uk-report*

Turner, A., Eccles, F., Keady, J., Simpson, J., and Elvish, R. (2017). *The use of the truth and deception in dementia care amongst general hospital staff. Aging & Mental Health 21(8), 862–869.*

Recovery-focused care and safety planning assessment and management

Alan Simpson   Jessica Sears

Learning outcomes

By the end of this chapter, you should be able to:

1 Understand conceptualizations of recovery in mental health services

2 Consider some of the potential barriers to recovery-focused working

3 Explore aspects of the therapeutic process and recovery-focused ways of working with service users that will help them in their recovery journey.

▼ Introduction

Clinical recovery is an idea that has emerged from the expertise of mental health professionals and involves reducing or eradicating symptoms, restoring social functioning, and in other ways 'getting back to normal' (Slade, 2009).

Personal recovery is an idea that has emerged from the expertise of people with lived experienced of mental illness. It is recognizing that despite living with often long-term effects of mental distress or illness, people can live meaningful, rewarding, and fulfilling lives.

For mental health nurses, recovery means working alongside people to support them in adapting to and living with mental health problems, while encouraging and supporting them to work towards personal goals. At times, it may also mean the nurses carrying hope and optimism for the future when the person they are supporting is most challenged by the difficulties they face.

The importance of addressing service users' personal recovery is now supported across professional guidance and national policies. The new Community Mental Health Framework for Adults and Older Adults states that adoption of the framework will enable people with mental health problems to: 'Manage their condition or move towards individualised recovery on their own terms, surrounded by their families, carers, and social networks, and supported in their local community', and 'Contribute to and be participants in the communities that sustain them, to whatever extent is comfortable to them' (NHS England et al., 2019, p. 6).

▼ The CHIME framework

As part of a large study on recovery, Leamy et al. (2011) identified and reviewed 97 research papers that described studies conducted in 13 countries, including the US (n = 50), the UK (n = 20), Australia (n = 8), and Canada (n = 6). The conceptual framework they developed summarized the key features of personal recovery under headings that created the acronym CHIME, outlined in Box 10.1.

Leamy et al. (2011) acknowledged that people of Black and minority ethnic origin placed a greater emphasis on spirituality and stigma. This led to two additional themes: culturally specific facilitating factors, and collectivist notions of recovery.

Tuffour et al. (2019) further explored the experiences and understanding of recovery among Black African

Box 10.1 Conceptual framework for personal recovery (CHIME)

C: Connectedness
- Having good relationships and being connected in positive ways to others.
- Peer support between people with experience of mental health issues.
- Relationships with carers, friends, and family.
- Positive connections with health professionals and community involvement are also important.

H: Hope and optimism

Widely acknowledged as key to recovery. There can be no change without the belief that a better life is both possible and attainable. It includes:
- belief in recovery
- motivation to change
- hope-inspiring relationships
- positive thinking and valuing success
- having dreams and aspirations.

I: Identity
- Regaining a positive sense of self and identity.
- Overcoming stigma and being recognized as a whole person—rather than defined by illness.

M: Meaning
- Living a meaningful and purposeful life is important.
- Some find spirituality important, while others find meaning through employment or the development of stronger interpersonal or community links.
- Importance of feeling valued and contributing as active members of the community.

E: Empowerment
- Focusing on strengths, taking personal responsibility and control of your life.
- Social inclusion of people with experience of mental health issues in their communities and in decisions about their lives.
- Use of self-management techniques.

Adapted with permission from Leamy, M., Bird, V., Boutillier, C., Williams, J., & Slade, M. (2011). Conceptual framework for personal recovery in mental health: Systematic review and narrative synthesis. *The British Journal of Psychiatry*, 199(6), 445–452. doi:10.1192/bjp.bp.110.083733

service users. Participants conceptualized recovery as a pragmatic and subjective concept across a continuum of clinical, functional, and spiritual dimensions, resilience, identity, and their social and cultural backgrounds. Further analysis identified the importance of religion (Tuffour, 2020). It is critical that these components are embedded in recovery-oriented services for Black African service users.

The researchers that developed CHIME subsequently tested the validity and relevance of this framework. Bird et al. (2014) asked 48 mental health service users across seven focus groups in England about the meaning of personal recovery. The analysis broadly validated the CHIME categories. However, three key areas of difference were identified: practical support, a greater emphasis on issues around diagnosis and medication, and scepticism surrounding recovery.

Participants stressed the importance of practical support to improve their material circumstances, access wider life opportunities, or simply to get through the days when they were less able to manage, so that they could move forward with their recovery. Some also placed more emphasis on the importance and choice of medication, and how being diagnosed—and sometimes misdiagnosed—had a big part to play in their recovery. Finally, the idea of recovery as a driver for services was met with some scepticism by service users who had experienced cuts to services. Such findings have been reported in other studies of recovery-focused care (Simpson et al., 2016).

A subsequent study was more critical of the limitations of CHIME. Stuart et al. (2016) employed a method known as best-fit framework synthesis to assess the extent to which CHIME accommodated the findings on personal recovery in 18 papers. The authors concluded that CHIME was over-optimistic and failed to acknowledge the considerable challenges inherent in living with and overcoming mental distress. They suggested CHIME-D: a simple expansion of the recovery model which more explicitly acknowledged 'Difficulties'. Many of these are underpinned by social inequality and the authors make a strong case for researchers and practitioners to be more concerned with understanding these realities and actively challenging them.

▼ Evidence base

Two large mixed methods studies conducted in England and Wales report important findings that can inform recovery-focused care planning, risk and safety planning, and care coordination. The first focused on support provided by community mental health teams (Simpson et al., 2016); the second on acute inpatient mental healthcare (Coffey et al., 2019).

Both studies found staff trying to work in recovery-focused ways, but this was frustrated by several factors including:

- restructuring/reorganization of services
- lack of staff
- high workloads
- competing or contradictory policies
- differing understandings of recovery, including views that 'Recovery is not appropriate here/for these people'.

In community services, Simpson et al. (2016) found that service users valued therapeutic relationships and saw these as central to their recovery, yet often had insufficient contact with staff. The burdensome administrative elements of care coordination and care plans reduced staff opportunities for recovery-focused work. There were few common understandings of recovery, which limited shared decision-making and agreed goals. Risk assessments were central to clinical concerns but were rarely discussed with service users or families. Multidisciplinary team discussions and decisions tended to occur 'behind closed doors', thus limiting the potential involvement of service users and carers. A reluctance to engage in dialogue may prevent genuine involvement of the person in their own recovery and work against opportunities for positive risk-taking as part of recovery-focused work (Coffey et al., 2016).

In the acute inpatient study (Coffey et al., 2019), a relationship was found between service users reporting high quality of care, better therapeutic relationships, and a focus on recovery on wards. For staff, there was a moderate correlation between recovery orientation and quality of therapeutic relationships, with considerable variability. Interestingly, across six organizations and 19 wards, staff consistently rated the quality of therapeutic relationships higher than service users did. Similarly, staff accounts of routine collaboration with service users in developing care plans contrasted with a more mixed picture in service user accounts—and in the examination of documentation.

Understandings of recovery varied, as did views of hospital care in promoting recovery. Some ward staff doubted that 'recovery' was 'appropriate' for people in severe distress, whereas service users saw hospital admission and often the administration of medication as an important period of stabilization before embarking on the next tentative steps in their recovery. As in the community study, managing risk was a central issue for staff. Service users were aware of measures being taken to keep them safe, although their involvement in safety discussions was less apparent. Overall, recovery ideas were evident in inpatient services, but ambivalence remained concerning their relevance.

Evidence from practice suggests a huge potential in adopting recovery-focused approaches but this can be hampered by structural, organizational, and perhaps professional barriers too. In the next section, we outline approaches that can help you provide recovery-focused care.

▼ Recovery-focused practice

The key principle to recovery is that it is a personal process. One aspect is about alleviating symptoms of distress, but it is also about engagement in an active life, personal autonomy, social identity, meaning and purpose in life, and a positive sense of self. We now explore the steps you will take with service users to help their recovery journey.

1 Engagement

The first step is engagement based on mutual understanding and trust. To do so, we need to recognize the genuine fears a service user may harbour about mental health care. These could include:

- stigma; feelings of guilt and shame

Box 10.2 Engagement tips

- If the service user is unsure about engaging with services, try to understand the reasons why, listen, and show understanding.

- A warm and friendly approach will help service users feel more at ease about talking to you.

- Give reassurance where appropriate while also being honest and transparent.

- Explain what the service user can expect from your service and what types of interventions/support are available (e.g. talking therapy, social prescribing, peer support, social support, medication, formulation, and psychoeducation).

- Ask the service user about the type of support they think would be helpful and their goals.

- Sometimes the service user may want help with social issues (housing, finances) as this is the most important thing for them at that point in time.

- Offer the service user choice in how they engage (e.g. meeting online or in person, suitable times, etc.).

- Give positive affirmation for their courage in seeking help.

Box 10.3 Assessment tips

- Put the service user at ease: use open body language, smile, be polite, ensure their comfort, and provide a space that safeguards privacy.

- Explain the assessment process (e.g. how long it takes, what is it used for) and ask who they are willing to share information with.

- Use an assessment structure (your workplace will have a standard template for assessments) to guide the conversation, but use it flexibly, that is, if the service user veers naturally to another part of the assessment, you can follow their lead and return to the missing sections later.

- Use active listening skills be non-judgemental, give verbal and non-verbal feedback, ask open questions, reflect what is said to ensure you have understood, seek clarification, and summarize.

- Explore the person's strengths and skills as well as their current difficulties to get a better understanding of the person and what will help their recovery.

- At the end, thank them for their time and for sharing their story with you. Explain the next steps, such as team input, the formulation process, letter with the outcome of the assessment, care planning, and follow-up appointments.

- lack of culturally sensitive care
- difficulty recognizing and expressing mental health concerns
- difficulty accessing help
- lack of trust in authority figures; concerns about confidentiality.

Nevertheless, the tips outlined in Box 10.2 can improve engagement.

Aim to work in partnership with service users through mutual participation and shared decision-making.

2 Assessment

A range of factors impact mental health, so it is vital that your assessment is holistic and covers a range of issues that are important to the service user: consider what is happening in their life now and what has happened to them previously. Box 10.3 contains some useful principles to follow.

3 Formulation

Formulation is the process of developing an understanding of what is happening for a person and why, to inform treatment options.

This process is not an exact science and can be subject to bias depending on your own knowledge, skills, and personal experience. It is often useful to discuss your assessment and initial formulation with your multidisciplinary team to gain a range of perspectives and insights. Below are some key theories which will help develop your formulations:

Biopsychosocial model

The biopsychosocial model proposes that biological, social, and psychological factors are interlinked and contribute to the development and maintenance of mental health difficulties. For example:

- **biological factors** include age, sex, genetic vulnerabilities, health conditions, immune response, medication effects and side effects, and temperament
- **psychological factors** include core beliefs, perceptions, attachments, self-esteem, coping skills, and personality
- **social factors** include family circumstances, social networks, school, culture, religion, poverty, housing, and employment.

Attachment theory

People's early attachments can impact their ability to form trusting, reciprocal relationships, therefore some interventions may focus on building healthy relationships.

As professionals we should also role model healthy relationships by treating others with respect and warmth, listening, and being authentic and honest.

Stress vulnerability model

The stress vulnerability model (Zubin et al., 1977) proposes that we are all vulnerable to mental health difficulties when faced with distressing events and prolonged periods of stress.

The stress vulnerability bucket (adapted from Brabban and Turkington, 2002) is a psychoeducational tool clinicians can use with service users to gain a shared understanding of what is happening for them.

The idea is that water in a bucket symbolizes someone's stress levels, which will overflow if they experience extreme mental distress (Figure 10.1).

Rocks representing someone's predisposing vulnerabilities take up space at the bottom of the bucket. These may include genetics, early traumatic experiences, or social factors such as poverty or racism.

Coping strategies are depicted as a tap in the bucket which lets the water out. These may include spending time with friends, talking to trusted people, doing sports or exercise, or eating and sleeping well.

Unhelpful coping strategies that may give short-term relief but ultimately add to stress levels—such as heavy drinking or drug use, avoidance, and withdrawal—are shown as a tap with a hose which returns water into the bucket.

See the practice example in Box 10.4.

4 Care planning

Assessment and formulation should enable you to have a good understanding of what matters to the service user, what they are struggling with, what strengths and resources they have which will aid their recovery, and which interventions recommended in National Institute for Health and Care Excellence guidelines are in line with your agreed formulation. You can then co-produce a care plan through a process of shared decision-making (National Institute for Health and

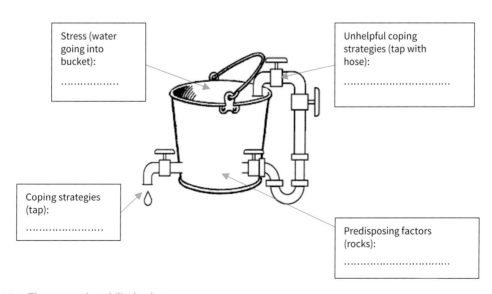

Stress (water going into bucket):

....

Unhelpful coping strategies (tap with hose):

....

Coping strategies (tap):

....

Predisposing factors (rocks):

....

Figure 10.1 The stress vulnerability bucket

Box 10.4 Practice example: stress vulnerability bucket

Use an example from your own clinical practice and think about how you would fill out the different sections of the stress vulnerability bucket (Figure 10.1) with a service user.

Here are some example questions which you may find helpful when using this tool:

1 Is there anything from your family history, early life experiences, or health conditions which you think might make you more vulnerable to mental health difficulties (the rocks at the bottom of the bucket)?

2 What sorts of things are causing you stress now (the water going into the bucket)?

3 What helps you to cope with this stress (the tap)?

4 What can help in the short term but can lead to more stress (the tap with the hose)?

5 What happens when the stress is too much to cope with (over-flowing bucket)?

Care Excellence, 2021). It is vital that this care plan is personalized and in the service user's own words. Ensure they have a copy.

Care planning tools

Dialog+ (Priebe et al., 2007) is an assessment and care planning tool which allows service users to rate themselves on eight life domains. This facilitates meaningful therapeutic conversations with the service user about what is important to them and can guide the care planning process. You can use Dialog+ at regular intervals so that service users can review their progress and update their care plan goals accordingly. Free resources are available (https://www.elft.nhs.uk/dialog/resources).

5 Safety planning

When someone is in crisis, they are likely to feel out of control and unsafe. Safety plans can ground service users with coping strategies and interventions they have identified as being helpful for them at such times.

Part of safety planning will be to work with the service user to think about what increases their feelings of safety. Coping mechanisms could be mindfulness, breathing exercises, grounding exercises, positive affirmations, talking to trusted people, creative activities, walking, or practising yoga, to name a few.

Crisis/safety plan

Someone in a mental health crisis may find decision-making or explaining what support is helpful difficult, but trust can break down if clinicians make decisions quickly to reduce the risk of harm without involving the service user or their families.

Drawing up an advance crisis plan or advanced choice document collaboratively with service users means that in times of crisis there is a shared understanding of which support is helpful, who to involve, and what each person's role is. See the practice example in Box 10.5.

6 Community and partnership working

The NHS Long Term Plan and community mental health transformation framework set out a vision of mental health services embedded in the community (NHS England et al., 2019). Voluntary sector, community organization, and social enterprises services can play a key role in helping people recover and stay well. They offer a range of services, activities, and places for people to go where they can connect with others and make a positive contribution to their community.

Many general practitioner surgeries now have social prescribers or community connectors to help people reconnect with their local community and find friendship, a sense of purpose, and enjoyment in life. Community support should be tailored to the individual and their interests.

When exploring community support options with service users it may be helpful to think of the 'Five Ways to Wellbeing' (Aked et al., 2008):

• Connect—meet friends, family, join a group

• Be active—walk, dance, run, swim

• Take notice—look at nature, mindfulness

Box 10.5 Practice example: case study and crisis plan

Gemma is 19 years old. She lives with her mum and suffers with severe anxiety, low mood, and suicidal thoughts. Gemma and her mum are close, but they have a volatile relationship and hurtful things are sometimes said when they row. When Gemma is feeling stressed or angry, she sometimes steals alcohol from her mum's cupboard and cuts herself as an emotional release. This became much worse during COVID-19 lockdowns as she was cut off from her support networks and felt there was no escape.

Gemma had good friends from school who she could confide in about her feelings but has found it difficult to re-establish these friendships since the COVID-19 pandemic. She has set up a small business making and selling jewellery. She finds going for walks alone relaxes her and helps her to think clearly. She wants to go to university but is worried about getting into debt and failing the course.

Think about how you would co-produce a crisis plan with Gemma. You may want to consider:

- if and how you would involve family members or friends?

- is there anything else that would be helpful to know about?

- what questions could you ask Gemma to find out this information?

Below is a sample structure for a personalized safety or crisis plan:

When I am in a crisis

> I will feel like …
> I will have thoughts like …
> I will have urges like …
> I will act like …

What I will do to keep myself safe

> Things I will tell myself …
> Things I will do …
> People I can speak to or places I will go to keep safe …
> What friends, family, and professionals should do to help keep me safe …
> What people should say …
> What they should do if I am behaving in certain ways …

- Keep learning—take a course, learn a new skill
- Give—volunteer, help a friend.

These five evidence-based actions can improve well-being if practised regularly.

Peer support

Peer support is based on people drawing on their own experience to help each other. Many find it helpful to meet with someone who has gone through similar experiences (Gillard et al., 2013). Different types of peer support are available in the community, in crisis services, and in inpatient settings.

The charity Mind outlines some of the key aspects of peer support and why people find it helpful (see https://www.mind.org.uk/). Reasons cited include:

- brings together people with shared experiences to support each other

- provides a space where people feel accepted and understood
- treats everyone's experiences as being equally important
- involves both giving and receiving support.

Service users may find leaflets or links to websites useful so they can explore these options themselves while others might prefer that you link them into a local service.

Recovery colleges

Recovery colleges enable people with lived experience and professional expertise to co-produce educational opportunities. People attend recovery colleges as 'students' not 'patients' or even 'service users' and attend classes and courses that can cover a wide range of topics such as managing your finances or learning various coping strategies. Many find it beneficial (Thériault et al., 2020). Peer support is often a key component.

▲ Conclusion

The concept of recovery is a complex and contested one, with research and lived experience developing our understanding over time. However, key aspects of the CHIME framework resonate with most service users and staff, while recognizing the need to be alert to specific needs when working with people from various cultural backgrounds. This amplifies the personalized nature of a recovery-focused approach to care. We have summarized some of the key approaches to working in such a person-centred way.

The huge pressures on mental health services due to financial and other factors such as staffing levels create barriers and difficulties for mental health nurses aiming to work collaboratively with service users, but it is a worthwhile focus for our work, and it is valued by service users. Staff need to ensure they find the support and supervision necessary to maintain a recovery-orientated mindset to support service users who want to be involved in discussions and decisions about their care, who want to live meaningful and rewarding lives, and who value mental health nurses that take the time and effort to work collaboratively and sensitively to help them achieve their goals—even while still battling with the effects of mental illness.

✖ Tips from service users

1 Spend time building a therapeutic relationship; this is key so that people have trust in you and in the recovery journey.

2 Listen without judgement and check you have understood.

3 Provide a safe and non-threatening environment and give reassurance that people are welcome to be open and honest about their experiences.

W Companion website

For extra resources on the topics covered in this chapter, visit the companion website at: www.oup.com/mhns

✚ References

Aked, J., Mark, N., Cordon, C., and Thompson, S. (2008). *Five Ways to Wellbeing. New economics foundation. Available at: https://neweconomics.org/uploads/files/five-ways-to-wellbeing-1.pdf*

Bird, V., Leamy, M., Tew, J., Le Boutillier, C., Williams, J., and Slade, M. (2014). *Fit for purpose? Validation of a conceptual framework for personal recovery with current mental health consumers. Australian & New Zealand Journal of Psychiatry 48(7), 644–653.*

Brabban, A. and Turkington, D. (2002). *The search for meaning: detecting congruence between life events, underlying schema, and psychotic symptoms. In: A.*

P. Morrison, Ed., A Casebook of Cognitive Therapy for Psychosis, pp. 59–75. New York: Routledge.

Coffey, M., Cohen, R., Faulkner, A., Hannigan, B., Simpson, A., and Barlow, S. (2016). *Ordinary risks and accepted fictions: how contrasting and competing priorities work in risk assessment and mental health care planning. Health Expectations 20(3), 471–483.*

Coffey, M., Hannigan, B., Barlow, S., Cartwright, M., Cohen, R., Faulkner, A., Jones, A., and Simpson, A. (2019). *Recovery-focused mental health care planning and co-ordination in acute inpatient mental health settings: a cross national comparative mixed methods study. BMC Psychiatry 19, 115.*

Gillard, S. G., Edwards, C., Gibson, S. L., Owen, K., and Wright, C. (2013). *Introducing peer worker roles into UK mental health service teams: a qualitative analysis of the organisational benefits and challenges. BMC Health Services Research 13, 188.*

Leamy, M., Bird, V., Le Boutillier, C., Williams, J., and Slade, M. (2011). *Conceptual framework for personal recovery in mental health: systematic review and narrative synthesis. British Journal of Psychiatry 199(6), 445–452.*

National Institute for Health and Care Excellence (2021). *Shared Decision Making. Available at: https:// www.nice.org.uk/about/what-we-do/our-programmes/ nice-guidance/nice-guidelines/shared-decision-making*

NHS England, NHS Improvement, and National Collaborating Central for Mental Health (2019). *Community Mental Health Framework for Adults and Older Adults. London: NHS England, and NHS Improvement/National Collaborating Central for Mental Health.*

Priebe, S., McCabe, R., Bullenkamp, J., Hansson, L., Lauber, C., Martinez-Leal, R., Rössler, W., Salize, H., Svensson, B., Torres-Gonzales, F., van den Brink, R., Wiersma, D., and Wright, D. J. (2007). *Structured patient-clinician communication and 1-year outcome in community mental healthcare: cluster randomised controlled trial. British Journal of Psychiatry 191, 420–426.*

Simpson, A., Hannigan, B., Coffey, M., Barlow, S., Cohen, R., Jones, A., Všetečková, J., Faulkner, A.,

Thornton, A., and Cartwright, M. (2016). *Recovery-focused care planning and coordination in England and Wales: a cross-national mixed methods comparative case study. BMC Psychiatry 16, 147.*

Slade, M. (2009). *Personal Recovery from Mental Illness: A Guide for Mental Health Professionals. Cambridge: Cambridge University Press.*

Stuart, S. R., Tansey, L., and Quayle, E. (2016). *What we talk about when we talk about recovery: a systematic review and best fit framework synthesis of qualitative literature. Journal of Mental Health 26(3), 291–304.*

Thériault, J., Lord, M.-M., Briand, C., Piat, M., and Meddings, S. (2020). *Recovery colleges after a decade of research: a literature review. Psychiatric Services 71(9), 928–940.*

Tuffour, I. (2020). *'There is anointing everywhere': an interpretative phenomenological analysis of the role of religion in the recovery of Black African service users in England. Journal of Psychiatric and Mental Health Nursing 27(4), 352–361.*

Tuffour, I., Simpson, A., and Reynolds, L. (2019). *Mental illness and recovery: an interpretative phenomenological analysis of the experiences of Black African service users in England. Journal of Research in Nursing 24(1–2), 104–118.*

Zubin, J. and Spring, B. (1977). *Vulnerability: a new view of schizophrenia. Journal of Abnormal Psychology 86(2), 103–126.*

(11) Key skills in telemental health

Mary Munro   **Billy Ridler**

Learning outcomes

By the end of this chapter, you should be able to:

1 Recognize the increased use of telemental health care within mental health nursing settings

2 Evaluate service user and clinician experiences of telemental health care

3 Identify the strengths, barriers, and considerations for the use and implementation of telemental health

4 Appy key considerations and steps pre, during, and post implementation of telemental health care.

▼ Introduction

This chapter will focus on the concepts of telemental health within mental health nursing care. The fundamentals of mental health nursing suggest that the ability to communicate and form therapeutic relationships is key to providing the best possible care for service users. Furthermore, the mental health nursing role is ever evolving, as are the modes in which clinicians engage in consultations and forms of communication. Telemental health has been used for over two decades, but the COVID-19 pandemic has fast-tracked its use tenfold. Telemental health has been utilized more frequently over recent years and looks to be a common option that is here to stay for the future of mental health care. However, it is essential that both staff and service users are confident and comfortable with its use, and it is provided as an alternative to face-to-face communication, and not the only option. This chapter will explore the use of telemental health pre and post the COVID-19 pandemic, both service user and clinician experiences of its use, and considerations for and barriers to its use.

▼ Mental health nursing: a relational profession

The role of the mental health nurse has developed over the past 20 years and has often been difficult to define (Chambers, 2017). Pilgrim (2019) refers to the core fundamentals of mental health nursing as building effective relationships and enabling person-centred and recovery-focused care with service users who use mental health services alongside their relatives and/or carers. A recent review of mental health nursing in England recommended a reclaiming of this focus by emphasizing that mental health nurses must enhance the therapeutic relationship, by valuing experimental knowledge while recognizing and working to overcome power differentials that can exist in relationships between nurses and service users (Health Education England, 2022). These concepts are not new. Hildegard Peplau was a renowned nursing theorist who would challenge mental health nurses to thrive through the development of the profession and to provide a continued commitment to the nurse–service user relationship, engagement in evidence-based practice, and support of competence in information technology (Peplau, 1988). Peplau's theory of interpersonal relations emphasized the importance of the nurse–service user relationship and how the two work together towards the common goal of wellness. Peplau's theory provides guidance for nurses on how to interact with people so that they are empowered to be in control of their care. As the nursing role and how engagement and communication with service users have evolved, remembering the mental health nursing fundamental principles and Peplau's interpersonal theory is key to delivering the best possible care, particularly when thinking about commencing, continuing, or ending care in online and eHealth environments.

The concept of eHealth

The term 'eHealth' has been commonly used within health care services since the year 2000, and there are some differing opinions on what exactly it is. However, all definitions make reference that eHealth is the use of information and communication technologies for health (World Health Organization, 2021). See Table 11.1 for a glossary of terms relating to eHealth. Brørs et al. (2020) suggest that there is more to eHealth than just technology, as it incorporates using, recording, managing, and transmitting information to support health settings, in particular to make decisions collaboratively about patient care, and that computers (and other information and communication technology devices) are merely the technology that enables this to happen. eHealth can cover:

* electronic care records (including assessment)
* electronic communication (email, SMS texting, and telephone)
* telehealth (including video consultations)
* information governance (confidentiality and system security)
* personal health records.

Telemental health

Telemental health, a subset of telemedicine, can involve providing a range of services including mental health assessment and reviews, therapy (individual therapy, group therapy, family therapy), education, and medication management (Whaibeh et al., 2020). Telemental health can involve direct interaction between a mental health professional and the service user. Mental health care can be delivered in a live, interactive communication and is used in a variety of different settings, including private practice, community and outpatient clinics, hospitals, prison and forensic settings, schools, nursing homes, and military treatment settings (Barnett et al., 2021).

Telemental health has been used in one form or another for over 60 years, but more prominently since 1990 with the expansion of the internet making it more accessible globally. A developing evidence base identified that for some, telemental health care may be preferable to in-person care, for example, people with severe anxiety disorders and individuals with physical limitations may find remote consultations particularly useful (Madigan et al., 2021). By allowing service users to receive care in their homes, it can reduce barriers such as travel time, costs, and stigma associated with receiving mental health care in person (Connolly et al., 2020).

Table 11.1 Glossary of terms relating to eHealth

eHealth (also known as digital health)	The use of information and communications technology in support of health and health-related fields
mHealth	The use of mobile wireless technologies for health
Telehealth (also known as telemedicine)	The use of telecommunications and virtual technology to deliver health care outside of traditional health care facilities

Source: data from World Health Organization (2021).

▼ COVID-19 response: expansion and rapid adoption of telemental health care

The use of digital technology has played an important role in addressing the contemporary health care needs of the population within health and social care settings and has been seen as a mechanism to overcome or mitigate some of the barriers and challenges that are experienced (Mishkind et al., 2021). Despite this, prior to the COVID-19 pandemic, uptake of telemental health had been quite fragmented, with studies suggesting telemedicine was used by about 17% of clinicians daily prior to the pandemic (Zhu et al., 2024). During the pandemic this increased to 40% of clinicians using it daily (Zhu et al., 2024) with some authors describing the near-overnight implementation, and adoption of telemental health structures to support clinical care (Hong et al., 2021). For mental health care and support services, many clinicians and service users had to quickly adapt to the challenges posed both by the pandemic and by the public health measures to control it (Steidtmann et al., 2021). Consequently, many mental health care, treatment, and support services made the decision early on during the pandemic to restrict face-to-face contact with vulnerable population groups, including older people, people who use substances, and those with coexisting physical health problems. Triage of referrals was introduced for many services nationally and where appropriate, telephone assessments or video conferencing were offered in lieu of face-to-face assessments.

Research exploring the increased use of telemental health care during the pandemic reported that it has become an attractive option for some clinicians and service users, owing to a combination of increased acceptability, feasibility, and cost-effectiveness (Zhu et al., 2024). The use may have been born out of necessity, but it appears telemental health may remain a standard approach to care delivery in some mental health settings going forward. To optimize its use, it is essential that both staff and service users feel confident and equipped to utilize telemental health (Juan et al., 2021). While some fundamental training on system delivery, understandably, may have been missed or fast-tracked during the pandemic owing to the reactive nature and need for service delivery change, it is important that in areas where telemental health will remain standard practice that staff and service users can engage with training and development. Furthermore, many of the digital technologies utilized were done so without input from service users, family members, and carers. Therefore, it is essential that an understanding of service user experience and quality of care is reviewed.

▼ Contemporary experiences of telemental health

Research exploring telemental health prior to the pandemic suggested that it may be an effective, acceptable, and feasible tool to support mental health care, with the highest acceptability being evidenced where its use was well designed and planned (Barnett et al., 2021). The evidence available was assessed as being of relatively low quality, with limited information looking at medium- to long-term outcomes, sample groups were homogeneous in nature, and there was limited exploration of concepts such as digital exclusion—with many participants having opted into this form of care in the studies (Barnett et al., 2021). Several studies have been conducted on service experiences during the pandemic. Benudis et al. (2022) explored service user experiences of telemental health during the COVID-19 pandemic. Results suggested that 70% of respondents reported that the quality of care via video conferencing or telephone was equally good or much better than in-person visits and were somewhat or very satisfied with telemental health overall. For service users respondents who reported that they preferred telehealth over in-person visits (65%), the reasons provided were no or less travel time, appointments were easier to attend and reschedule, and appointments were less expensive. However, for the 35% of respondents who preferred in-person visits, they stated that it was easier to talk more openly, there was better quality of care in person, they were used to in-person treatment, and they found the use of technology challenging. Although overall service user experience remained favourable to telemental health, service users reported issues securing private space for sessions and concerns about internet privacy and confidence using technologies.

These findings were similar in Shah et al's (2022) qualitative study exploring what had changed for people with mental ill health accessing care and treatment during the pandemic. While many participants described reduced access to or quality of support from NHS mental health services during the pandemic, some participants found it helped them to look for alternatives which they might not have previously considered to support their mental health, including online support groups, digital forums and social media, mobile apps, and meditation. However, although use of alternative or new forms of support was helpful for many participants, for some there was a sense of having to rely on them because no other options were available. Furthermore, many participants felt that they were digitally excluded owing to lack of access to equipment or did not have the skills or offering of training to use the platforms provided, removing the choice of preference; older populations felt particularly left behind by the quick transition to online services.

The evidence to date of service user experiences of telemental health, although limited, suggests that there are advantages to telemental health care and some individuals have found it to be a preferable option than face-to-face appointments, which has helped them explore other supports, saved time, reduced costs, and has been more convenient overall. However, it must be noted that this is not the experience for all individuals and although telemental health should be offered as an option, it is important to explore service user preference and ability to engage in telemental health, to make sure that individuals are not digitally excluded, and that care and support is person-centred.

The experience of UK mental health care staff has also been explored during the pandemic. Johnson et al. (2020) surveyed over 2,000 staff from a range of sectors and professions and sought to explore the impact on mental health care, and on mental health services of the pandemic. The findings identified a range of key points, describing what was working well in telehealth and what can prevent, or was preventing, telehealth from working. These are summarized in Table 11.2. The points identified are only from one perspective but do reflect the findings within other studies conducted.

A limitation of the evolving evidence base for telemental health care may be the context in which the wider-spread implementation of the services has taken place. Studies have explored the acceptability of telemental health care, and comparisons have been made to acceptability versus face-to-face contact but in the context of the pandemic, where face-to-face support was reduced dramatically, acceptability and experience may reflect that some care, and support, in whatever form, is preferable to none (Juan et al., 2021). Lived experience commentary written by Beverley Chipp and Karen Machin warns that 'gratitude for any contact under the circumstances, and satisfaction within this context should not be used to justify any narrowing of choice in future provisions' (Juan et al., 2021, p. 5).

Table 11.2 What is working well, and what is preventing telemental health from working

What is working well in telehealth	What can prevent telehealth from working
Efficiency of remote working • Allows prompt responses • Saves travelling time • Is better for the environment • May be more convenient for both staff and service users • Allows staff to connect easily with each other, even if based in different places and different teams • Allows home working	**Inadequate resources** • Equipment and internet connections of low quality • Processes and preferred platforms not clearly established • Staff may lack training and confidence **Impacts on communication and therapeutic relationships** • May be harder to establish and maintain a good therapeutic relationship • May be harder to make an assessment, especially at first contact • May be challenging for longer, more in-depth sessions
Best alternative for now • Remote working is allowing services to keep going despite infection control restrictions • Innovative use of IT and digital tools can allow group programmes or individual therapies to continue successfully	**Digital exclusion** • People who lack equipment and resources to connect • People who do not have skills or confidence to connect (including people with cognitive impairments) • People lacking a suitably private environment for remote appointments
Benefits for some service users • Some service users are happy with video-call technology and even prefer it • Access is improved for some people, especially if travel and public places are challenging • May be an efficient way of helping people with less complex needs	**Service user preferences** • Some service users strongly prefer confidential conversations to be face to face, or may feel suspicious or anxious about remote means • If they do accept remote contacts, some prefer simpler phone or messaging modalities • Some service users do not engage with remote contacts

▼ **Implementation of telemental health: key considerations**

Relationship

As discussed above, mental health nursing is a relational profession, with the therapeutic relationship being a central mechanism to enable optimal care, support, and experience for service users. Some service users, and staff, have concerns that telemental health, especially that facilitated via telephone or video conferencing technology, is more impersonal compared with face-to-face contact and that this can make it more challenging to establish rapport (Juan et al., 2021; Painter, 2021). Noticing non-verbal communication and body language were highlighted as aspects which may be more challenging when connecting with a service user via video conferencing. These concerns are not universal but there does appear to be a general theme within the literature that establishment of rapport, and progression to a therapeutic relationship using telemental health, is to some extent inferior when compared to face-to-face contact. Factors that appear to influence the quality of care, and therapeutic relationship, specifically include service provider's confidence, and competence in using the technology that is facilitating the telemental health care; people not being familiar with the technology being used, or mistrusting the technology; and quality of the contact, that is, image quality, audio quality, and connection reliability (Juan et al., 2021).

Glass and Bickler (2021) explored the ways in which marriage and family therapists adapted to telemental health care during the pandemic and their work highlighted some key tools and approaches that may support in facilitating the establishment of a therapeutic relationship. They described the strengths associated with telemental health care, identifying that some service users felt more comfortable being vulnerable, and able to express more freely aspects of their life. Optimizing telemental health care may involve the service provider recognizing the strengths and distinct nature of telemental health care, to enable all opportunities to be taken to optimize this mode of contact. Tool and techniques that may facilitate establishment of rapport and development of the therapeutic relationship are highlighted in Table 11.3.

Choice

Factors that influence and inform preference regarding telemental health care for service users are dynamic and include the reason and purpose of contact with the care provider, the relationship with the care provider, and the ability, of both parties, to use the technologies required to facilitate telemental health care (Juan et al., 2021). Juan et al. (2021) revealed that experiences and preferences in relation to telemental health are essentially personal, and that it is not possible to make assumptions about individual's preferences. Given this, it is essential that choice is a key consideration within telemental health care. Adopting co-production as a framework for the implementation and use of telemental health, at both an individual and system level, may support in placing choice at the centre. This would be consistent with contemporary values, and policy, within mental health care (Health Education England, 2022). Choice will be central to the development and roll-out of blended models of telemental health care. Painter et al. (2021) reported a study in which 13 participants took up the offer of an online consultation rather than an in-person consultation. Overall, participants' satisfaction was high, with almost all willing to receive further video calls in the future. Participants felt they were able to share information as freely as they would have done if it were face to face. Blended approaches that offer individuals choice and include different types of remote and face-to-face contacts may support in enhancing service user satisfaction and experience. Service providers should aim to provide personalized, flexible options as these attributes were found to be valued by service users (Juan et al., 2021). This approach may involve an evolution in thought and discussion around telemental health provision (and other forms of remote care). Rather than discussing remote care versus face-to-face care, the strengths and limitations of both should be considered in the context of each service and individual, and a hybrid model adopted offering aspects of both. In this context, telemental health should be viewed as an evolution of care that can be offered rather than a replacement. Table 11.4 suggests an approach that could be taken when approaching telemental health care.

Table 11.3 Tools and techniques to optimize the therapeutic relationship within telemental health care

Cues	Service providers need to be more in tune with cues. These cues may come in verbal, non-verbal, auditory, and/or visual forms. Awareness of tone of voice, facial expressions, and eye contact—both those of the service provider and service user facilitate the establishment of rapport
Own environment	Telemental health via video conferencing provides the opportunity to see the service user in their own environment, and comment on elements of the environment. Rapport can be established through discussion of pictures/posters, musical instruments, presence, or pictures of family. Additionally, the service provider may be able to see how the service user interacts with their environment and systems within the environment, i.e. family relations
Comfort	Where in person, the service provider may lean forward, provide a tissue, or other forms of non-verbal comfort. Within the telemental health space, a focus on verbal comfort, and expression of empathy via intentional use of tone, language, and eye contact are key
Structure	Identifying the purpose for the contact, planning ahead, and having goals were all identified as important to enhance the telemental health session
Understanding of technology	Service providers having a good understanding of the technology and being able to support troubleshooting when issues arise optimizes contact
Video conference etiquette	Ensuring lighting is in front of the camera, and not behind, to optimize view of face, a camera position that allows face to be in the middle of the screen, and an appropriate background can all optimize experience
Validation	Validating the service user's opinions of telemental health including any challenges experienced is key. Additionally, validation is a way of exploring power imbalances and inequities when they present within telemental health
Self-awareness	The service provider's awareness of self is critical to establishing therapeutic relationships. The service provider needs to be aware of, and acknowledge, their own biases to allow for an environment of authenticity and sensitivity

Source: data from Glass, V. Q. and Bickler, A. (2021). Cultivating the therapeutic alliance in a telemental health setting. *Contemporary Family Therapy*, 43(2), 189–198.

Table 11.4 Step-by-step guide to telemental health consultation

Step 1	**Consider acceptability in partnership** As this chapter has highlighted, telemental health has its advantages for both clinicians and service users; however, it does not meet all service users' needs. Therefore, the first step should be to consider the appropriateness for telemental health for the aims of the contact. It is important to explore with the service user what their contact preference would be and provide options including initial face-to-face, hybrid, or telemental health consultation
Step 2	**Choice and access** Offer choice of telehealth platforms where possible and levels of comfort of utilizing the chosen format. Identify any training needs for clinician, and service user, so that both can engage in confidence with the chosen platform. Are there 'how-to guides' or 'troubleshooting' guides that could be available before, and during the contact? Furthermore, ensure that the service user has access to the necessary technology to access the telemental health platform
Step 3	**Initial contact—plan and discuss** At the beginning of the telemental health contact, the clinician and service user should discuss, and agree, on the aim of the contact from a therapeutic perspective, but also discuss factors unique to telemental health contact such as what will happen if someone's technology does not work, is there a backup form of contact? What are expectations around privacy within the environment, are there other people present or nearby? If so, how may this impact the contact? Are there any distractions within the environment that may take someone's attention, and how will the other person be aware when this happens? How will distress or discomfort be communicated, and what support will be provided if this occurs? What steps will be taken if contact is lost, and not re-established? Allow time during the initial period to discuss perspectives, beliefs, and, if appropriate, concerns around the use of telemental health
Step 4	**Review and reflect** As the contact is ending, time should be spent reviewing the therapeutic work that has taken place as well as an explicit review of the use of the mode of contact—how acceptable was it? Was information shared freely, or were there barriers? How might telemental health be used going forward within the relationship? The clinician should reflect on aspects such as their beliefs around the nature of the contact, how the contact met expectations or plans, is self-awareness impacted, what interpersonal skills were utilized, and which of these needed to be adapted or enhanced to use within telemental health care?

▲ Conclusion

It is envisaged that telemental health care will form a significant part of mental health care going forward. The evidence suggests that, for some, telemental health care is an agreeable way to receive care, and in some situations may be preferable to face-to-face contact. However, the factors that influence acceptability for service users of this form of contact are varied and unique. So, rather than being viewed as a direct replacement for face-to-face contact within services, telemental health care should be seen as one tool within a hybrid service that offers a range of mechanisms to facilitate contact. Choice, planning, confidence, and competence all appear to be essential to optimize the experience of telemental health care.

✖ Tips from service users

1 Offer choice wherever possible, and if telemental health is the only choice at any given time, do not assume acceptability is the same as preference.
2 Enable optimal use of the technology facilitating telemental care by ensuring the necessary technology is available, that instructions on its use are available, and that the service provider can provide support, especially for commonly encountered challenges.
3 Actively seek feedback on the experience of telemental health contact, and reflect on how the mode of contact is facilitating the achievement of therapeutic outcomes.

W Companion website

For extra resources on the topics covered in this chapter, visit the companion website at: www.oup.com/mhns

✚ References

Barnett, P., Goulding, L., Casetta, C., Jordan, H., Sheridan-Rains, L., Steare, T., Williams, J., Wood, L., Gaughran, F., and Johnson, S. (2021). *Implementation of telemental health services before COVID-19: rapid umbrella review of systematic reviews. Journal of Medical Internet Research 23(7), e26492.*

Benudis, A., Re'em, Y., Kanellopoulos, D., Moreno, A., and Zonana, J. (2022). *Patient and provider experiences of telemental health during the COVID-19 pandemic in a New York City academic medical center. Psychiatry Research 311, 114496.*

Brørs, G., Norman, C. D., and Norekvål, T. M. (2020). *Accelerated importance of eHealth literacy in the COVID-19 outbreak and beyond. European Journal of Cardiovascular Nursing 19(6), 458–461.*

Chambers, M. (2017). *Psychiatric and Mental Health Nursing: The Craft of Caring, 3rd ed. New York: Routledge Taylor and Francis Group.*

Connolly, S. L., Miller, C. J., Lindsay, J. A., and Bauer, M. S. (2020). *A systematic review of providers' attitudes toward telemental health via videoconferencing. Clinical Psychology: Science and Practice 27(2), e12311.*

Glass, V. Q. and Bickler, A. (2021). *Cultivating the therapeutic alliance in a telemental health setting. Contemporary Family Therapy 43(2), 189–198.*

Health Education England (2022). *Commitment and Growth: Advancing Mental Health Nursing Now and for the Future. Available at: https://www.hee.nhs.uk/sites/ default/files/documents/Commitment%20and%20 Growth%20Advancing%20Mental%20Health%20Nurs ing%20Now%20and%20for%20the%20Future.pdf*

Hong, J. S. W., Sheriff, R., Smith, K., Tomlinson, A., Saad, F., Smith., T., Engelthaler, T., Phiri, P., Henshall, C., Ede, R., Denis, M., Mitter, P., D'Agostino, A., Cerveri, G., Tomassi, S., Rathod, S., Broughton, N., Marlow, K., Geddes, J., and Cipriani, A. (2021). *Impact of COVID-19 on telepsychiatry at the service and individual patient level across two UK NHS mental health Trusts. Evidence Based Mental Health 24(4), 161–166.*

Johnson, S., Dalton-Locke, C., Juan, N. V. S., Foye, U., Oram, S., Papamichail, A., Landau, S., Olive, R. R., Jeynes, T., Shah, P., Rains, L. S., Lloyd-Evans, B., Carr, S., Killaspy, H., Gillard, S., and Simpson, A. (2020). *Impact on mental health care and on mental health service users of the COVID-19 pandemic: a mixed methods* survey of UK mental health care staff. *Social Psychiatry and Psychiatric Epidemiology 56(1), 25–37.*

Juan, N. V. S., Shah, P., Schlief, M., Appleton, R., Nyikavaranda, P., Birken, M., Foye, U., Lloyd-Evans, B., Morant, N., Needle, J. J., Simpson, A., Lyons., Rains, L. S., Dedat, Z., and Johnson, S. (2021). *Telemental health during the COVID-19 pandemic: a co-produced framework analysis. PLoS One 16(9), 1–20.*

Madigan, S., Racine, N., Cooke, J. E., and Korczak, D. J. (2021). *COVID-19 and telemental health: benefits, challenges, and future directions. Canadian Psychology 62(1), 5.*

Mishkind, M. C., Shore, J. H., Bishop, K., D'Amato, K., Brame, A., Thomas, M., and Schneck, C. D. (2021). *Rapid conversion to telemental health services in response to COVID-19: experiences of two outpatient mental health clinics. Telemedicine and e-Health 27(7), 778–784.*

Painter, J., Turner, J., and Procter, P. (2021). *Understanding and accommodating patient and staff choice when implementing video consultations in mental health services. CIN: Computers, Informatics, Nursing 39(10), 578–583.*

Peplau, H. (1988). *Interpersonal Relations in Nursing: A Conceptual Frame of Reference for Psychodynamic Nursing. New York: Palgrave Macmillan.*

Pilgrim, D. (2019). *Key Concepts in Mental Health, 2nd ed. London: Sage Publishing.*

Shah, P., Hardy, J., Birken, M., Foye, U., Olive, R. R., Nyikavaranda, P., Dare, C., Stefanidou, T., Schlief, M., Pearce, E., Lyons, N., Machin, K., Jeynes, T., Chipp, B., Chhapia, A., Barber, N., Gillard, S., Pitman, A., Simpson, A., … Lloyd-Evans, B. (2022). *What has changed in the experiences of people with mental health problems during the COVID-19 pandemic: a coproduced, qualitative interview study. Social Psychiatry and Psychiatric Epidemiology 57(6), 1291–1303.*

Steidtmann, D., McBride, S., and Mishkind, M. C. (2021). *Experiences of mental health clinicians and staff in rapidly converting to full-time telemental health and work from home during the COVID-19 pandemic. Telemedicine and e-Health 27(7), 785–791.*

Whaibeh, E., Mahmoud, H., and Naal, H. (2020). *Telemental health in the context of a pandemic: the COVID-19 experience. Current Treatment Options in Psychiatry 7(2), 198–202.*

World Health Organization (2021). *Global Observatory for eHealth. Available at: https://www.who.int/observatories/global-observatory-for-ehealth*

Zhu, D., Paige, S. R., Slone, H., Gutierrez, A., Lutzky, C., Hedriana, H., Barrera, J. F., Ong, T., and Bunnell, B. E. (2021). *Exploring telemental health practice before, during, and after the COVID-19 pandemic. Journal of Telemedicine and Telecare 30(1), 72–78.*

12 The essence of physical health care

Michael Nash
Roupmatee Joggyah

Christine Kakai

Learning outcomes

By the end of this chapter, you should be able to:

1 Identify key risk factors for poor physical health in people living with mental health problems

2 Explain the concept of health screening

3 Examine side effect assessment as a way of screening physical health

4 Explain how stigma and diagnostic overshadowing can impact physical health.

▼ Introduction

Improving the physical health of service users and reducing premature death was a key policy goal of *No Health Without Mental Health* (Department of Health, 2011). This led onto the *Five Year Forward View for Mental Health* (NHS England, 2016), where the policy commitment to improving the physical health of service users remains a key target. The reason why specific policies were required can be found in evidence of poor physical health and poor physical health outcomes in people with severe mental illness (SMI), which are manifested in three key ways:

1 **Higher mortality (death) rates**: Olfson et al. (2015) found adults living with schizophrenia were more than 3.5 times as likely to die compared with adults in the general population, with cardiovascular disease the highest mortality rate.

2 **Early mortality**: people with SMI die as much as 20 years prematurely than the general population. This mortality gap has been described as one of the greatest health inequalities in England (NHS England, 2016).

3 **High levels of comorbidity**: people with schizophrenia tend to have three or more coexisting medical conditions (Smith et al., 2013). This moves the issue from comorbidity (e.g. schizophrenia and type 2 diabetes), to one of multimorbidity (e.g. schizophrenia, type 2 diabetes, obesity, and hypertension).

Causes of poor physical health in people with SMI are complex and multifactorial, for example, people with SMI may have difficulties communicating symptoms or health needs owing to psychotic symptoms such as thought disorder. Therefore, while standard explanations of 'lifestyle' factors or medication side effects are important contributors to poor physical health, the 'parity of esteem' agenda illustrates other factors such as:

- stigma and negative attitudes of other health professionals

- diagnostic overshadowing (where clinically diagnostic symptoms are attributed to the mental illness diagnosis and go untreated, e.g. a person with schizophrenia complains of hearing strange noises and this is attributed to auditory hallucinations and not tinnitus due to an ear infection)

- insufficient integration of physical and mental health care

- lack of specialized care pathways (e.g. diabetes care pathways for people with psychotic disorders) are emerging as additional reasons (Nash, 2018).

The report entitled *Improving the Physical Health of People with Mental Health Problems: Actions for Mental Health Nurses*

(Department of Health and Public Health England, 2016) highlights eight key areas for focusing practice on physical health such as quitting smoking, tackling obesity, improving physical activity, and medication optimization. These are important factors in a little-addressed area of mental health nursing practice—preventative health screening. Screening is emerging as a frontier aspect of practice and is a boundary that mental health nurses must push to extend practice. This chapter will examine types of screening that mental health nurses can get involved in, such as screening for:

- physical conditions

- physical health risk factors
- complications
- preventative interventions
- medication side effects.

We must also be mindful of two other important things:

- Barriers to screening in people with SMI
- The importance of following up on screening to ensure that appropriate treatment is instigated for any diagnosed physical conditions.

▼ What is preventative health screening?

Preventative health screening, or screening, is the process of identifying illness early so that prompt intervention can be given to prevent more serious illness occurring. Sometimes a person may not have symptoms of an illness or symptoms go unnoticed, so screening can identify conditions early. However, screening needs to be a proactive process, waiting until symptoms appear is not really screening.

▼ Screening for physical conditions

Taking blood for analysis is a way of screening for a range of physical conditions such as anaemia (low number of red blood cells), infection (raised number of white blood cells), increased blood glucose concentration (diabetes) or high cholesterol levels. Blood tests also screen for system functioning, such as the renal (kidney) function test and liver function test, which are important in mental health as the liver and kidneys play a key role in metabolizing psychotropic medication, which can be toxic to service users prescribed this medication. The liver function test is also an important parameter for practitioners working with people who misuse alcohol owing to the impact that this has on a person's liver. Furthermore, blood monitoring is a requirement for certain medications such as lithium (to detect toxicity) or clozapine (to monitor white blood cell count).

glucose) (Diabetes UK, n. d.). Table 12.1 outlines blood glucose levels and their relationship to diabetes. Risk factors for prediabetes include age (being over 45 years), family history of diabetes, being overweight or obese, smoking, being physically inactive, having conditions such as high blood pressure, and ethnic minority status, especially South Asian, African Caribbean, or Black African. Service users face increased exposure to these risk factors compared to the general population (Nash, 2014) and when medication side effects are added, the importance of screening for prediabetes (and diabetes) becomes paramount.

Exploring family history (parents and siblings) is another important aspect of screening as some physical conditions, such as diabetes, may have a genetic component. Therefore,

Screening example: prediabetes

Holt and Mitchell (2015) report that diabetes prevalence is two to three times higher in people with SMI, affecting around 12% of people receiving antipsychotics. Therefore, screening for diabetes is an important aspect of physical health care. When blood glucose levels are above the normal range, but not high enough for a diagnosis of diabetes, the person is in the stage of prediabetes (also referred to as impaired fasting

Table 12.1 General range of fasting blood glucose levels and diabetes

'Normal' blood glucose	Prediabetes	Diabetes
<5.5 mmol/L	5.5–6.9 mmol/L	≥7 mmol/L

Source: data from https://www.diabetes.co.uk/fasting-plasma-glucose-test.html

while a person may be asymptomatic, a family history should be a red flag in terms of targeted physical health monitoring.

Benefits of early detection

Prediabetes does not have any clinical symptoms, so it often goes unrecognized. This serves as a missed opportunity for early intervention. When conditions are diagnosed, early interventions may not need to be invasive. For example, in prediabetes, modifications to diet and physical activity can help manage blood glucose levels. However, when missed, the risk of developing full-blown diabetes is increased and this may mean more invasive treatment such as taking medication and daily blood glucose monitoring **as well as** modifications to diet and physical activity. Furthermore, diabetes will only get

Table 12.2 Self-assessment exercise: screening for behavioural risk factors (see answers at end of chapter)

Diet	What are the recommended daily calorie intakes for men and women?
Physical activity	What is the government recommended level of physical activity per week?
Alcohol	What are the recommended maximum numbers of alcohol units per week for men and women?

Source: data from https://www.nhs.uk/live-well/

progressively worse if unidentified because if left untreated it may result in serious complications (see later in chapter).

▼ Screening for physical health risk factors

In mental health care, language is a powerful tool for inclusion but also a powerful weapon of exclusion. Embracing a public health approach to screening is a way of promoting less judgemental language such as 'unhealthy' behaviour. Therefore, avoid using terminology such as 'lifestyle factors' which might be interpreted as judgemental because it implies there is a choice. However, in many instances service users have little choice owing to social determinants of health such as exclusion, homelessness, unemployment, poverty, and deprivation. Therefore, service users may not be able to adopt a 'healthy' lifestyle, because they cannot afford it.

Certain behaviours increase the risk of particular conditions, for example, smoking is a behaviour that increases the risk of cancer. Therefore, using 'behavioural risk factor', instead of lifestyle factor, is less judgemental as the focus is on the behaviour and not the person. Important behavioural risk factors recognized as harmful in SMI include:

- smoking (including vaping)
- unbalanced diet—high in fat and low in fibre

- lack of physical activity
- alcohol/substance use
- risky sexual activity.

Screening for risk factors is important because we know that some are modifiable—they can be reduced or eliminated by early intervention, health education, and health promotion; for example, people can stop smoking with the help of smoking cessation interventions. See Table 12.2 for a screening self-assessment exercise.

Identifying risk factors will probably occur during physical health monitoring, for example, if a service user is admitted into hospital or if they are having a recommended annual physical health check (National Institute for Health and Care Excellence, 2014). Using the Modified Early Monitoring System (MEWS) is not screening in a traditional sense. This is because not everyone will be on this, as it targets those who may need physical observations recorded periodically throughout the day. Therefore, it only 'screens' for a select group and only a defined set of parameters.

▼ Screening for complications of physical conditions: type 2 diabetes

People with SMI are at greater risk of physical conditions such as hypertension or type 2 diabetes. Physical health issues in

SMI usually remain undiagnosed for long periods so when they are finally diagnosed, complications may be evident and may even be the reason for diagnosis. In type 2 diabetes, service users require more than blood glucose monitoring; they also require regular review to ensure that they do not have complications. Screening for complications of type 2 diabetes is very important for both the quality of life of service users and their overall physical health outcomes. Complications of type 2 diabetes can be:

- **life-threatening**—diabetic ketoacidosis where insulin levels are dangerously low and blood glucose becomes dangerously high

- **acute**—hyperglycaemia (high blood glucose) or hypoglycaemia (low blood glucose)

- **long term**—(among others) cardiovascular problems such as hypertension and stroke, kidney problems such as nephropathy (reduced kidney function), lower limb amputation, and opportunistic yeast infections such as *Candida* (thrush) due to high blood glucose promoting oral or genital yeast growth.

Peripheral neuropathy

A significant complication of type 2 diabetes is peripheral neuropathy. This is a type of nerve damage that arises as a long-term complication of high blood glucose concentrations. Small blood vessels and capillaries get damaged over time and harden, restricting blood flow to tissue and nerves. This leads to less tissue perfusion with oxygen resulting in tissue death (necrosis) and nerve damage. An example of this is lower limb peripheral neuropathy where blood flow (e.g. below the knee) is restricted and can lead to a diabetic leg ulcer or, in more severe cases, gangrene of the toes, which can result in amputation. In screening for peripheral neuropathy, mental health nurses must be able to recognize early signs that the person may report such as numbness in the hands and feet (which can be painful), pins and needles sensation in fingers or toes, tingling feelings in the extremities or extremities being cold to touch, and they may appear very pale/white.

Nerve damage can also lead to disorders such as erectile dysfunction in men due to damage to the small blood vessels of the penis or retinopathy (damage to the retina of the eye) leading to early blindness. The UK has a free, annual diabetic retinopathy screening programme for anyone aged 12 and over with a diabetes diagnosis. Therefore, mental health nurses do not have to perform this screening, but be facilitators, or advocates, for service users' access.

It is also worth remembering that eye problems (blurred vision) and sexual dysfunction (impotence due to high levels of prolactin) are side effects of antipsychotic medications. If service users with SMI and type 2 diabetes report such symptoms, mental health nurses should not automatically assume they are medication side effects without investigating whether they are actually complications of type 2 diabetes.

▼ Screening for uptake of public health interventions

People with SMI are at greater risk of dying from infections, with research suggesting this could be five times higher than the general population (Piatt et al., 2010; Bertolini et al., 2023). Therefore, another way that screening can be used is to identify the uptake of public health interventions, such as vaccinations. Consent and autonomy are important, so discussing vaccinations requires tact and respect, especially if matters of cultural or religious identity are relevant. Examples of vaccinations include:

- winter flu jab

- COVID-19

- pneumococcal vaccine

- human papillomavirus vaccine in adolescents aged 12–13 years (may be of interest to practitioners in child and adolescent mental health)

- hepatitis B—for people who inject drugs.

In addition to vaccinations, mental health nurses could be screening for uptake of smoking cessation and if it is low, they could engage in a health education and promotion drive around tobacco reduction. Another important area for screening from which people with SMI face exclusion is cancer screening. Research shows that service users have lower rates of cancer screening for breast, cervical, and prostate cancer when compared to the general population (Solmi et al., 2020). Therefore, as with diabetic retinopathy, mental health nurses will not have to perform the actual cancer screening but be facilitators and advocates for service user access. Table 12.3 summarizes UK national cancer screening programmes and inclusion criteria.

There are no specific national screening programmes for men regarding testicular or prostate cancer, but mental

Table 12.3 National UK cancer screening programmes

Screening	Inclusion criteria	Frequency
Breast	Women aged 50–70	Every 3 years
Cervical screening	All women and people with a cervix aged 25–64	Age 25–49: every 3 years Age 50–64: every 5 years
Bowel screening	Everyone aged 60–74 People 75 or over can self-request a test kit	Every 2 years

Source: data from https://www.nhs.uk/conditions/nhs-screening/

health nurses need to be aware of the drive for increasing prostate health in men aged over 50 years. Prostate Cancer Risk Management (NHS, 2021) is an informed choice programme where men aged 50 or over can discuss having a prostate-specific antigen test with their general practitioner.

Screening is beneficial for early detection of illness and better health outcomes. Yet, it is a matter of choice—people in the general population choose not to get screened, which is often because they have not been given adequate information to allow them to make an informed decision. Therefore, mental health nurses must be knowledgeable about screening programmes so that they can educate service users about their benefits and what screening entails. This can reassure people that screening is not painful and empower them with knowledge to make positive decisions.

▼ Medication monitoring: screening for side effects

Medication monitoring is an important aspect of mental health nursing practice, which should be more than checking compliance because it offers nurses another avenue for physical health screening by identifying side effects. Medication side effects can contribute to lower quality of life and are a unique risk factor for poor physical health in service users because the general population do not take them. They are a double-edged sword, as they can cause weight gain and obesity, and sedation and movement disorders, such as tremor or unsteady gait, which may limit the service user's ability to participate in physical activity required to lose weight.

All mental health nurses have a role in medication monitoring, but nurse prescribing offers a way of increasing the physical health outcomes of service users by ensuring medication regimens are reflective of current needs (e.g. reducing medication or discontinuing medications that are no longer required). However, there is the issue of prescribing for physical conditions which may fall outside the scope of practice for prescribers. Nonetheless, prescribers can effectively monitor physical health side effects such as weight gain, or constipation.

Prescribers will also need to be aware of contraindications of medications prescribed for physical conditions in people with SMI. For example, medications such as angiotensin-converting enzyme inhibitors, diuretics, and non-steroidal anti-inflammatory drugs (such as ibuprofen) can increase lithium serum concentrations and need to be carefully monitored if prescribed to someone who is taking lithium (Malhi et al., 2020). This is because these types of medications can decrease lithium excretion causing lithium levels to build up, leading to lithium toxicity. Prescribers should caution service users about taking over-the-counter medications such as ibuprofen and should routinely assess this.

Constipation is a common side effect of antipsychotics but is less studied even though it can be severe and lead to complications such as paralytic ileus, bowel occlusion, and death (DeHert et al., 2011). In a Scottish primary care study of differences in physical conditions in people with schizophrenia and the general population, Smith et al. (2013) found one of the most common physical conditions in schizophrenia was constipation.

Signs and symptoms of constipation to look for include:

- headache
- feeling bloated and nauseous
- abdominal pain
- confusion
- decrease in stool volume and frequency.

Screening for constipation:

- Assess bowel habits:
  - Time/amount/frequency of stool
  - Consistency of stool (using Bristol Stool Chart; see 'Screening tools')
  - Bleeding on defecation
  - History of laxative use.
- Assess lifestyle:
  - Fibre content in diet
  - Daily fluid intake
  - Exercise patterns
  - Recently stopping smoking
  - Alcohol/drug consumption
  - Current medications
  - Anxiety/depression/stress.

Constipation risk is increased in SMI due to factors such as:

- medications—notably antipsychotic medication such as clozapine
- 'physical health' medication such as a diuretic
- type 2 diabetes
- unbalanced diet
- low levels of hydration
- low levels of physical activity
- lack of screening or side effect monitoring.

Screening is important for increasing physical health outcomes for people with SMI. However, screening is one thing, intervention following screening is equally important. Intervention will require interprofessional working, within the multidisciplinary team, but also across traditional health care boundaries (e.g. with primary care and secondary adult general health services). Creating screening pathways that incorporate comorbidity treatment plans is worth considering because the issues associated with physical health and SMI are complex and will only exacerbate if there is no structured way of navigating two complex health care services. Care pathways can also promote communication and liaison across boundaries so that key information and changes to care are not lost or delayed in bureaucratic systems.

▼ Inclusive screening and physical health monitoring

Service users reflect the composition of society, so our physical health monitoring needs to be inclusive and reflect this. In terms of sex, a low-risk waist:hip ratio is different between women (≤0.80) and men (≤0.90). Ethnicity is important in low-risk waist circumference and differs between White European, Black African, Middle Eastern, and mixed origin men (>94 cm/ >37 inches) and African Caribbean, South Asian, Chinese, and Japanese origin Asian men (>90 cm/>35 inches).

Religion also requires sensitivity in physical health monitoring where fasting may be an obligation (e.g. during the holy month of Ramadan). Muslim service users may feel obligated to fast, but if they have type 2 diabetes this will present obvious problems. We should work closely with all religions to draw up sensitive guidelines because fasting is a common and recurring aspect of religious practice, where observance needs to be facilitated safely.

In terms of gender identity, we need to be mindful of cancer screening for trans* service users (trans* = all types of gender self-identification). While individuals may self-identify their gender, there may be a need for them to remain engaged with sex-based cancer screening. This may be a distressing

experience for them as they are being recognized in screening by the sex they do not identify with.

The advice that we should 'screen the target organ, not the gender' is safest. For example, if a transgender man (an individual born female who has transitioned or is transitioning to be a man) still has a cervix, they should continue with cervical screening for early identification of cervical cancer (PULSE, 2019). This advice may change in those who have had a hysterectomy. Likewise, a trans woman or non-binary person assigned male at birth can get prostate cancer. Therefore, as with non-trans men, prostate screening should be offered. Liaison with general practitioner services to ensure gender identity is accurately recorded to prevent exclusion from screening is important, but mental health nurses need to get service user consent as there may be a cultural or religious reason why they may feel they cannot disclose this information. Screening is, therefore, not just about the physical taking of samples—there may be complex issues which require tact and compassion on the part of nurses as professionals and as advocates for access to screening services for transgender service users.

▼ Screening and intervening

Following screening it is important that an intervention follows, if required. This may take the form of health education and promotion advice as a form of primary prevention if no physical health issues are found, which could prevent or delay the onset of conditions. However, if a physical health issue is found then secondary prevention is required to intervene early to improve health outcomes—preventing more serious complications arising. Interventions may be non-pharmacological in nature (i.e. not requiring drug treatment) such as changes to diet, increasing physical activity, tobacco, and alcohol reduction. Pharmacological interventions may be required if conditions are more advanced (e.g. an oral hypoglycaemic for type 2 diabetes or a statin for high cholesterol levels). In the event of severe complications, tertiary prevention may be required to improve the quality of life in people who have required invasive interventions for serious conditions (e.g. if someone has had a stroke, or required an amputation owing to diabetes). Increasing quality of life by improving physical functioning can contribute to longer life expectancy. However, this type of care is complex and requires an interdisciplinary approach as the skill sets may be beyond the scope of practice for mental health nurses.

A good guide for both screening and intervening is the updated Lester Positive Cardiometabolic Health Resource (Perry et al., 2023).This tool addresses screening related to issues covered in this chapter. It can also facilitate closer links between mental health and primary and secondary health care services regarding prevention, increased screening, and interventions.

▲ Conclusion

Screening is a preventative health care activity that occurs across health and social care services. In mental health care there is evidence of service users having less access to screening compared to the general population, which can contribute to later identification of physical conditions and poorer physical health outcomes. Resources are scarce, so screening must be targeted and strategic. We have explored how some medications can lead to weight gain and obesity. Therefore, targeting drug naïve service users (people who have not taken antipsychotics before) is a proactive way that mental health nurses can identify an at-risk group and intervene with co-produced lifestyle programmes as a way of slowing down the rate of weight gain. Lastly, mental health nurses may also need to be advocates for service users in accessing screening services. This may entail challenging negative stereotypes and stigma that may be present in acute and secondary care services, but in mental health services also.

✖ Tips from service users

1   I would like to be treated as a whole person and health-care professionals to use a holistic care approach.
2   I would like healthcare professionals to explain what health promotion is rather than handing out leaflets without an explanation.
3   I'd like help to make sure I was having all the check-ups I needed, nurses could help me and remind me to keep my appointments.

W   Companion website

For extra resources on the topics covered in this chapter, visit the companion website at: www.oup.com/mhns

✚ Useful websites

Lester adaptation of the cardiometabolic health resource: https://www.rcpsych.ac.uk/docs/default-source/improving-care/ccqi/national-clinical-audits/ncap-library/eip-2024/ncap-lester-tool-intervention-framework.pdf?sfvrsn=21e45dbd_17

Making Every Contact Count (MECC): https://www.england.nhs.uk/wp-content/uploads/2016/04/making-every-contact-count.pdf

National Health Service (2021). Breast screening (mammogram): https://www.nhs.uk/conditions/breast-screening-mammogram/

National Health Service (2021). Prostate-specific antigen testing: https://www.nhs.uk/conditions/prostate-cancer/psa-testing/

✚ Screening tools

Calorie counting: https://assets.publishing.service.gov.uk/government/uploads/system/uploads/attachment_data/file/528193/Eatwell_guide_colour.pdf

Assessment/diagnosis of constipation: https://cks.nice.org.uk/topics/constipation/diagnosis/assessment/

https://cks.nice.org.uk/topics/constipation/management/adults/

British Stool Chart: https://www.nice.org.uk/guidance/cg99/resources/cg99-constipation-in-children-and-young-people-bristol-stool-chart-2

Clinical Toolkit: https://www.rcgp.org.uk/clinical-and-research/resources/toolkits.aspx

Alcohol withdrawals: https://www.nice.org.uk/guidance/cg100/chapter/Recommendations#acute-alcohol-withdrawal

Clozapine interactions: https://www.drugs.com/drug-interactions/clozapine.html

https://bnf.nice.org.uk/drug/clozapine.html

Answers to Table 12.2 self-assessment exercise

- The recommended daily calorie intake for males is 2,500 and for females 2,000.

- The government-recommended physical activity level is at least 150 minutes of moderate-intensity activity five times a week or 75 minutes of vigorous-intensity activity per week.

- The recommended maximum number of alcohol units per week for men and women is 14 standard units.

✚ References

Bertolini, F., Witteveen, A. B., Young, S., Cuijpers, P., Ayuso-Mateos, J. L., Barbui, C., . . . Sijbrandij, M. (2023). Risk of SARS-CoV-2 infection, severe COVID-19 illness and COVID-19 mortality in people with pre-existing mental disorders: an umbrella review. BMC Psychiatry 23(1), 181.

DeHert, M., Hudyana, H., Dockx, L., Bernagie, C., Sweers, K., Tack, J., Leucht, S., and Peuskens, J. (2011).

Second-generation antipsychotics and constipation: a review of the literature. European Psychiatry 26(1), 34–44.

Department of Health (2011). No Health Without Mental Health: A Cross-Government Mental Health Outcomes Strategy for People of All Ages. London: Department of Health.

Department of Health and Public Health England (2016). *Improving the Physical Health of People with Mental Health Problems: Actions for Mental Health Nurses. London: NHS England.*

Diabetes UK (n. *d.). Prediabetes. Available at: https://www. diabetes.org.uk/preventing-type-2-diabetes/prediabetes*

Harris, E. C. and Barraclough, B. (1998). *Excess mortality of mental disorder. British Journal of Psychiatry 173, 11–53.*

Holt, R. I. and Mitchell, A. J. (2015). *Diabetes mellitus and severe mental illness: mechanisms and clinical implications. Nature Reviews Endocrinology 11(2), 79–89.*

Malhi, G. S., Bell, E., Outhred, T., and Berk, M. (2020). *Lithium therapy and its interactions. Australian Prescriber 43(3), 91–93.*

Nash, M. (2014). *Physical Health and Well-Being in Mental Health Nursing: Clinical Skills for Practice. Milton Keynes: Open University Press.*

Nash, M. (2018). *The physical healthcare of people with mental health problems. In: I. Norman and I. Ryrie, Eds., The Art and Science of Mental Health Nursing: Principles and Practice, pp. 626–644. Milton Keynes: Open University Press.*

National Institute for Health and Care Excellence (2014). *Psychosis and Schizophrenia in Adults: Prevention and Management. Clinical Guideline [CG178]. Available at: https://www.nice.org.uk/guidance/cg178*

NHS (2021). *PSA Testing: Prostate Cancer. Available at: https:// www.nhs.uk/conditions/prostate-cancer/psa-testing/*

NHS England (2016). *Five Year Forward View for Mental Health. London: NHS England.*

Olfson, M., Gerhard, T., Huang, C., Crystal, S., and Stroup, T. S. (2015). *Premature mortality among adults with schizophrenia in the United States. JAMA Psychiatry 72(12), 1172–1181.*

Perry, B. I., Holt, R. I. G., Chew-Graham, C. A., Tiffin, E., French, P., Pratt, P., Byrne, P., and Shiers, D. E. (2023 update). *Positive Cardiometabolic Health Resource: an intervention framework for people experiencing psychosis and schizophrenia. Royal College of Psychiatrists, London.*

Polcwiartek, C., O'Gallagher, K., Friedman, D. J., Correll, C. U., Solmi, M., Jensen, S. E., and Nielsen, R. E. (2024). *Severe mental illness: cardiovascular risk assessment and management. European Heart Journal ehae054.*

PULSE (2019). *Transgender Patients Are Missing Out on Cancer Screening, Warns Health Minister. Available at: https://www.pulsetoday.co.uk/news/politics/transgen der-patients-are-missing-out-on-cancer-screening-warns-health-minister/*

Smith, D. J., Langan, J., McLean, G., Guthrie, B., and Mercer, S. W. (2013). *Schizophrenia is associated with excess multiple physical-health comorbidities but low levels of recorded cardiovascular disease in primary care: cross-sectional study. BMJ Open 3(4), e002808.*

Solmi, M., Firth, J., Miola, A., Fornaro, M., Frison, E., Fusar-Poli, P., Dragioti, E., Shin, J. I., Carvalho, A. F., Stubbs, B., Koyanagi, A., Kisely, S., and Christoph, U. (2020). *Disparities in cancer screening in people with mental illness across the world versus the general population: prevalence and comparative meta-analysis including 4 717 839 people. Lancet Psychiatry 7(1), 52–63.*

(13) Low-intensity cognitive behavioural therapy interventions (guided self-help)

Marie Chellingsworth

Learning outcomes

By the end of this chapter, you should be able to:

1 Demonstrate an understanding of the nature and context of low-intensity cognitive behavioural therapy (guided self-help)

2 Demonstrate an understanding of the evidence base

3 Identify the key skills involved in the delivery and support of low-intensity cognitive behavioural therapy for anxiety and depression

4 Apply knowledge and skills of low-intensity guided self-help interventions for anxiety and depression to your nursing practice.

▼ Introduction

Depression and anxiety disorders frequently occur as a main presenting problem, or as a comorbidity alongside other mental and physical health conditions. These disorders are often collectively termed 'common mental health problems' (CMHPs) owing to their high prevalence. They cause significant distress and suffering, and have far-reaching social and economic impacts for the person, their loved ones, and wider society. CMHPs are a major public health problem, and it is essential that appropriate treatment is provided and prioritized.

In the UK, NHS treatments for CMHPs are recommended in clinical guidelines via the National Institute for Health and Care Excellence (NICE) (2004, 2005, 2011a, 2011b, 2013, 2018, 2022). These guidelines propose a stepped care approach for the effective and efficient management of CMHPs with multiple access points and levels of entry to psychological treatments (Bower and Gilbody, 2005; Lovell and Richards, 2000; Richards et al., 2010; Scogin et al., 2003; Van Straten et al., 2015). Stepped care is aimed to enable service delivery to be least restrictive, with the treatment most likely to benefit the person offered first, such as low-intensity interventions, and higher intensity interventions offered only if there is not an adequate response or there is clinical justification, often called 'stepping-up' (Bower and Gilbody, 2005). Low-intensity interventions have demonstrated that they can be delivered by mental health clinicians or paraprofessionals with training and supervision (Richards et al., 2012, 2017).

▼ What is low-intensity cognitive behavioural therapy guided self-help?

Cognitive behavioural therapy (CBT) is a 'talking therapy' that is based on the belief that physical sensations (feelings), actions (behaviour), and our thoughts (cognitions) are all interlinked (Williams and Chellingsworth, 2010). These symptoms can make it difficult for the person to want to engage in usual activities and they may begin to avoid them to try to manage their symptoms, forming a vicious cycle (Williams and Chellingsworth, 2010). CBT is offered at two levels in the stepped care model. High-intensity CBT (step 3) is delivered by a trained and supervised CBT therapist over a period of usually up to 26 sessions. Low-intensity CBT (step 2) is a CBT intervention delivered via a guided self-help package such as a workbook, book, group, class or webinar, digital app, or an online computerized programme that does the work of the CBT with minimal support from a trained clinician or practitioner (Box 13.1).

Despite the first NICE guideline being published in 2004, it was still very difficult for people to access the psychological treatments NICE recommended, with many individuals waiting months or even years to receive psychological treatment (Anderson et al., 2005; Lovell and Richards, 2000). Despite CMHPs accounting for a third of all disability, it attracted only 2% of NHS funding for mental health, with most of the expenditure being on severe and enduring mental health (Layard, 2006). There was also wide variation in the skills of the workforce to deliver NICE guideline-recommended treatments, with workforce skills poorly informed by the evidence base (Ngui et al., 2010). In 2006, Lord Richard Layard from the London School of Economics and Political Science published the seminal *Depression Report* which set out a strong economic argument for change (Layard, 2006). The analysis showed that the cost to society of anxiety disorders and depression was £12 billion per year in terms of loss of revenue, 1% of national income, and a cost of £7 billion to the taxpayer, and that providing NICE-approved therapies such as low- and high-intensity CBT would cost £0.6 billion and, therefore, pay for itself. As a result, the Improving Access to Psychological Therapies (IAPT) programme was successfully piloted and then rolled out across England in 2008. In 2020–2021, there were 1.46 million referrals, with 90% of people accessing the service within 6 weeks and 606,192 people completing a course of treatment, and 51.4% of those receiving treatment moved to recovery. By 2023/2024, the aim is for 1.9 million people to be able to access treatment per year (NHS Digital, 2021). This is, however, still the tip of the iceberg. The current commissioning level is only for 25% of need, which means there are still many people with CMHPs unable to access these treatments through the services and who may be under the care of mental health nurses in primary, secondary, or tertiary care settings who require access to these interventions.

Mental health nurses have been supporting CBT self-help interventions in primary, secondary, and tertiary care for many years and are well placed to deliver this intervention. The first UK-based university-accredited low-intensity CBT course was the Structured Psychosocial InteRventions (SPIRIT training) course based at Glasgow Caledonian University. The training started in 2001 and is still available as an online course via the Living Life to the Full website (https://llttf.com/free-resources/). It was based on the Five Areas CBT model (Williams, 2001; Williams and Chellingsworth, 2010; Williams et al., 2010) and was attended by many mental health nurses and clinicians to implement a CBT approach into their practice (Garland and Chellingsworth, 2006; Garland et al., 2002; Williams and Garland, 2002; Williams et al., 2010; Wright et al., 2002).

Box 13.1 Underlying principles of low-intensity CBT guided self-help

- Based on CBT principles mediated through a workbook, book, internet programme, app, or other form of health technology.

- The intervention is focused on the service user applying CBT change methods into practice between sessions, with the nurse or practitioner reviewing progress, problem-solving any difficulties, and making a new plan in 'a plan, do, review approach cycle' (Williams and Chellingsworth, 2010).

- Review sessions should usually consist of 15–30 minutes with up to 3 hours of total contact with the health professional.

▼ The evidence base of low-intensity CBT guided self-help interventions

There are currently over 30 systematic reviews and 50 randomized controlled trials that demonstrate evidence of the efficacy of low-intensity CBT guided self-help interventions (Cuijpers et al., 2019; Delgadillo, 2018). Delgadillo (2018) argues that this form of treatment is highly efficient, considering its low-intensity (brief), low-cost, flexible, and accessible nature. The results of a meta-analysis (2,470 service users living with depression) comparing low-intensity interventions with usual care by Bower et al. (2013) suggested that service users who are more severely depressed at baseline demonstrate larger treatment effects, so more severely depressed clients show at least as much clinical benefit from low-intensity interventions, demonstrating their utility across the full care spectrum, not just primary care.

▼ Assessing for suitability

'Anxiety' is an informal umbrella term. There are a range of different anxiety disorders, each with a different evidence-based treatment protocol. As anxiety disorders have shared features such as avoidance, arousal symptoms of the adrenalin response, worry, and negative predictions, it is essential that the nurse is familiar with the different symptomology of each of the anxiety-based disorders to initiate the correct treatment pathway. Panic attacks may be experienced as panic disorder, but also as a specifier symptom in other anxiety disorders that do not meet the criteria for panic disorder.

This type of assessment begins with the present symptoms in the here and now, not the chronological order of the service user history. The autonomic physical, behavioural, and cognitive symptoms experienced at times when they feel particularly down/anxious are gathered using recent examples. A suggested outline for a semi-structured, service user-centred interview for suitability for a low-intensity CBT guided self-help approach is shown in Box 13.2. This is not a prescribed list; the assessor should weave between these questions repeatedly, gathering recent examples of ABC symptom clusters in situations and using the 'W' questions to confirm details on their presentation and variances until the nurse feels that a disorder-specific understanding has been reached. See Box 13.3 for an overview of the different disorders as a guide to disorder-specific recognition.

Once the assessment has been completed and the service user has been given some brief information about the problem, the recommended treatment should be introduced. This decision should be based upon NICE guidelines. A key role of the nurse in the initial assessment and first treatment session is building a positive relationship and engendering hope that change is possible. It should also be discussed that the work that they put into place between sessions is the agent of change. This ensures that the service user is aware of the importance of the between-session tasks and attributes change to their own actions. Regular reviews are essential, focusing on reviewing the tasks, problem-solving any difficulties, and making a new plan (Williams and Chellingsworth, 2010). Towards the end of the intervention, and as the service user begins to improve, it is also important that relapse prevention planning is completed.

▼ Selecting low-intensity CBT guided self-help material

The assumption of low-intensity interventions is that the technical CBT information is fully contained in the materials (University College London, 2015). A systematic review suggested that the actual type of health technology used in guided self-help may not be critical to effectiveness (Gellatly et al., 2007) and should be based on service user preference in conjunction with the specific types of technology available. Ensuring it contains the correct disorder-specific CBT protocol is essential (Table 13.1 provides an overview). Accessibility is a key consideration because of the challenges posed by functional literacy levels (Anderson et al., 2005; Williams and Chellingsworth, 2010,) and impaired concentration and motivation in CMHPs. The reading age of any text needs to be inclusive (Martinez et al., 2008). Good materials should state their readability scores within them and have an associated clinician's guide to support the material. With

Box 13.2 Format for a service user-centred semi-structured assessment

ABC and the 'four Ws'

- What is the main current problem?

  o Autonomic: autonomic physical symptoms (when and where they occur/do not occur and what makes the difference, current ways of managing them).

  o Behavioural: behaviours (e.g. avoidance, escaping from situations to make them end more quickly, things they have reduced or stopped because of the problem and why, if they can ever do these things, things they have started doing more of as a result of the problem and why, can they manage without these things, if so, what happens, etc.).

  o Cognitive—what mood congruent thoughts they notice before/during/ after a recent example of the problem, in other situations where the problem occurs, and at times their mood is particularly affected.

- Where does the problem occur/not occur and what makes the difference, what do they do to try to manage this/get relief from their symptoms?

- When does the problem happen, are there times it does not happen, if so, what makes the difference, are there any places or situations they no longer attempt as the problem would occur there?

- With whom is the problem better or worse and what makes the difference?

Current triggers

- Is there anything else that particularly triggers the problem on a day-to-day basis, such as time of day, specific events, etc. (not the historical onset that is gathered in development and maintained later)?

Impact

- The consequences of the problem in key life areas. Specific effects of the problem on various aspects of the person's current lifework, home, social, private leisure, and family/relationship functioning.

Risk assessment and routine outcome measures

- If the person is experiencing thoughts of self-harm or suicide then this should be funnelled to ascertain the content of the thoughts, when they last occurred, how frequently they occur, how intensively they occur, how long they have been experiencing them, and what tends to trigger them.

- Have they made any plans?

- Have they taken any actions towards implementing/researching their plans?

- What protective factors keep them from acting on thoughts of self-harm or suicide (or would keep them safe from acting on any thoughts if they were to experience them and are not currently)?

- How stable is the relationship(s) with protective factors (e.g. partner is a protective factor but there are relationship difficulties, has children but restricted seeing them by partner or care services etc., or pet dog is a protective factor but it is old and unwell)?

- See also Chapter 21 for further information regarding risk assessment and Chapter 23 for further information on self-harm and suicide.

Other important information

- Modifying factors: things that make the current problem worse or better.

- Onset of current episode and course of the problem over its duration.

- Service user expectations and goals for working on the current problem.

- Past episodes and any previous treatment.

- Prescription and over-the-counter drug use, when they take it/do not take it, and side effects; alcohol use and if this has increased or decreased as a result of the current problem; and caffeine use and if this has increased or decreased as a result of the current problem.

- Any other relevant information the client wishes to discuss.

Box 13.3 Disorder-specific recognition guide

Obsessive–compulsive disorder

C: cognitive theme = responsibility for harm to self or others. Frequent intrusive, abhorrent, and unwanted obsessional thoughts, images, urges, or impulses.

A: active fear defence cascade (fight or flight) with high distress. Panic attack specifier symptoms can occur.

B: compulsive activities aimed to prevent harm likelihood and reduce distress (neutralizing behaviours). The person does not want to carry out the compulsions but cannot resist the urge.

Generalized anxiety disorder

C: cognitive theme = future-focused apprehensive worry about situations that are uncertain, uncontrollable, or unpredictable in life domain areas: health, work/studies, finances, family, relationships. Type II metacognitive worries (worries about worrying). Worry thoughts are experienced as a verbal linguistic (chains of words) with imagery less likely.

A: predominantly passive fear defence cascade (freeze-based response) with tension and secondary physical symptoms of tension such as aches, pains, gastrointestinal upset, sleep disturbances, headaches, and concentration difficulties. Panic attack specifiers less likely.

B: worrying, attempts to gain control, certainty, and predictability in life, avoiding situations that feel uncertain, uncontrollable, or unpredictable, trying to control worry.

Panic disorder (with or without agoraphobia)

C: cognitive theme = catastrophic misinterpretation of (adrenalin-based) bodily sensations as a sign of imminent harm to self (e.g. 'My heart is racing, I am having a heart attack').

A: active fear defence cascade (fight or flight) experienced from both a calm or anxious state, these attacks, therefore, may seem to come 'out of the blue' to the person. Adrenalin symptoms build to a peak quickly, usually within 10 minutes.

B: attempts to avoid future attacks/escape quickly from situations that bring on symptoms, safety-seeking behaviours to try to bring down symptoms artificially (e.g. carrying water to manage a dry mouth or using a trolley to lean on if fearful of collapse in a supermarket).

Health anxiety

C: cognitive theme = catastrophic misinterpretation of benign-based bodily sensations as a sign of illness imminent or in the future (e.g. 'I have a lump on my arm, what if I have cancer?').

A: active fear defence cascade in situations when threat is nearer, passive fear defence cascade in situations where there are apprehensive worries about symptoms and illness in future situations. Panic attack specifiers possible.

B: attempts to seek certainty regarding health status/avoid checking/checking/prevent signs of illness.

Social anxiety disorder

C: cognitive theme = fear of negative evaluation by others and/or performance failure as a focus of thinking (can be all social situations or a specific social performance like presentations, toileting, talking on the telephone, etc.).

A: active fear defence cascade in situations when threat is nearer (e.g. a social event), passive fear defence cascade in situations on a build-up to a social event. Panic attack specifiers possible.

B: attempts to avoid social situations or performance/escape quickly from situations that have been entered or endure with high distress.

Post-traumatic stress disorder

C: cognitive theme = recurrent unwanted reliving of unprocessed traumatic event live with full sensory experience. Difficulty disengaging from threat-related information.

A: active fear defence cascade. Panic attack specifiers possible.

B: attempts to avoid reliving triggers/escape quickly from situations that have been entered or endure with high distress.

Depression

C: cognitive theme = actual or perceived loss, hopelessness and helplessness, rumination on negative thoughts and depression.

A: depression 'As' (concentration, sleep, appetite, energy, motivation, etc.).

B: avoidance (negatively reinforced) of activities that exacerbate symptoms to reduce symptoms/no longer give positive reinforcement.

Table 13.1 Recommended low-intensity CBT interventions

Disorder	Recommended low-intensity CBT self-help intervention	Free self-help material
Depression	Behavioural activation or CBT self-help for depression	Chellingsworth, M. (2021). *Get Back to Being You with Behavioural Activation*. The CBT Resource. Available at: https://mchellingsworth.wixsite.com/thecbtresource/our-english-self-help-booklets Williams, C. (2001–2022). Living Life to the Full free online course: Available at: https://llttf.com/free-resources/
Generalized anxiety disorder	Worry management CBT	Chellingsworth, M. (2021). *Worry Less, Live More with Generalised Anxiety Disorder*. The CBT Resource. Available at:https://mchellingsworth.wixsite.com/thecbtresource/our-english-self-help-booklets
Panic disorder with/without agoraphobia	Exposure and habituation	Chellingsworth, M. (2021). *Fears Conquered with Exposure and Habituation*. The CBT Resource. Available at: https://mchellingsworth.wixsite.com/thecbtresource/our-english-self-help-booklets
Specific phobias	Exposure and habituation	Chellingsworth, M. (2021). *Fears Conquered with Exposure and Habituation*. The CBT Resource. Available at: https://mchellingsworth.wixsite.com/thecbtresource/our-english-self-help-booklets
Obsessive–compulsive disorder	Exposure and response prevention	Lovell, K. and Gega, L. (2011). *Obsessive Compulsive Disorder: A Self-Help Book*. The University of Manchester. Available at: https://cedar.exeter.ac.uk/media/universityofexeter/schoolofpsychology/cedar/documents/liiapt/OCDSelf_Help_Workbook.pdf
Social anxiety disorder	Not recommended in NICE guidelines to be treated with low-intensity interventions. Step up to high-intensity CBT	
Post-traumatic stress disorder	Not recommended in NICE guidelines to be treated with low-intensity interventions. Step up to high-intensity CBT/eye movement desensitization and reprocessing	

(continued)

Table 13.1 Continued

Disorder	Recommended low-intensity CBT self-help intervention	Free self-help material
Health anxiety	Not recommended to be treated with low-intensity interventions. Step up to high-intensity CBT for exposure and response prevention	

all materials it is essential that the nurse is familiar with the material, knows its content, and understands it to assist the service user (University College London, 2015).

An example of someone who has used low-intensity CBT in practice is provided in Box 13.4.

Box 13.4 Practice example: Afework

Afework, 65 years old, is experiencing moderate depression. During initial assessment he described feeling down and exhausted with early morning waking. He said he has lost interest in many previously enjoyed activities such as socializing, walking his dog (Abai), gardening, and films. He feels he has made a 'mess' of his life and has achieved nothing and worries that his husband 'must be fed up with me'. He spends most of his day sitting on the sofa doing 'nothing' with the curtains still closed. His depression began 9 months ago after his other dog (Ajani) died suddenly, and his best friend went into a nursing home. Afework has been taking an antidepressant (sertraline) for 4 months with no side effects. He feels they have 'possibly helped a little'. Afework stated he did not have any plans or actions in place regarding taking his own life or harming himself, although reported he sometimes had fleeting thoughts that his husband would be 'better off without me' but stated these were infrequent and he would never act on them. His husband and dog were strong protective factors. Afework had the following goals:

1 'To play crown green bowls once each week with friends.'

2 'To walk Abai each day.'

3 'To have an evening meal ready for my husband once a week.'

The mental health nurse offered a low-intensity guided self-help intervention called behavioural activation using the *Get Back to Being You with Behavioural Activation* self-help guide (Chellingsworth, 2021) and gave him a rationale of how this could help to lift his mood by reversing the vicious cycle of symptoms he was experiencing using the examples within the guide. The nurse ensured that he understood the rationale for behavioural activation then began to work with Afework to plan a routine regulation time for eating and sleeping/waking based on his current reported symptoms. Then they worked with Afework to create a hierarchy of avoided previously pleasurable, routine, and necessary activities, breaking these into easier tasks at the bottom of the hierarchy, with more difficult and most difficult tasks at the top, and with a mix of each type in each level. He began with easier routine tasks such as opening the curtains and taking the dog out into the garden. Over the next three phone contact sessions, Afework had built back a routine and structure in his day and gradually increased his activity levels up the hierarchy each week. His mood had started to improve. Once his depression lifted, relapse prevention was discussed with Afework, and together they drew up an individual plan for staying well using the workbook.

The companion website for this chapter contains another practice example that you can work through yourself.

▲ Conclusion

Low-intensity CBT guided self-help is firmly established as a service user-focused approach that can be delivered by the mental health nurse. The key role of the mental health nurse (and other mental health workers) using this approach is to work collaboratively with service users to assess, support, guide, and monitor their use of an appropriate disorder-specific low-intensity CBT intervention.

✖ Tips from service users

1 If you live in England, you can access free psycho-logical therapy at your nearest NHS-funded service. You can find your nearest service here: https://www.nhs.uk/service-search/mental-health/find-an-NHS-talking-therapies-service/

2 Guided low-intensity CBT, much like high-intensity CBT, is an active form of treatment. It is what you do between sessions, putting the skills into practice in your daily life, that brings about change.

3 Try to honestly share thoughts and emotions with your practitioner. The thoughts you may be experiencing can be very distressing, scary, or unpleasant, but your practitioner is trained to support and understand these. They will have worked with many others who may have experienced similar thoughts.

4 Try to set aside time regularly to work on your tasks to get the most out of the treatment.

5 If you are not sure about anything, ask your practitioner—they will never mind responding to questions.

6 There are different forms of psychological therapies. At an assessment your practitioner will work with you collaboratively to see which is the most useful option for the difficulty you are currently experiencing.

W Companion website

For extra resources on the topics covered in this chapter, visit the companion website at: www.oup.com/mhns

✚ References

Anderson, L., Lewis, G., Araya, R., Elgie, R., Harrison, G., Proudfoot, J., Schmidt, U., Sharp, D., Weightman, A., and Williams, C. (2005). *Self-help books for depression: how can practitioners and patients make the right choice? British Journal of General Practice 55(514), 387–392.*

Bower, P. and Gilbody, S. (2005). *Stepped care in psychological therapies: access, effectiveness, and efficiency. British Journal of Psychiatry 186(1), 11–17.*

Bower, P., Kontopantelis, E., Sutton, A., Kendrick, T., Richards, D., Gilbody, S., Knowles, S., Cuijpers, P., Andersson, G., Christensen, H., Meyer, B., Huibers, M., Smit, F., van Straten, A., Warmerdam, L., Barkham, M.,

Bilich, L., Lovell, K., and Liu, E. (2013). *Influence of initial severity of depression on effectiveness of low intensity interventions: meta-analysis of individual patient data. BMJ 346, f540.*

Chellingsworth, M. (2021). *Get Back to Being You with Behavioural Activation. The CBT Resource. Available at: https://mchellingsworth.wixsite.com/thecbtresource/our-english-self-help-booklets*

Cuijpers, P., Noma, H., Karyotaki, E., Cipriani, A., and Furukawa, T. A. (2019). *Effectiveness and acceptability of cognitive behavior therapy delivery formats in adults with depression: a network meta-analysis. JAMA Psychiatry 76(7), 700–707.*

Delgadillo, J. (2018). *Guided self-help in a brave new world. British Journal of Psychiatry 212(2), 65–66.*

Garland, A. and Chellingsworth, M. (2006). *Living life to the full. Interview by Clare Lomas. Nursing Times 102(40), 20–21.*

Garland, A., Fox, R., and Williams, C. (2002). *Overcoming reduced activity and avoidance: a Five Areas approach. Advances in Psychiatric Treatment 8, 453–462.*

Gellatyly, J., Bower, P., Hennessy, S., Richards, D., Gilbody, S., and Lovell, K. (2007). *What makes self-help interventions effective in the management of depressive symptoms? Meta-analysis and meta-regression. Psychological Medicine 37(9), 1217–1228.*

Layard, R. (2006). *The Depression Report: A New Deal for Depression and Anxiety Disorders. Centre for Economic Performance special papers (CEPOP15). London: Centre for Economic Performance, London School of Economics and Political Science.*

Lovell, K. and Richards, D. (2000). *Multiple access points and levels of entry (MAPLE): ensuring choice, accessibility, and equity of CBT services. Behavioural and Cognitive Psychotherapy 28(4), 379–91.*

Martinez, R., Whitfield, G., Dafters, R., and Williams C. J. (2008). *Can people read self-help manuals for depression? A challenge for the stepped care model and book prescription schemes. Behavioural and Cognitive Psychotherapy 36(1), 89–97.*

National Institute for Health and Care Excellence (2004). *Depression in adults: recognition and management. Clinical guideline [CG113]. [Replaced by NG22.]*

National Institute for Health and Care Excellence (2005). *Obsessive–Compulsive Disorder and Body Dysmorphic Disorder: Management. Clinical guideline [CG31]. Available at: https://www.nice.org.uk/guidance/cg31*

National Institute for Health and Care Excellence (2011a). *Generalised Anxiety Disorder and Panic Disorder in Adults: Management. Clinical guideline [CG113]. [Last updated June 2020.] Available at: https://www.nice.org.uk/guidance/cg113*

National Institute for Health and Care Excellence (2011b). *Common Mental Health Problems: Identification and Pathways to Care. Clinical guideline [CG123]. Available at: https://www.nice.org.uk/guidance/cg123*

National Institute for Health and Care Excellence (2013). *Social Anxiety Disorder: Recognition, Assessment, and Treatment. Clinical guideline [CG159]. Available at: https://www.nice.org.uk/guidance/cg159*

National Institute for Health and Care Excellence (2018). *Post Traumatic Stress Disorder. Clinical guideline [CG116]. Available at: https://www.nice.org.uk/guidance/cg116*

National Institute for Health and Care Excellence (2022). *Depression in Adults: Treatment and Management. NICE guideline [NG222]. Available at: https://www.nice.org.uk/guidance/ng222*

Ngui, E. M., Khasakhala, L., Ndetei, D., and Roberts, L. W. (2010). *Mental disorders, health inequalities and ethics: a global perspective. International Review of Psychiatry 22(3), 235–244.*

NHS Digital (2021). *Psychological Therapies, Annual Report on the Use of IAPT Services, 2020–21. Available at: https://digital.nhs.uk/data-and-information/publications/statistical/psychological-therapies-annual-reports-on-the-use-of-iapt-services/annual-report-2020-21/data-quality-statement*

Richards, D. A., Chellingsworth, M., Hope, R., Turpin, G., and Whyte, M. (2012). *National Programme Supervisor Materials to Support the Delivery of Training for Psychological Wellbeing Practitioners Delivering Low Intensity Interventions. London: Rethink.*

Richards, D. A., Rhodes, S., Ekers, D., McMillan, D., Taylor, R. S., Byford, S., Barrett, B., Finning, K., Ganguli, P., Warren, F., Farrand, P., Gilbody, S., Kuyken, W., O'Mahen, H., Watkins, E., Wright, K., Reed, N., Fletcher, E., Hollon, S. D., Moore, L., … Woodhouse, R. (2017). *Cost and Outcome of BehavioRal Activation (COBRA): a randomized controlled trial of behavioural activation versus cognitive-behavioural therapy for depression. Health Technology Assessment 21(46), 1–366.*

Richards, D. A., Weaver, A., Utley, M., Bower, P., Cape, J., Gallivan, S., Gilbody, S., Hennessy, S., Leibowitz, J., Lovell, K., Owens, L., Pagel, C., Paxton, R., Pilling, S., Simpson, A. E., Tomson, D., and Vasilakis, C. (2010). *Developing Evidence-Based and Acceptable Stepped Care Systems in Mental Health Care: An Operational Research Project. Final report. Southampton: NIHR Service Delivery and Organisation Programme.*

Scogin, F., Hanson, A., and Welsh, D. (2003). *Self-administered treatment in stepped-care models of depression treatment. Journal of Clinical Psychology 59(3), 341–349.*

University College London (2015). *Guide to evaluating self-help material for anxiety and depression. PWP Training Review. Available at: https://www.ucl.ac.uk/pals/sites/pals/files/7_guide_to_evaluating_self-help_materials.pdf*

van Straten, A., Hill, J., Richards, D. A., and Cuijpers, P. (2015). *Stepped care treatment delivery for depression: a systematic review and meta-analysis. Psychological Medicine 45(2), 231–246.*

Williams, C. (2001). *Overcoming Depression and Low Mood: A Five Areas Approach. London: Hodder Arnold.*

Williams, C. and Chellingsworth, M. (2010). *CBT: A Clinician's Guide to Using the Five Areas Approach. London: Hodder Arnold.*

Williams, C., and Garland, A. (2002). *A cognitive-behavioural therapy assessment model for use in everyday clinical practice. Advances in Psychiatric Treatment 8(3), 172–179.*

Williams, C., Martinez, R., Dafters, R., Ronald, L.H., and Garland, A. (2010). *Training the wider workforce in cognitive behavioural self-help: the SPIRIT (Structured Psychosocial InteRventions in Teams) training course. Behavioural and Cognitive Psychotherapy 39, 139–149.*

Wright, B., Williams, C., and Garland. A. (2002). *Using the Five Areas cognitive–behavioural therapy model with psychiatric patients. Advances in Psychiatric Treatment 8(4), 307–315.*

14 Key skills for delivering psychosocial interventions in dementia care

Juanita Hoe

Rachel Thompson

Learning outcomes

By the end of this chapter, you should be able to:

1 Explain the different psychosocial interventions for people with dementia

2 Appraise the skills needed to plan and conduct psychosocial therapeutic activities in dementia

3 Describe the impact of specific psychosocial interventions on different health outcomes for people with dementia and their family carers

4 Identify relevant psychosocial interventions appropriate to the needs of your service users.

▼ Introduction

Globally, the number of people living with dementia is increasing because of the ageing population (Livingston et al., 2020). This means most nurses will care for someone living with dementia and their families at some stage in their career (Hoe and Thompson, 2010). Caring for people effectively can be difficult, as dementia is a complex and multifaceted disorder and requires an adequately trained workforce that can support integrated, culturally appropriate, person-centred, psychosocial care (World Health Organization, 2017). Accordingly, nurses working within dementia care should be able to provide evidence-based, culturally sensitive interventions appropriately tailored to the needs of this population.

Evidence supporting the use of psychosocial interventions in dementia care has increased significantly over recent years and focuses on cognitive, psychological, and social aspects of well-being (Whitty et al., 2020). Interventions include individualized counselling, cognitive-based strategies, reminiscence, life story work, and creative approaches such as music, dance, and art. Interventions for family carers involving psychoeducation and emotional support are also well established and the use of dyadic or group interventions are encouraged (National Institute for Health and Care Excellence, 2018; World Health Organization, 2017). In this chapter, we focus on three well-established cognitive-based psychosocial interventions that are recommended for use with people living with dementia. We will explore the knowledge and skills needed to deliver these interventions either individually or as a group.

▼ Background

Dementia is characterized by advancing cognitive and functional decline leading to loss of autonomy and independence with performing activities of daily living. Consequently, this degenerative disease, often coupled with additional health and social needs, can significantly impact individuals and its management is complex (Livingston et al., 2020; National Institute for Health and Care Excellence, 2018). The absence of a cure or disease-modifying pharmacological treatments to prevent or delay dementia has led to the development of non-pharmacological (psychosocial) interventions that seek to reduce cognitive decline, increase independence, and improve well-being (Orrell et al., 2012; Whitty et al., 2020). Accordingly, the evidence for psychosocial interventions in dementia care such as therapeutic activities, education, and psychological support has seen significant growth over the last two decades (Whitty et al., 2020). However, the use of evidence-based interventions in practice is variable (Clemson et al., 2018).

Participating in meaningful activity is important to the physical and mental well-being of people living with dementia, while inactivity has a detrimental effect and is associated with the presence of depression and behaviour that can be challenging (Maruta et al., 2020; Wenborn, 2017). National and global policy now recommend access to cognitive-based interventions for people living with dementia within both community and institutional settings (National Institute for Health and Care Excellence, 2018; World Health Organization, 2017). Examples of cognitive-based interventions include cognitive stimulation therapy (CST) (Spector et al., 2003), reminiscence therapy (Woods et al., 2018), and life story work (McKeown et al., 2010). These therapeutic activities help to improve and maintain cognitive function, promote environmental engagement and social interaction, encourage independence, provide enjoyment, and increase psychological well-being (Hoe and Thompson, 2010).

Box 14.1 Guiding principles for facilitating cognitive stimulation therapy sessions

1   Mental stimulation

2   New ideas, thoughts, and associations

3   Using orientation, both sensitively and implicitly

4   Opinions rather than facts

5   Using reminiscence as an aid to the here and now

6   Providing triggers to aid recall

7   Continuity and consistency between sessions

8   Implicit (rather than explicit) learning

9   Stimulating language

10 Stimulating executive functioning

11 Person-centredness

12 Respect

13 Involvement

14 Inclusion

15 Choice

16 Fun

17 Maximizing potential

18 Building/strengthening relationships.

Reproduced from Spector, A., Thorgrimsen, L., Woods, R. T., and Orrell, M. (2006). *Making a difference: an evidence-based group programme to offer Cognitive Stimulation therapy (CST) to people with dementia*. Hawker Publications.

▼ Selecting a psychosocial intervention

How dementia impacts individuals varies significantly. Determining the appropriateness for psychosocial interventions requires individualized assessment of the person's cognitive abilities and other psychological and physical symptoms, the progression of their condition, and the need to involve others in decision-making (Moniz-Cook and Rewston, 2020). Involving family carers wherever possible and continued engagement in social and leisure activities are important, even at later stages of the condition (Menne et al., 2012). Moniz-Cook and Rewston (2020) advise that practitioners first gather information about potential vulnerabilities, such as how the current situation has affected both the person living with dementia and their carer. Then identify strengths such as interests, close relationships, and cultural network resources, which can balance out vulnerabilities and be used to select which interventions may be most helpful (Clare et al., 2012).

▼ Cognitive stimulation therapy

CST consists of various group or individual activities and exercises undertaken to improve cognitive and social functioning. Founded on the 'use it or lose it' maxim, it reinforces the protective nature of doing mental exercises to maintain brain health (Orrell et al., 2012). Guiding principles underpin the delivery of CST sessions based on principles of person-centred care in dementia that promote respect, inclusivity, collaboration, choices, and enjoyment (Spector et al., 2006) (Box 14.1).

The focus is on implicit learning and information processing through using multisensory stimulation and reality orientation techniques (Spector et al., 2003). Cognitive activities include word and number games, quizzes, arts and crafts, sports, board games, and discussions about current affairs, designed to stimulate thinking and memory, improve concentration, enhance language and problem-solving skills, and provide social engagement (Spector et al., 2003). CST programmes are provided in community and residential settings and delivered as a group or individual activity (Orrell et al., 2012). In addition, family carers can be trained to conduct individual CST sessions with their relatives (Orrell et al., 2017).

Benefits of cognitive stimulation therapy

CST consistently produces both short-term and long-term benefits for people living with dementia through improving cognitive function, language skills, and quality of life and is a useful and cost-effective intervention for people with mild to moderate dementia (Lobbia et al., 2019). It has the strongest evidence for cognitive benefits in dementia, when compared with other psychosocial approaches, and has been adapted

for use in several languages and is used in several countries worldwide (Alzheimer's Disease International, 2011; Lobbia et al., 2019).

Planning and facilitation of cognitive stimulation therapy sessions

- CST facilitators can be nurses, allied health professionals, care staff, or volunteers. Facilitators have usually received training, but manuals exist that provide detailed guidance for facilitating group or individual CST sessions (Aguirre et al., 2012; Spector et al., 2006; Yates et al., 2015).
- Group CST sessions typically involve two facilitators and six to eight people with mild and moderate dementia.
- Initial twice-weekly sessions are delivered over 7 weeks. Then ongoing 'maintenance CST' sessions can be offered through weekly sessions for a longer-term period.
- Sessions typically last for 45 minutes (Table 14.1), but longer may be needed to prepare materials and gather participants together.

Table 14.1 Outline plan for a cognitive stimulation therapy session

Activity	Structure of CST session	Time allocated
Introduction and warm-up activities	• Group name chosen • Sing theme song • Reality orientation board • Discuss current event (use newspaper or photograph/screenshot from social media)	10 minutes
Main activity	• Adapt group programme to participants' abilities and preferences • Offer a choice of activities which target different levels of ability (level A or level B—level B activities are less demanding)	25 minutes
Closing	• Thank group members individually for their participation • Sing theme song • Give reminder about next session (time and theme) • Farewells	10 minutes
Progress monitoring	Complete a session record for each member	Post session, 15–30 minutes

Content and structure of cognitive stimulation therapy sessions

- Sessions consist of structured activities and discussions about topics that can be adapted culturally and include food, childhood, sounds, physical exercises, famous faces, word games, number games, and current affairs.

- Each CST session begins with warm-up activities, for example, playing catch with a soft ball while participants introduce themselves; discussing the date, weather, and location or a current news event; and singing the group theme song. These activities are designed to encourage group interaction and increase alertness. They also promote orientation, stimulate participation, and encourage cohesion and group identity.

- The aim is for people to feel empowered rather than de-skilled and CST activities should focus on the strengths of the person living with dementia rather than areas of difficulty.

- Facilitators should not dominate the discussion but encourage contributions from all participants and support diversity in opinions.

Monitoring progress in cognitive stimulation therapy sessions

Record the attendance and level of interest, communication, enjoyment, and mood shown during the session of the person living with dementia. This enables facilitators to monitor progress and modify the programme if needed.

▼ Reminiscence therapy

Reminiscence occurs naturally as people age and share stories about significant life experiences and memories from the past (Butler, 1963). It is used therapeutically to strengthen elements of cognition and promote self-acceptance and well-being (Pinquart and Forstmeier, 2012). People living with dementia often have good and intact memories for past events, and reminiscence draws on preserved abilities rather than emphasizing their difficulties. It improves communication and social inclusion and promotes a sense of competence as the person uses retained skills (Woods et al., 2018).

Reminiscence therapy consists of three approaches: simple reminiscence, life review, and life review therapy (Westerhof et al., 2010). Simple reminiscence is unstructured and facilitates conversations using autobiographical storytelling aimed at remembering and sharing memories of past events to enhance communication and positive feelings (Pinquart and Forstmeier, 2012; Westerhof et al., 2010). Life review and life review therapy contributes to successful ageing by helping with problem-solving and overcoming past traumatic experiences (Butler, 1963). It is more structured, covers the lifespan, and focuses on re-evaluating positive and negative life events to promote psychological well-being and alleviate symptoms of depression (Pinquart and Forstmeier, 2012; Westerhof et al., 2010). Reminiscence therapy can be undertaken as a group or individual activity and include family carers. Joint reminiscence programmes, such as Remembering Yesterday, Caring Today (Schweitzer and Bruce, 2008) showed improvements in relationships between people living with dementia and their family carer (Charlesworth et al., 2016).

Benefits of reminiscence therapy

Reminiscence is a well-established intervention consistently shown to be effective for older people living with dementia (Woods et al., 2018) and for those experiencing depression (Bohlmeijer et al., 2007; Pinquart and Forstmeier, 2012). Other benefits include improvements to emotional well-being, self-mastery, cognitive function, and life satisfaction (Bohlmeijer et al., 2007). Still, evidence regarding the therapeutic effect of reminiscence remains inconclusive with inconsistent results reported for different settings, modes of delivery, and impact on health-related outcomes. Woods et al.'s (2018) review of reminiscence therapy in dementia found improvements to cognition, communication, mood, and quality of life, with the greatest effect being shown in care home-based studies. Group and community settings were associated with improvements in communication, while individual reminiscence therapy is associated with greater benefits for cognition and mood (Woods et al., 2018).

Facilitating group reminiscence therapy sessions

- Get to know about the people with dementia attending the reminiscence group. Learn about their histories, hobbies, and interests beforehand and identify any topics to avoid.

Box 14.2 Suggested reminiscence discussion topics

Themes reflect key milestones and shared experiences in people's lives:

- Family life
- Childhood
- Teenage years
- Early career
- Seasons
- School days
- Major life events (e.g. graduation, wedding, birth of children)
- Military career
- Holidays
- Historical events (e.g. the Queen's coronation or Silver/Gold Jubilee)
- Sporting events/achievements
- Music
- Pets
- Sensory sensations
- Local neighbourhood.

- Reminiscence therapy can be conducted once or twice per week, with sessions typically lasting 30–60 minutes. Group sessions may be offered as a 4–12-week programme or conducted as a regular ongoing activity.
- The facilitator role is to cultivate and guide discussions and to keep topics relevant to the participants present. See Box 14.2 for suggested reminiscence discussion topics.
- Involve all participants in the reminiscence activity and ensure that everyone has an opportunity to contribute.

Planning group reminiscence therapy activities

- Choose appropriate themes that are culturally relevant and reflect key stages of people's lives which they can share with others (e.g. family or working life, childhood, or school days).
- The use of multisensory activities helps prompt memories, with those using a combination of senses being most effective (e.g. presenting something you can touch, smell, and taste like a piece of fruit).
- Ensure a mix of activities using different mediums and familiar items to trigger memories and promote discussion such as household or workplace objects, food, sweets, music, newspaper clippings, archive film clips or adverts, books, and old photographs.

Communicating effectively and avoiding challenges

- Some life events such as school days or wartime events may arouse unhappy memories so allow participants to opt out of discussions if preferred.
- Some people living with dementia may be unable to immediately recall information and find direct factual questions challenging, such as 'How old were you when you got married?' Avoid asking questions that are too probing and allow people sufficient time to respond.
- Keep questions short and open ended (Table 14.2). The facilitator can share their own memories of past events to help initiate or keep the discussion going.

▼ Life story work

Life story work enables delivery of individualized, person-centred care through exploring the biography of a person. Like reminiscence and life review, it provides an opportunity to talk about life experiences. The process involves 'the recording of individual information to produce a tangible product such as a life story book, story board or multimedia resource to inform care delivery' (Murphy, 2000, p. 57). A template is used covering significant episodes in people's lives such as childhood, family, work, and life events as well as current information about who is important and preferences for care. Multiple formats are available, with digital versions becoming increasingly used, including pictures, photographs, video clips, and music (Thompson, 2011). Life story work enables those providing care to understand and ensure the person's needs are met. Information is used to enhance staff's understanding of the person, their history, factors influencing their likes and dislikes,

Table 14.2 Suggested questions to stimulate a reminiscence therapy discussion

Life stage	Trigger question
Childhood	What was life like when you were young?
	Which was your best subject at school?
	Who was your favourite teacher?
Adolescence	Did your family have any traditions?
	How did you celebrate your birthdays?
	Who were your best friends growing up?
Adulthood	What was your first job?
	Where is your most favourite place in the world?
	How did you feel when you got married?
Retirement	What were you plans for retirement?
	What do you miss most about work?
	What new skills or hobbies have you learnt since retiring?
General	What values and beliefs are important to the way you live your life?
	Do you have any regrets about your life?
	What advice would you give to young people to help them be successful in life?

and what supports their well-being. This becomes particularly significant when the person's cognitive function declines and they are unable to share important biographical information and express preferences.

Life story work is grouped under the headings of narrative, chronological, care-focused, or hybrid (Gridley et al., 2016). A crucial consideration is appropriateness of the format to the setting in which life story work is implemented. In hospitals, brief care-focused formats such as personal profiles or passports may be most useful (Thompson, 2017). Whereas in residential care settings, a more biographical or hybrid approach may be possible (Metcalfe, 2017). In earlier stages of dementia, a more narrative approach may be used either individually or as a group therapeutic intervention (Jennings, 2014). Choice of format is influenced by personal preference. An increasing variety of formats are available with electronic versions offering flexibility and the ability for continuous updating (Kindell et al., 2014; Thompson, 2011). Notably, McKeown et al. (2015) highlight the importance of ownership of life story work and recommend checking previous preferences for sharing information for those less able to contribute. A framework for understanding different models of life story work, their purpose, and the process involved may help with determining the approach needed (Gridley et al., 2016) (Table 14.3).

Benefits of life story work

People living with dementia require care and support in a range of community and institutional settings. Life story work enhances person-centred care by allowing nurses to make the link between past and present and promote understanding of the person's preferences for care (McKeown et al., 2010). It can help with understanding the meaning behind what people say and how they behave, reinforce identity, and facilitate communication (Bruce and Schweitzer, 2014). Positive outcomes for people living with dementia include improvements in cognition and mood (Subramaniam et al., 2014; Woods et al., 2018) as well as enjoyment and improved self-worth (Gridley et al., 2016). Additional benefits for family carers include improved relationships with the person with dementia and reduced burden (Haight et al., 2003).

For life story work to be effective at improving person-centred care, time must be given for the education of staff, development of skills, and leadership to support a cohesive, planned approach (Cooney and O'Shea, 2019; Gridley et al., 2016; McKeown et al., 2015; Thompson, 2011). Additional research is needed to identify individual benefits and distinguish the merits of different approaches to life story work, but there are some clear benefits for its use. A sensitive approach is required which focuses on process as much as outcome, encourages staff to build relationships with families and understand the uniqueness of the people they care for, and use this to inform person-centred care.

Table 14.3 A framework for understanding different models of life story

Approach	Purpose	Focus	Suitability/who for?	Process	Format
Narrative	To illuminate the person's life and capture what makes them unique More in line with 'life review'	The person's interpretation of the facts and emotions rather than the accuracy are important	People who can actively contribute to the process and benefit from life review process/ telling their story	Fluid process of storytelling including past, present, and future wishes Facilitated and supported by a carer/staff	Format is determined by the person and/ or the person collating the information
Biographical/ chronological	To gather a chronological account of a person's life	Collection of facts, memory, and timelines rather than feelings and meaning May also involve significant others to help provide information	People who can recall and share relevant biographical information and benefit from reminiscence May need support in recalling specific details	Structured process charting the person's life from birth to current day using templates/ headings	Use of a template or guidance which follows a timeline and highlights key events, e.g. creating a life story for a person with dementia (Dementia UK, 2023)
Care focused	To learn about specific aspects of a person's life that will help staff understand the person, i.e. their behaviour/ preferences and enhance communication	Information may be drawn from many sources including assessment, observation, and interaction Often care staff or family will provide information	People who are less able to share life story information due to reduced cognitive abilities and/or physical illness benefit from care staff understanding their needs	Dependent on the stage or extent of abilities of the person and is often shaped by the care- setting Less biographical information gathered	Use of a brief template/ personal profile/ passport which identifies key information such as roles, relationships, and likes/dislikes

Table 14.3 Continued

Approach	Purpose	Focus	Suitability/who for?	Process	Format
Hybrid	Combination of a care focus with a narrative or biographical element	Mainly focused on life story work in care settings but narrative elements may be included in the development, e.g. person's perspective about what they want included is important and information may be gathered from others	People who require support from families/care staff but can contribute to shaping and determining content May be helpful in enhancing identity, supporting reminiscence/ life review, and identifying needs	Various formats may be used according to the preference of the person, family, and/or care setting	Use of a template which enables adaptation and inclusion of the person's narrative/ perspective

Source: data from Gridley, K., Brooks, J. C., Birks, Y. F., Baxter, C. R., and Parker, G. M. (2016). Improving care for people with dementia: development and initial feasibility study for evaluation of life story work in dementia care. *Health Services and Delivery Research* 4(23), i–300.

Conducting life story work

- Life story work is a complex intervention involving multiple people, varying formats, and different settings. Care is required to clarify the aims and purposes of life story work and adapt the approach used to the situation and needs of the person and their family.

- Before embarking on life story work, undertake an assessment of the person's abilities, needs, and preferences, including their willingness to be involved.

- Not everyone will want to share their life story and although certain information may be shared in the context of a caring or therapeutic relationship, it may not be appropriate for recording. Table 14.4 uses the analogy of a chest of drawers to illustrate different information that might be appropriate for sharing (Brooker, 2010).

Table 14.4 Guidance for sharing personal information

Drawer	Type of personal information
Top drawer	Information freely available about a person such as demographics, jobs, family members, interests/hobbies, and preferences
Middle drawer	Information the person may choose to share in a friendship or caring relationship such as thoughts, feelings, beliefs, and more personal memories
Bottom drawer	Information that may be private or shared with a few close others such as family secrets, private or traumatic memories

Source: data from Brooker, D. (2010, 12 February). The VIPS model and the importance of life story work. Presentation at the First National Life Story work Conference, Leeds, UK.

▲ Conclusion

Therapeutic and stimulating psychosocial activities are important in dementia care and should be provided for people living with dementia regularly and planned around their individual abilities and interests. Everyone has an inbuilt need to engage in purposeful and meaningful activity that does not diminish with age. This need has enabled psychosocial interventions to be designed that are underpinned by the principles of person-centred care and are well tolerated and acceptable to people living with dementia. Furthermore, there is growing evidence of the therapeutic benefits of these interventions in maintaining and enhancing cognition, increasing independence, and improving quality of life. However, further research is needed to strengthen the evidence by evaluating their effectiveness using different modes of delivery, settings, and stages of the illness. Successful features of interventions such as CST are the structured approach to the design and delivery of the programme, and the same level of rigour should be applied in practice. Appropriate training and resources are required for nurses to acquire the skills and knowledge needed to facilitate activities and ensure ongoing delivery of therapeutic psychosocial interventions in dementia care.

✖ Tips to support implementation in practice

1. Discuss the purpose of gathering personal life story information with the individual where possible, and/or their family carer and clarify its use.
2. Assess the person's capacity to share information and ensure that information sharing is in the person's best interests.
3. Consider the best format according to the needs of the person and its suitability for the setting.
4. Involve the person and their family carers in gathering relevant information and ensure it will support the person's care.
5. Provide education, training, and involve all staff in understanding the benefits for using life story work in practice.
6. Provide clear information and resources to support its use and ensure a copy is kept in the patient's records in case of readmission.
7. Ensure the life story is kept in an easily accessible and visible place.
8. Provide clear leadership and ongoing support in the continued use of life story information to promote the delivery of person-centred care.
9. Regularly review and gather feedback from all those involved including people living with dementia and family carers.

W Companion website

For extra resources on the topics covered in this chapter, visit the companion website at: www.oup.com/mhns

✚ References

Aguirre, E., Spector, A., Streater, A., Hoe, J., Woods, B., and Orrell, M. (2012). *Making a Difference 2: An Evidence-Based Group Programme to Offer Maintenance Cognitive Stimulation Therapy (CST) to People with Dementia: The Manual for Group Leaders. London: Journal of Dementia Care/Hawker Publications Ltd.*

Alzheimer's Disease International (2011). *World Alzheimer Report 2011: The Benefits of Early Diagnosis and Intervention. London: Alzheimer's Disease International.*

Bohlmeijer, E., Roemer, M., Cuijpers, P., and Smit, F. (2007). *The effects of reminiscence on psychological* well-being in older adults: a meta-analysis. Aging and Mental Health 11(3), 291–300.

Brooker, D. (2010, 12 February). The VIPS model and the importance of life story work. Presentation at the First National Life Story work Conference, Leeds, UK.

Bruce, E. and Schweitzer, P. (2014). Working with life history. In: M. Downs and B. Bowers, Eds., Excellence in Dementia Care: Research into Practice, 2nd ed., pp. 203–219. Buckingham: Open University Press.

Butler, R. N. (1963). The life review: an interpretation of reminiscence in the aged. Psychiatry 26, 65–76.

Charlesworth, G., Burnell, K., Crellin, N., Hoare, Z., Hoe, J., Knapp, M., Russell, I., Wenborn, J., Woods, B., and Orrell, M. (2016). Peer support and reminiscence therapy for people with dementia and their family carers: a factorial pragmatic randomised trial. Journal of Neurology, Neurosurgery & Psychiatry 87(11), 1218–1228.

Clare, L., Nelis, S. M., Martyr, A., Roberts, J., Whitaker, C. J., Markova, I. S., Roth, I., Woods, R. T., and Morris, R. G. (2012). The influence of psychological, social and contextual factors on the expression and measurement of awareness in early-stage dementia: testing a biopsychosocial model. International Journal of Geriatric Psychiatry 27(2), 167–177.

Clemson, L., Laver, K., Jeon, Y. H., Comans, T. A., Scanlan, J., Rahja, M., Culph, J., Low, L. F., Day, S., Cations, M., and Crotty, M. (2018). Implementation of an evidence-based intervention to improve the wellbeing of people with dementia and their carers: study protocol for 'Care of People with dementia in their Environments (COPE)' in the Australian context. BMC Geriatrics 18(1), 1–11.

Cooney, A. and O'Shea, E. (2019). The impact of life story work on person-centred care for people with dementia living in long-stay care settings in Ireland. Dementia 18(7–8), 2731–2746.

Dementia UK (2023). Creating a Life Story for a Person with Dementia. Available at: https://www.dementiauk.org/information-and-support/living-with-dementia/creating-a-life-story/

Gridley, K., Brooks, J. C., Birks, Y. F., Baxter, C. R., and Parker, G. M. (2016). Improving care for people with dementia: development and initial feasibility study for evaluation of life story work in dementia care. Health Services and Delivery Research 4(23), i–300.

Haight, B. K., Bachman, D. L., Hendrix, S., Wagner, M. T., Meeks, A., and Johnson, J. (2003). Life review: treating the dyadic family unit with dementia. Clinical Psychology & Psychotherapy: An International Journal of Theory & Practice 10(3), 165–174.

Hoe, J. and Thompson, R. (2010). Promoting positive approaches to dementia care in nursing. Nursing Standard 25(4), 47–56.

Jennings, L., Ed. (2014). Welcome to our world. In: A Collection of Life Writing by People Living with Dementia, pp.15–19. Canterbury: Kent and Medway Forget-Me-Nots.

Kindell, J., Burrow, S., Wilkinson, R., and Keady, J. D. (2014). Life story resources in dementia care: a review. Quality in Ageing and Older Adults 15(3), 151–161.

Livingston, G., Huntley, J., Sommerlad, A., Ames, D., Ballard, C., Banerjee, S., Brayne, C., Burns, A., Cohen-Mansfield, J., Cooper, C., and Costafreda, S. G. (2020). Dementia prevention, intervention, and care: 2020 report of the Lancet Commission. Lancet 396(10248), 413–446.

Lobbia, A., Carbone, E., Faggian, S., Gardini, S., Piras, F., Spector, A., and Borella, E. (2019). The efficacy of cognitive stimulation therapy (CST) for people with mild-to-moderate dementia: a review. European Psychologist 24(3), 257–277.

Maruta, M., Makizako, H., Ikeda, Y., Miyata, H., Nakamura, A., Han, G., Shimokihara, S., Tokuda, K., Kubozono, T., Ohishi, M., and Tomori, K. (2020). Associations between depressive symptoms and satisfaction with meaningful activities in community-dwelling Japanese older adults. Journal of Clinical Medicine 9(3), 795.

McKeown, J., Clarke, A., Ingleton, C., Ryan, T., and Repper, J. (2010). The use of life story work with people with dementia to enhance person-centred care. International Journal of Older People Nursing 5(2), 148–158.

McKeown, J., Ryan, T., Ingleton, C., and Clarke, A. (2015). 'You have to be mindful of whose story it is': the challenges of undertaking life story work with people with dementia and their family carers. Dementia 14(2), 238–256.

Menne, H. L., Johnson, J. D., Whitlatch, C. J., and Schwartz, S. M. (2012). Activity preferences of persons with dementia. Activities, Adaptation & Aging 36(3), 195–213.

Metcalfe, V. (2017). *Life story work in care homes. In: P. Kaiser and R. Ely, Eds., Life Story work with People with Dementia: Ordinary Lives, Extraordinary People, pp. 165–177. London: Jessica Kingsley Publishers.*

Moniz-Cook, E. and Rewston, C. (2020). *Choosing psychosocial interventions for people with dementia and their families. In: J. Manthorpe and E. Moniz-Cook, Eds., Timely Psychosocial Interventions in Dementia Care: Evidence-Based Practice, pp. 30–47. London: Jessica Kingsley Publishers.*

Murphy, C. (2000). *Crackin' Lives: An Evaluation of a Life Story Book Project to Assist Patients from a Long Stay Psychiatric Hospital in their Move to Community Care Situations. Stirling: Dementia Services Development Centre.*

National Institute for Health and Care Excellence (2018). *Dementia: Assessment, Management, and Support for People Living with Dementia and their Carers. NICE Guideline [NG97]. Available at: https://www.nice.org.uk/guidance/ng97*

Orrell, M., Yates, L., Leung, P., Kang, S., Hoare, Z., Whitaker, C., Burns, A., Knapp, M., Leroi, I., Moniz-Cook, E., and Pearson, S. (2017). *The impact of individual cognitive stimulation therapy (iCST) on cognition, quality of life, caregiver health, and family relationships in dementia: a randomised controlled trial. PLoS Medicine 14(3), e1002269.*

Orrell, M., Woods, B., and Spector, A. (2012). *Should we use individual cognitive stimulation therapy to improve cognitive function in people with dementia? BMJ 344, e633.*

Pinquart, M. and Forstmeier, S. (2012). *Effects of reminiscence interventions on psychosocial outcomes: a meta-analysis. Aging & Mental Health 16(5), 541–558.*

Schweitzer, P. and Bruce, E. (2008). *Remembering Yesterday, Caring Today: Reminiscence in Dementia Care: A Guide to Good Practice. London: Jessica Kingsley Publishers.*

Spector, A., Thorgrimsen, L., Woods, R. T., and Orrell, M. (2006). *Making a Difference: An Evidence-Based Group Programme to Offer Cognitive Stimulation Therapy (CST) to People with Dementia. London: Hawker Publications.*

Spector, A., Thorgrimsen, L., Woods, B., Royan, L., Davies, S., Butterworth, M., and Orrell, M. (2003). *Efficacy of an evidence-based cognitive stimulation therapy programme for people with dementia: randomised controlled trial. British Journal of Psychiatry 183(3), 248–254.*

Subramaniam, P., Woods, B., and Whitaker, C. (2014). *Life review and life story books for people with mild to moderate dementia: a randomised controlled trial. Aging and Mental Health 18(3), 363–375.*

Thompson, R. (2011). *Using life story work to enhance care. Nursing Older People 23(8). 16–21.*

Thompson R. (2017). *Life story work for people with dementia in acute general hospitals; an alternative model for care. In: P. Kaiser and R. Ely, Eds., Life Story Work with People with Dementia: Ordinary Lives, Extraordinary People, pp. 153–164. London: Jessica Kingsley Publishers.*

Wenborn, J. (2017). *Meaningful activities. In: S. Schüssler and C. Lohrmann, Eds., Dementia in Nursing Homes, pp. 5–20. Cham: Springer.*

Westerhof, G. J., Bohlmeijer, E. T., and Webster, J. D. (2010). *Reminiscence and mental health: a review of recent progress in theory, research and interventions. Aging & Society 30(4), 697–721.*

Whitty, E., Mansour, H., Aguirre, E., Palomo, M., Charlesworth, G., Ramjee, S., Poppe, M., Brodaty, H., Kales, H. C., Morgan-Trimmer, S., and Nyman, S. R. (2020). *Efficacy of lifestyle and psychosocial interventions in reducing cognitive decline in older people: systematic review. Ageing Research Reviews 62, 101113.*

Woods, B., O'Philbin, L., Farrell, E. M., Spector, A. E., and Orrell, M. (2018). *Reminiscence therapy for dementia. Cochrane Database of Systematic Reviews 3(3), CD001120.*

World Health Organization (2017). *Global Action Plan on the Public Health Response to Dementia 2017–2025. Geneva: World Health Organization.*

Yates, L., Orrell, M., Leung, P., Spector, A., Woods, B., and Orgeta, V. (2015). *Making a Difference 3: Individual Cognitive Stimulation Therapy: A Manual for Carers, Vol. 3. London: Hawker Publications Ltd.*

(15) Behavioural activation

Maria Filip   Tim Carter

Learning outcomes

By the end of this chapter, you should be able to:

1 Understand the theoretical basis for behavioural activation

2 Describe the evidence base for behavioural activation

3 Understand how behavioural activation is implemented with a service user experiencing depression

4 Support a service user experiencing depression using the principles of behavioural activation.

▼ Introduction

What is behavioural activation?

Behavioural activation (BA) is a practical, structured, behaviourally oriented therapeutic approach to treating depression. BA is centred on the idea that depression is maintained by a person's context or environment and that changes in their context/environment can help alleviate symptoms of depression. BA works on the premise that the physical, cognitive, and emotional symptoms of depression often result in people experiencing increasingly punishing and less rewarding day-to-day lives, leading to understandable but problematic avoidance behaviour. BA works by identifying and reducing avoidance behaviour, re-establishing a helpful daily and weekly routine, and encouraging a service user to re-engage with life.

The evidence for behavioural activation

Over the previous three decades, a substantial and impressive evidence base has emerged for BA, demonstrating it as an effective and well-tolerated, acceptable treatment for depression. The evidence base for BA includes multiple high-quality randomized controlled trials demonstrating its effectiveness across the life span (Orgeta et al., 2017; Tindall et al., 2017) and across the spectrum of depression severity (Lorenzo-Luaces et al., 2019). BA is recommended by the National Institute for Health and Care Excellence (2022) as a primary treatment approach for depression. Importantly, the research suggests that BA can be easily taught to non-therapy-trained mental health professionals, and can be as effective in such circumstances as full cognitive behavioural therapy (Richards et al., 2016).

Rationale for behavioural activation

Life stressors are often a precursor to the development of depression. These can include the loss of a loved one, social exclusion, and loss of purpose, but also more chronic stressors such as financial or relationship difficulties. Once individuals become depressed, most of their behaviours serve as avoidance from painful thoughts, feelings, and additional stressors. Day-to-day activities may start to feel overwhelming and people cope by pulling back from life. The less people do, the lower their motivation to engage in meaningful activities becomes. In addition, the initial stressors tend to worsen, further contributing to low mood (Martell et al., 2001). Initially, this withdrawal can give people a sense of relief from the emotional pain and physical strain of engaging with life. However, once this cycle sets in, symptoms of depression exacerbate. People might feel more tired, lack energy, have reduced motivation, experience difficulty concentrating, and become more irritable. Sleep and appetite can also be affected. As a result, this leads to even less engagement in activities, worsening of mood, and a further exacerbation of symptoms.

Key principle for behavioural activation

Service users are encouraged to engage with activity regardless of their mood, that is, if they feel demotivated, they should still engage with a scheduled activity. This is based on the idea that motivation comes after action. If service users wait to feel motivated, it is likely that their depression will be prolonged.

▼ A guide to supporting service users with depression using the principles of behavioural activation

Step 1: giving the rationale

Behavioural activation is a way of helping service users to break the vicious cycles of avoidance and to reconnect with a sense of enjoyment and achievement in their lives, thereby alleviating depressive symptoms. The first step is to support them in recognizing the cycle of depression, its impact on their behaviour, and how disengaging from life exacerbates ongoing stressors. Although behavioural activation focuses on changing service users' behaviours, acknowledging the life stressors which have led to depression brings an attitude of compassion and helps to normalize why service users started to reduce their activities. This strengthens the rationale for beginning to engage with activities again, as not only will it help to alleviate symptoms of depression, but it will also help to reduce the impact of the initial stressors. For instance, a service user struggling with the loss of a loved one might stay indoors more and stop socializing, which is likely to increase feelings of loneliness, making the loss more acute. Thus, supporting them in contacting friends might boost their mood and increase feelings of connection, thereby softening the impact of the loss.

Step 2: creating a collaborative understanding of the service user's depression

To support service users in understanding this cycle, the Five Areas model (Greenberger and Padesky, 1995) is completed collaboratively. Here, we take an example (situation) where the person felt down and explore the thoughts, emotions, physical sensations, and how they coped (behaviours) at the time. A key feature of depression is that thinking becomes more negative, leading to withdrawal from activities. This model reflects how all these areas interlink with one another: emphasizing that the less people do, the less motivation people have, the more tired and depleted they feel, feeding into critical thoughts about the self, which ultimately lead to them doing less and disengaging from life. A template for the Five Areas model can be found in Figure 15.1 and used to photocopy to share with service users.

Step 3: establishing a baseline of current activities

The next step is to ask service users to keep a diary of their current activities for a week. This gives you and the service user an overall picture in order to make links between behaviours and mood. We would generally ask service users to break this down into morning, afternoon, and evening activities. It is helpful for service users to rate their mood at the time, on a scale from 0 to 10, where 0 represents being at their lowest. At the following session, the diary is used to reflect on patterns in low mood. For instance, a service user might find their mood is at its worst when coming back from work and staying on the sofa for the rest of the evening, feeling disconnected from the world. When reflecting on the baseline diary, it is important to support the service

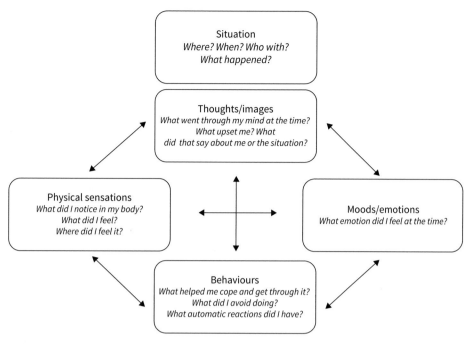

Figure 15.1 The Five Areas model

user in understanding the links between reduced activity and impact on their mood. The diary might evoke feelings of sadness when service users realize how little they are doing, or just how much things have changed for them. Thus, offering empathy and compassion while supporting them in starting to think about what they miss in life is paramount. A template of the baseline diary can be found in Table 15.1.

Table 15.1 Baseline diary of activities

	Monday	Tuesday	Wednesday	Thursday	Friday	Saturday	Sunday
Morning							
Record activity (what)							
Record time (when)							
Rate mood 0–10							
Afternoon							
Record activity (what)							
Record time (when)							
Rate mood 0–10							
Evening							
Record activity (what)							
Record time (when)							
Rate mood 0–10							
Overall patterns—what did you notice from keeping the diary?							

Step 4: identifying activities to reintroduce

Following on from the baseline diary, the emphasis in the next session is on identifying activities which are meaningful for service users. Previous literature recommends looking at activities in the following categories: routine, necessary, and pleasurable (Pasterfield et al., 2014). Routine activities might involve eating, washing, and establishing a sleep routine. Necessary activities reflect those where there can be a consequence for not doing them, such as paying bills. Pleasurable activities are usually reduced first, thus a discussion about their hobbies can help service users to reconnect with activities which might have previously given them a sense of enjoyment. Some service users might notice they still engage with routine and necessary activities but that they stopped engaging in pleasurable activities. Highlighting the impact of this on their mood, in that routine and necessary activities continue to deplete energy levels, is important. Using a battery analogy here can help service users make sense of the impact: when depressed, their energy levels are low, thus at the minus end of a battery; continuing to do necessary and routine activities requires energy of them, keeping them at the low end of the battery; and pleasurable activities can be seen as 'positive charge' to the battery therefore allowing them to buffer the impact of other tasks.

Step 5: daily routine

Special consideration needs to be given to supporting service users to look after themselves more by ensuring they eat, wash, and work towards establishing a sleep routine. Before any other activities can be introduced, it is key to work with service users to highlight that their energy levels would naturally be depleted if their diet or sleep are affected. Jacobson et al. (2001) highlight that 'disruption of these routines can cause us to be out of sync with our environments and can contribute to the exacerbation of depression' (p. 259). In summary, the focus at this stage would be on dovetailing a self-care routine with other activities the service user has been avoiding.

Step 6: making activities manageable

Due to the physical symptoms of depression, particularly lethargy, lack of motivation, and difficulty concentrating, service users might find it difficult to begin engaging in activities. In addition, they might place blame on themselves for not being able to get on with seemingly straightforward tasks and experience guilt. An attitude of validation and highlighting the impact of symptoms of depression help service users to attribute this to the condition rather than think of themselves as lazy (Kinsella and Garland, 2008). Service users might attempt to perform at the same level as they did prior to being depressed and expect to complete tasks in similar timeframes.

To help service users manage this, it is recommended to grade activities as this enhances motivation (Macdonald et al., 2008). Grading activities involves working with the person to break down tasks into parts which are achievable either in terms of length of time or of how much they do. For instance, if a service user has been putting off ironing and now this feels too big a task, we would help them to break this into manageable chunks. For example, getting the iron and ironing board out one day, and then ironing for 5 minutes the next day. A useful analogy for grading activity is to think of a marathon runner who has suffered an injury. They would need to pace themselves to reach the required level of fitness to run the marathon. Being consistent and gradually increasing the amount they run is likely to help them build their stamina again in the same way that behavioural activation can help service users create momentum in their lives. An exploratory discussion about the impact of doing part of an activity in comparison to none at all might help to highlight the benefits of engaging with the technique. Most often, service users report that even doing small parts of a task gives them a sense of achievement, relief, and motivation.

Step 7: establishing routine through scheduling activity

Once you and the service user have an overview of which activities they would like to reintroduce and how to make this manageable, beginning to schedule these activities is the next step. A diary should be used here to help allocate a specific time and day for activities to be treated as appointments with themselves as this can enhance engagement (Veale, 2008). Service users can use a diary similar to the baseline in Table 15.1 or they can use other aids they rely on to organize their day (e.g. paper diary or phone calendar). The key here is to make these resources as accessible as possible to facilitate service users in implementing changes in their lives.

Things to consider:

- Only change an activity when there is an external factor (e.g. a friend cancels a meeting).
- If an activity has to be changed, then service users should schedule something different to do.

Step 8: ongoing review of activity

The majority of sessions would be devoted to this stage of the process. This involves reviewing activities and exploring any barriers to engagement which might arise during treatment. Service users might find that some weeks are more difficult to continue to practise this technique, thus the sessions can focus on discussing patterns they have noticed and what makes it more likely that they would engage with the technique. For example, one service user might find it easier to go out for a run if they change into their gear before leaving work. If changes to their schedule disrupt this, it can be beneficial to collaboratively discuss ways to re-establish this routine and pre-empt barriers.

▼ Common pitfalls

Ambivalence about change

> While change inevitably has disadvantages (we may have to tolerate distress and endure discomfort in our efforts), they may be outweighed by the price we pay for staying as we are.
>
> (Smith, 2022, p. 93).

It can be common for service users to face difficulties in making changes and engage in treatment. They might agree with the rationale and acknowledge the potential benefits of behavioural activation, but still feel stuck in terms of making a change. Revisiting the rationale and exploring any fears or anxieties service users might have about treatment can enhance their motivation. If ambivalence is still present, research recommends approaching this by helping service users to understand their own ambivalence about change and to collaboratively resolve it (Westra, 2004). A decisional balance exercise which involves listing the pros and cons of changing versus staying the same can be useful here. It is recommended to do this in session with the service user, allowing them to make their own mind up about whether to make a change. It is often the case that, when faced with the reasons written out, that service users are able to balance what is important about making a change with some of the discomfort this may bring. It is a powerful exercise because we are not trying to convince the service user one way or another, we are simply helping them to make a decision based on what they value in life and how treatment taps into this. In practice, this might mean that the service user will feel more motivated to 'drive' the treatment and engage fully with behavioural activation. Ultimately, this is the gold standard in treatment as we are a mere vehicle to service users' recovery. Focusing on enhancing their motivation and self-efficacy will help them to consolidate the changes made after the sessions come to an end.

Difficulty identifying meaningful activity

When service users have experienced depression for some time, it may seem impossible to identify meaningful activities. There has been considerable research looking into how to support service users to engage with this stage of treatment. Most of this research centres around identifying what service users value in life and supporting them in finding activities in line with their core values (Harris, 2019). Finding meaning in life surpasses the idea of goals. Goals can help us achieve and keep us motivated. However, what research is showing is that when we work in accordance with our values, we are much more likely to feel fulfilled and identify activities and associated goals (Farchione et al., 2017). If service users are struggling to identify meaningful activities, spending one session exploring their values would provide a context for this and facilitate a sense of empowerment in choosing activities which most closely align with what matters for them. Box 15.1 gives a list of common values which can be used in session and also as homework for the service user to reflect on their values. After you have collaboratively identified the values most important to them, ask service users to rate on a scale from 0 to 10 how much they are living in line with each value. For example, if someone identifies looking after their health and fitness as very important but they rate living in line with this as 2/10, it can provide an opportunity to think of ways to live a life more aligned with this. Starting small and grading activity is important. Service users might set a big goal, such as doing a park run. This is a great goal to work towards; however, when we think of value-based activities, we would like to encourage implementing something small each day which means they are living in line with this value. In this example, it might be going for a 20-minute walk or joining a running group. These types of activities are likely to keep service users motivated because even if they reach their goal of doing a park run, it surpasses this goal and it orients them towards living a meaningful life long term.

Box 15.1 Identifying which values matter to you

Values are a set of ideas and beliefs about how you want to live your life and the kind of person you aspire to be. Values guide behaviour. Sometimes, life stressors get in the way of us living a life in keeping with our core values. Clarifying your values can help to give meaning to the things we do each day. For example, someone who values family, might spend more time at home and choose to reduce their working hours. If someone values their health and fitness, they might invest time every day doing something towards looking after their health such as going for a walk. Below is a list of common life values. Identify five to ten values which are most important to you. You can rate them in order of importance from 0 to 10. This list is not exhaustive. You can write a list of other values which are meaningful to you. These could reflect the following life domains: family, friendships, work, hobbies, personal growth, health and well-being, spirituality, and education.

Love and affection	Respect
Wealth	Nature
Lifelong learning	Health
Reliable	Fun
Sustainability	Fairness
Honesty	Adventure
Independence	Connection
Curiosity	Ambition
Kindness	Self-awareness
Open-mindedness	Patience.

Box 15.2 Practice example: David

David was a 38-year-old man who at the time had just been discharged from an acute admission ward where he was a voluntary patient following a suicide attempt. David's attempted suicide followed the breakdown of his marriage after he found his partner was being unfaithful. David had a diagnosis of depression (and a long-standing history of depression) and was now under the care of a community mental health team. He was assigned a mental health nurse (MHN) as his care coordinator.

Following three visits to David's home, the MHN decided that David could be supported with his depression through the use of BA as it was clear that David had very little structure to his week, had stopped engaging in most sociable and pleasurable activities, and his mood had started to deteriorate further.

The first step for the MHN was to provide a strong rationale for David. Essentially, the MHN had the difficult task of selling the idea that the less David did (and the more he avoided), the worse his symptoms became and the more difficult life became. The MHN used the model (Figure 15.1) to demonstrate to David how avoidance behaviour, although understandable, has the unintended consequence of increasing physical symptoms, while also making him feel more guilty, and more self-critical. It also gave David much more time to ruminate on the loss of his marriage, which further decreased his mood, motivation, and increased feelings of hopelessness. The MHN then presented the idea that David might be able to help alleviate his depression by starting to engage rather than avoid and start to do things, even when he doesn't want to.

David understood the principle but felt it would be extremely difficult to start doing things that he just didn't want to do and felt that he needed to feel better before he could do anything. The MHN asked David to keep the model for the week and start to notice the impact on his mood and motivation when he avoided something, or gave something up. David was also asked to keep a basic diary of his activity throughout the week.

At the next home visit, David reported that he noticed he was doing very little day to day and that

Box 15.2 Continued

his life mainly consisted of staying indoors watching TV and thinking about his marriage. David was reluctant to agree to the idea of re-engaging with things as he felt it would be too difficult and that he wouldn't be able to do anything. The MHN did a pros and cons list with David about starting to re-engage with things, she also suggested to David that motivation tends to come after action—an idea that David was dubious but intrigued about.

David and the MHN then generated a list of activities that David could start to plan in his week. David offered very little here and the MHN had to give some ideas based on what she knew of David. The MHN encouraged a mix of things that David was avoiding such as things that used to give him some pleasure, things that used to give him some satisfaction or achievement, and things that could give him some structure and routine to his week. Once a few things had been decided, the MHN encouraged David to pick two things to plan in the week. David was dubious about the point of only doing two things and expressed he thought it might be a waste of time. The MHN used the analogy of a marathon runner who had a serious injury and that when they were recommencing their training, they would likely start very slowly to avoid re-injuring themselves and causing a setback, or doing too much and demotivating themselves when they realize they cannot currently do what they used to. David agreed to stick to the plan of only doing two things and was encouraged to write each down in detail on a blank diary sheet, outline what he would do, and when he would do it. David decided to call his brother on the Wednesday at 7 pm, and to read a book he used to enjoy on Friday at 4 pm. The principle of engaging with the activity regardless of his mood and motivation at the time was stressed to David by the MHN.

At the next visit David reported he had undertaken both the two activities as planned. He said it was useful to call his brother who he had been avoiding talking to since his suicide attempt and from that phone call had planned to meet with him later in the week. David was surprised by how much his brother seemed to want to meet with him as he assumed his brother was fed up with him. David reported that the reading did not go as well as he was unable to concentrate and gave up after 10 minutes. The MHN made sure to praise David for both activities, making it clear just how difficult it is to do these things when depressed. David was encouraged to schedule further activity this week, adding more things into the weekly plan. It was also agreed that the book David was reading was perhaps not helpful given his concentration was affected currently, so it was agreed that David would read a magazine he used to enjoy instead, as this allowed him to read shorter articles. The MHN and David also agreed on a weekly routine as it was clear that David's sleeping and waking times were very inconsistent, as was his eating routine. The pros and cons of changing were once again explored and ultimately an agreement was made that David would get out of bed by 10 am every day. He would also eat at least twice a day, even if not hungry at the time (David was often going 24 hours without eating as he had a reduced appetite).

The next several visits to David consisted of reviewing the planned activities that David and the MHN had scheduled and exploring any impact the engagement in each activity may have had. Each visit would also focus on what David would schedule for the upcoming week, often based on what he got out of the week before. Over the weeks, David noticed his motivation to engage with things was improving and that he was even starting to enjoy things. David gradually increased his activity levels and started ultimately to look for volunteer work. As this was a big task, David and the MHN broke it down in manageable chunks for David to schedule. This was applied to other large tasks that started to emerge as David re-engaged with life. Over time, the frequency of the visits from the MHN reduced as David's mood improved and he started to schedule activity independently and spontaneously.

▼ Case vignette

For a detailed practice example, see Box 15.2.

▲ Conclusion

BA is a highly effective treatment approach for depression with a substantial evidence base and strong theoretical underpinnings. It has been shown to be effective for severe depression and the principles of the approach can be readily incorporated into mental health nursing practice. This person-centred, behavioural approach to alleviating depression gives MHNs a strong rationale and structured approach to help a service user overcome depression through meaningful and graded re-engagement with life.

✖ Tips from service users

1 'I'm somebody who likes things done a certain way. It was hard having to pace myself and not do too much as I felt I wasn't doing enough. Once I started to break things down, I noticed it got easier and I felt like I was achieving. This helped me feel better about myself. It's okay not to do it all in one go.'

2 'I can be really hard on myself for not getting things done. I found that once I started to be a bit more flex- ible and give myself time, I managed to do a lot more than in the beginning. Be kind to yourself.'

3 'I got frustrated with myself to begin with because the technique didn't seem to work. I was doing everything and I didn't feel any better. I realized that it takes some time for things to fall into place and that motivation comes from practising these activities more and more. Stick with it.'

W Companion website

For extra resources on the topics covered in this chapter, visit the companion website at: www.oup.com/mhns

✚ References

Farchione, T. J., Boswell, J. F., and Wilner, J. G. (2017). *Behavioral activation strategies for major depression in transdiagnostic cognitive-behavioral therapy: an evidence-based case study. Psychotherapy 54(3), 225–230.*

Greenberger, D. and Padesky, C. A. (1995). *Mind Over Mood: A Cognitive Therapy Treatment Manual for Clients.* New York: Guilford Press.

Harris, R. (2019). *ACT Made Simple: An Easy-to-Read Primer on Acceptance and Commitment Therapy.* Oakland, CA: New Harbinger Publications.

Jacobson, N. S., Martell, C. R., and Dimidjian, S. (2001). *Behavioral activation treatment for depression: returning to contextual roots. Clinical Psychology: Science and Practice 8(3), 255–270.*

Kinsella, P. and Garland, A. (2008). *Cognitive Behavioural Therapy for Mental Health Workers: A Beginner's Guide.* Hove: Routledge.

Lorenzo-Luaces, L. and Dobson, K. S. (2019). *Is behavioral activation (BA) more effective than cognitive therapy (CT) in severe depression? A reanalysis of a landmark trial. International Journal of Cognitive Therapy 12(2), 73–82.*

Macdonald, W., Rogers, A., Blakeman, T., and Bower, P. (2008). *Practice nurses and the facilitation of self-management in primary care. Journal of Advanced Nursing 62(2), 191–199.*

Martell, C. R., Addis, M. E., and Jacobson, N. S. (2001). *Depression in Context: Strategies for Guided Action. New York: W. W. Norton & Company.*

National Institute for Health and Care Excellence (2022). *Depression in Adults: Treatment and Management. NICE guideline [NG222]. Available at: https://www.nice.org.uk/guidance/ng222*

Orgeta, V., Brede, J., and Livingston, G. (2017). *Behavioural activation for depression in older people: systematic review and meta-analysis. British Journal of Psychiatry 211(5), 274–279.*

Pasterfield, M., Bailey, D., Hems, D., McMillan, D., Richards, D., and Gilbody, S. (2014). *Adapting manualized behavioural activation treatment for older adults with depression. The Cognitive Behaviour Therapist 7, e5.*

Richards, D. A., Ekers, D., McMillan, D., Taylor, R. S., Byford, S., Warren, F. C., Barrett, B., Farrand, P. A.,

Gilbody, S., Kuyken, W., O'Mahen, H., Watkins, E. R., Wright, K. A., Hollon, S. D., Reed, N., Rhodes, S., Fletcher, E., and Finning, K. (2016). *Cost and Outcome of Behavioural Activation versus Cognitive Behavioural Therapy for Depression (COBRA): a randomised, controlled, non-inferiority trial. Lancet 388(10047), 871–880.*

Smith, J. (2022). *Why Has Nobody Told Me This Before? London: Michael Joseph.*

Tindall, L., Mikocka-Walus, A., McMillan, D., Wright, B., Hewitt, C., and Gascoyne, S. (2017). *Is behavioural activation effective in the treatment of depression in young people? A systematic review and meta-analysis. Psychology and Psychotherapy 90(4), 770–796.*

Veale, D. (2008). *Behavioural activation for depression. Advances in Psychiatric Treatment 14(1), 29–36.*

Westra, H. (2004). *Managing resistance in cognitive behavioural therapy: the application of motivational interviewing in mixed anxiety and depression. Cognitive Behaviour Therapy 33(4), 161–175.*

16 Behavioural family interventions for the self-harming and suicidal adolescent

Anita Henderson   Roy Litvin

Learning outcomes

By the end of this chapter, you should be able to:

1 Understand the fundamental concepts of dialectical behavioural therapy

2 Identify a wide range of behavioural skills to apply in practice when working with young people who self-harm and to share with parents and/or carers

3 Devise a risk management care plan which includes dialectical behavioural therapy strategies for both the young person and parent/carer.

▼ Introduction

Young people who struggle to regulate their emotional responses can often turn to self-harming behaviours to manage these emotions. They may also experience suicidal thoughts and even make attempts to end their own life. This can of course be anxiety provoking for the parent or carer as well as the mental health nurse whose role it is to support the family at this challenging time. Unfortunately, some of these young people would have encountered some form of difficulty during their childhood, but not all. These can be referred to as adverse childhood experiences and can include physical abuse, sexual abuse, emotional abuse, living with someone who abused drugs and/or alcohol, exposure to domestic violence, and losing a parent through divorce, death, or abandonment (Bellis et al., 2019). Adverse childhood experiences can impact the young person's attachment style and their ability to recognize and manage different emotions. This includes the capacity to make and keep healthy relationships and manage behaviour in a school setting (Young Minds, 2018). In addition, there has been an increase in the number of young people being bullied through the use of social media. This affects one in five children aged 10–15 years

in England and Wales (Office for National Statistics, 2020), and has been found to contribute to self-harming behaviour in young people (Eyuboglu et al., 2021).

Due to the young person's inherent temperament and some of the psychosocial factors mentioned above, some young people can struggle to navigate the world of interpersonal relationships and experience emotions with such intensity that they are often too overwhelming for them to cope with (Brown and Plener, 2017). Some of these emotions may be of chronic emptiness, guilt, shame, and a fear of abandonment (C. Chen, 2019). To manage or cope with these emotions young people may use self-harming behaviours (W.-L. Chen and Chun, 2019). Each young person may have their own reason for why they hurt themselves, for example, it can be a form of punishment, to get 'bad' feelings out of the body, or an attempt to feel something when they have detached themselves from an emotional situation (Peh et al., 2017). People around the young person will often struggle to understand their high levels of emotional responses to situations and the behaviour that they use to cope with these emotions. Consequently, the child can be labelled as being either oversensitive, dramatic, or manipulative. An adult presenting

Box 16.1 Emotional unstable personality disorder diagnosis criteria

According to the ICD-10, emotionally unstable personality disorder is characterized as:

a definite tendency to act impulsively and without consideration of the consequences; the mood is unpredictable and capricious. There is a liability to outbursts of emotion and an incapacity to control the behavioural explosions. There is a tendency to quarrelsome behaviour and to conflicts with others, especially when impulsive acts are thwarted or censored. Two types may be distinguished: the impulsive type, characterized predominantly by emotional instability and lack of impulse control, and the borderline type, characterized in addition by disturbances in self-image, aims, and internal preferences, by chronic feelings of emptiness, by intense and unstable interpersonal relationships, and by a tendency to self-destructive behaviour, including suicide gestures and attempts.

Reproduced from World Health Organization (1992). *The ICD-10 Classification of Mental and Behavioural Disorders*. World Health Organization.

with these types of symptoms would likely be diagnosed as suffering from emotionally unstable personality disorder which is also known as borderline personality disorder (BPD) (Box 16.1). In young people, emotionally unstable personality disorder is not often diagnosed as the set of symptoms are often similar to those experienced by typical adolescences whose parts of the brain which control their emotions and impulses are still developing (Butera, 2014). However, it is useful to consider behavioural patterns in BPD in order to understand some of the behaviours the young person may present with (Linehan, 1993) (Box 16.2).

Box 16.2 Behavioural patterns in borderline personality disorder

Emotional vulnerability: a pattern of pervasive difficulties in regulating negative emotions, including high sensitivity to negative emotions, including high sensitivity to negative emotional stimuli, heightened emotional intensity, and slow return to emotional baseline, as well as awareness and experience of emotional vulnerability. May include a tendency to blame the social environment for unrealistic expectations and demands.

Self-invalidation: tendency to invalidate or fail to recognize one's own emotional responses, thoughts, beliefs, and behaviours. Unrealistically high standards and expectations for self. May include intense shame, self-hate, and self-directed anger.

Unrelenting crisis: patterns of frequent, stressful, negative environment events and disruptions, and roadblocks—some caused by the individual's chaotic lifestyle, others by an inadequate social milieu, and many by fate or chance.

Inhibited grieving: tendency to inhibit and overcontrol negative emotional responses, especially those associated with grief and loss, including sadness, anger, guilt, shame, anxiety, and panic.

Active passivity: tendency towards passive interpersonal problem-solving style, involving failure to engage actively in solving own life problems, often together with active attempts to solicit problem solving from others in the environment; learned helplessness.

Apparent competence: tendency for the individual to appear deceptively more competent than she actually is; usually due to failure of competencies to generalize across expected moods, situations, and time, and failure to display adequate non-verbal cues of emotional distress.

Reproduced from Linehan, M. (1993). *Cognitive Behavioural Treatment of Borderline Personality Disorder*. New York: Guilford Press, p. 10.

✖ Tip

Emotional dysregulation is one of the core components of attention deficit hyperactive disorder a neurodevelopmental disorder. In 2016, 26% of all children who self-harmed had a diagnosis of attention deficit hyperactive disorder or conduct disorder (Public Health England, 2016).

When devising a care plan for the young person, mental health nurses tend to focus on the child, but often ask the parents to be part of the risk management plan. Nurses give advice on how to make the home environment safe and how to contact services if another crisis arises, but they rarely support the parents in identifying strategies that they can employ to support their child in crisis or to prevent one. Using a case study example (Box 16.3), this chapter will provide mental health nurses with the skills to be able to support parents during challenging times and establish an affective risk management plan.

Box 16.3 Practice example

Sarah is a 15-year-old British girl from a mixed Black Caribbean and White background. Sarah is presenting with symptoms of fluctuation in her mood. Sarah's natural father died of cancer when she was 16 months old. After this her mother became depressed and started to use alcohol and drugs as a way of managing these feelings. Her mother remarried when Sarah was 4 years old to a man who also abused drugs and alcohol. Sarah has an older half-sister and half-brother from this relationship. Sarah often experienced her mother and stepfather fighting and she felt tense and frightened in her home environment. Although the drug use had stopped, Sarah's mother and stepfather were still consuming large amounts of alcohol. When Sarah was 5 years old, her stepfather started to sexually abuse her. He would come to her bedroom at night when her mother was intoxicated.

While at primary school, Sarah presented as withdrawn and was finding it difficult to achieve in school. Sarah was often seen by the school nurse for recurrent abdominal pain. Sarah liked the school nurse who had been in post for many years, and she saw her regularly. She disclosed to the school nurse that her stepfather had come into her bedroom at night and made her do things she did not like. The school nurse made an immediate safeguarding referral to social services who in turn alerted the police. Sarah's stepfather was forced to leave the family home. Following an investigation by social services and by the police, Sarah's stepfather was charged and placed in prison for sexually abusing Sarah, and her older stepsister as well. Sarah and her siblings were allowed to remain with Sarah's mother and were allocated a social worker to support the family through this time.

Sarah found the transfer to secondary school challenging and struggled to make friends. While at secondary school, Sarah was seen by the school nurse for superficial self-harm, but there was a high turnover of staff and she found it difficult to engage with the various school nurses. Over the past year, Sarah has been bullied by a group of girls in her class. She has not spoken to anyone about this. Sarah was reviewed regularly by her social worker, Naomi, whom she had known for 8 years and who she had an overall good relationship with. About 8 months ago, Naomi left her post and Sarah was discharged from Social Services.

Over the past 6 months, Sarah has struggled with emotional dysregulation. She often experiences intense feelings of rage, shame, panic, and a chronic sense of emptiness. She has also started to self-harm more severely by cutting her arms and legs and taking repeated small overdoses. She has frequently used social media and chat rooms about self-harm and suicide. Sarah expresses that she self-harms as it helps her to deal with 'all this horrible stuff' and has thoughts of not wanting to be here anymore. Sarah constantly argues with her mother at home, and both feel unable to communicate with one another. Following a recent overdose Sarah has attended the Emergency Department. While there, she was reviewed by the Children and Adolescent Mental Health Services (CAMHS) Urgent Care Team (UCT) who discharged her with a follow-up appointment within 7 days of leaving the hospital. At her review meeting, the UCT have recommended Sarah to attend the CAMHS DBT programme. This means that she will be attending weekly individual and group DBT sessions. She will also have access to phone coaching with her DBT therapist when she has a wish or a need to overdose or cut herself.

Sarah's mum no longer abuses alcohol and feels guilty that her past substance misuse has affected Sarah and her two stepchildren. She blames herself for not being able to prevent the abuse of both her daughter and stepdaughter. She is very keen to try and support Sarah but struggles to understand Sarah's emotive responses and feels she is constantly 'walking on eggshells' around her. Sarah has a fairly good relationship with her stepsister Sisa, and her stepbrother Peter. Sisa, who is 22, still lives in the family home with Sarah and her mother. Peter, who is 24, has moved in with his partner but still lives locally. Sarah is artistic and likes drawing and photography. She has recently joined a photography group at school following encouragement by her art teacher who she likes. Sarah has got some insight into her difficulties and has decided that she does want help.

▼ Background

There has been a significant increase in the number of young people suffering from mental health problems (Young Minds, 2018). The number of children experiencing mental illness has now increased from one in ten in 2016 to one in six, with rates of attendance at Emergency Department for acts of self-harm rising (NHS Digital, 2021; Public Health England, 2016). Self-harming behaviours can increase the risk of a person committing suicide (Hawton et al., 2012). From April 2019 to March 2020, the National Child Mortality Database in 2021 found that 108 young people had killed themselves, equating to 1.8 per 100,000 of 9–17-year-olds, with suicides among boys slightly higher (2.2 per 100,000) when compared to girls (1.5 per 100,000) (Williams et al., 2021). In 80% of these cases the young person's ethnicity was recorded and from this figure 76% of the young people who ended their own life were of a white ethnic background and 21% from a Black, Asian, or mixed ethnicity. Moreover, sexual and gender minority adolescents also have higher rates of self-harm and attempted suicide compared to heterosexual adolescents (Litvin et al., 2020; Patalay and Fitzsimons, 2021). With the National Child Mortality Database (Williams et al., 2021) recording that 61% of these deaths took place in the home, it is imperative that mental health nurses support parents with knowledge and interventions which can be used to support their child who is self-harming.

Marsha Linehan established a therapy called dialectical behavioural therapy (DBT). Linehan first devised this therapy for adults following her own battle with BPD and later adapted DBT to support adolescents and their parents/carers (Miller et al., 2007). Linehan's approach is based on the biosocial DBT theory where self-harm is thought to be an emotional regulation coping strategy for those people who have a biological sensitivity to experiencing emotions when they are met with an invalidating environment (Neacsiu et al., 2014). For example, when a parent may say to a child, 'Why are you are overreacting?'

DBT is devised of a programme of individual therapy, group work, 24-hour phone coaching in a crisis, and a consult group for the therapists. Family members are included in the groups which consist of a skill-based programme focusing on mindfulness, distress tolerance, emotional regulation, interpersonal effectiveness, and walking the middle path (these are explained in Table 16.1). As part of the programme, a group called 'Walking the Middle Path' supports

Table 16.1 Characteristics of dysregulation and corresponding dialectical behavioural therapy skills modules

Some characteristics of dysregulation	DBT skills modules
Emotion dysregulation	**Emotional regulation**
Emotional vulnerability; emotional reactivity; emotional lability; angry outburst; steady negative emotional states such as depression, anger, shame, anxiety, and guilt; deficits in positive emotions and difficulty in modulating emotions	Learning how to name emotions, identify triggers, and develop problem-solving skills. Understanding how to self-validate and how to change emotions through techniques such as 'opposite urge' where the young person would act the opposite to the way they are feeling with the aim of changing a negative emotion to a positive feeling
Interpersonal dysregulation	**Interpersonal effectiveness**
Unstable relationships, interpersonal conflicts, chronic family disturbance, social isolation, efforts to avoid abandonment, and difficulties getting wants and needs met in relationships and maintaining one's self-respect in relationships	Here, the young person would learn how to respect their values, how to reach their goals, make and maintain relationships, set boundaries, and make assertive requests

(continued)

Table 16.1 Continued

Some characteristics of dysregulation	DBT skills modules
Behavioural dysregulation Impulsive behaviours such as cutting classes, blurting out in class, spending money, risky sexual behaviour, risky online behaviours, bingeing and/or purging, drug and alcohol abuse, aggressive behaviours, suicidal and non-suicidal self-injurious behaviour	**Distress tolerance** Learn skills of how to tolerate dysregulated emotions when an immediate solution is not apparent. These skills include: Distract with Wise Mind ACCEPTS (Activities, Contributing, Comparisons, Emotions, Pushing away, Thoughts, Sensations) Self-Soothe with Six Senses IMPROVE (Imagery, Meaning, Prayer, Relaxing, One thing in the moment, Vacation, Encouragement) the moment Pros and Cons TIPP (Temperature, Intense exercise, Paced breathing, Progressive relaxation)
Cognitive dysregulation and family conflict Non-dialectical thinking and acting (i.e. extreme polarized, or black-or-white thinking), poor perspective taking and conflict resolution, invalidation of self and others, difficulty in effectively influencing own and others' behaviours (i.e. obtaining desired changes)	**Walking the middle path** Here the young person and family members learn the importance of didactic thinking and the principles of behaviourism and how to change behaviour and use validation to improve relationships
Self-dysregulation Lacking awareness of emotions, thoughts, action urges; poor attentional control; unable to reduce one's suffering while also having difficulty accessing pleasure; identity confusion, sense of emptiness, and dissociation	**Core mindfulness** This is the core skill of DBT—the young person will understand how to observe, describe, and participate in the present moment without judgement and be effective and mindful in their reactions and interactions.

Reproduced with permission from Miller, A. L., Rathus, J. H. and Linehan, M. (2007). *Dialectical Behavior Therapy with Suicidal Adolescents*. Guilford Press, New York & London, Table 2.1, p. 36.

the young person and the parents to communicate effectively with one another through the understanding of dialectics, validation, and behaviourism. The facilitator helps the family to learn how they can problem-solve through respecting one another's point of view. While this is an intensive programme, there are techniques from this approach that the mental health nurse and the family can use to support the person in crisis (see Table 16.2 later in this chapter).

Table 16.2 Crisis plan

Crisis care plan for Sarah and her family

If you sometimes struggle with thoughts about harming yourself, follow the plan one step at a time until you are safe.
   Remember: **these feelings will pass**.

Keep copies of the plan where you can easily find them when you'll need it.

What I need to do to reduce the risk of me acting on thoughts about harming myself when I am feeling emotionally overwhelmed

- I will use the DBT skills I have learnt to manage my distress. Here, I will use some of my TIPP skills to change my body chemistry which helps me reduce my extreme emotion FAST!
- **'TIP my temperature'**: to calm down fast I will hold my breath, put my face in a bowl of cold water or cold pack and place this on my eyes and cheeks. I will do this for 30 seconds.
- **'Intense exercise'**: to calm down my body when it is revved up by emotion I engage in intense exercise and go running or walk really fast.
- **'Paced breathing'**: to pace my breathing by slowing it down I will breathe deep into my stomach and breathe out more slowly than I breathe in (5 seconds in and 7 seconds out).
- **'Paired muscle relaxation':** to calm down by pairing muscle relaxation with breathing out I will tense my body muscles when I breathe deep into my stomach. While breathing out I will say the work 'Relax' in my mind, I will get rid of the tension and notice the difference in my body.
- I know that one of the best things to do to manage these thoughts is being distracted by something/one else: I can use my distress tolerance skills—**WISE Mind ACCEPTS** with Activities. We can often be in one of these three states of mind: Emotional, Wise, and Reasonable. When in distress we are often in our emotional mind. Sarah will go into her Wise Mind and instead of reacting in emotional mind with unhealthy behaviours will concentrate on the following activities;
- I can draw.
- I can go out with my camera and take some pictures.
- I can ask someone in the photography club if they want to come out and take pictures with me.
- I can ask my sister Sisa to take me out somewhere.
- I can go and visit my brother Peter and his partner.
- I can ask mum if she would spend some time with me.
- I will **self-soothe with my six senses** and use the survival crisis kit I have made:
- Stress ball.
- Look at the album I have made with all my favourite places I have been and want to go.
- Watch my favourite movie: *The Goonies*.
- Listen to my favourite music that makes me feel better.
- Smell my mother's perfume which I have sprayed on my favourite material I like to touch and feel.
- Use my lavender hand lotion.
- If this does not work and I still want to harm myself I will let someone know when I am feeling like this. I will:
- Try and speak to my mum or my sister Sisa if I'm at home.
- If there is no one at home or I am outside I can phone my brother Peter or his partner.
- If I feel like I can't describe how I'm feeling to my family, I will use the traffic light system:
   Green = I'm ok; Amber = I might need extra support; Red = I'm struggling.
- Phone my mental health nurse and ask for skills coaching to stop me from self-harming.
- If I am at school, I can ask my teacher if I can call my nurse.
- If I don't think that I can keep myself safe, I will follow the plan on the back of this safety plan or go straight to the Accident and Emergency Department.

(*continued*)

Table 16.2 Continued

What I can do to help my mood in general:
- I need to make sure I attend my Appointment with my DBT mental health nurse.
- I also need to make sure I attend the weekly DBT skills group.
- If I need support to phone my mental health nurse for extra DBT skills coaching.
- If I want to be on my own, I understand that mum or Sisa may want to check on me.
- I will try to make new friends at the photography group.
- I will do things that I enjoy like art and photography.
- I will try and spend some time relaxing:
- Use my mindfulness app.
- Take a bath.
- Go for a walk.
- I will try and eat a balanced diet.
- I will try and get regular exercise.

Mum needs to ensure:
- All sharp objects, medications, and chemicals are locked away.
- That she keeps a close eye on me during this difficult time and has a low threshold for seeking additional advice from CAMHS.
- That she supports me in attending all of my CAMHS appointments and attends the 'Walking the Middle Path' DBT module.
- To show an interest on how my day has been and if I have a problem or difficulty not to minimize this but to listen and offer me support if I need it.
- Mum to spend time with me and do things we used to enjoy (cinema, picnics in the park) or new things that I enjoy (outings to take pictures and draw, exhibitions).

I need to be a cheerleader for myself:
- I will tell myself that I can make it through this and that I am resilient.
- I will remind myself that things **will** get better.

Emergency contact details

Monday to Friday 9 am to 5 pm	Contact my care coordinator in **CAMHS** If I cannot reach the CAMHS team and I am worried about my own safety, I can speak to my mum and/or telephone: • The CAMHS support line on ....……………… • My GP • NHS direct on 111 • Go to my local Accident and Emergency Department, **or** • Telephone 999
Other times (Anytime between 5 pm and 9 am during the week & from 5 pm on Friday to 9 am on Monday over the weekend and on bank holidays)	Outside of hours, if I need support or I am worried about my own or someone else's safety, I can speak to my mum and/or telephone: • The CAMHS support line on 0800 731 2864 • My GP • NHS direct on 111 • Samaritans on 08457 90 90 90 • Child line on 0800 1111 • Go to my local Accident and Emergency Department, OR • Telephone 999

▼ Behavioural interventions

Just under half of young people's first contact with mental health services is when presenting to the Emergency Department following an episode of self-harm. As we see in Sarah's story, some young people and their families would have experienced many difficulties beforehand. Sarah suffered from significant abuse, which is a predisposing factor for her self-harm, but the likely triggers for her current episode of self-harm is that she had no one to talk to about this experience, as well as being bullied at school. In an ideal situation, she would have received that support from her mother rather than her social worker. However, her relationship with her mother had become fragmented. Sarah's family had a traumatic past which can often be the cause of such relationship challenges (Fong et al., 2021). However, even parents who do not have such traumatic pasts, but whose child is emotionally dysregulated, will often find themselves in the same situation as Sarah's mother, where they feel helpless to support their child and have a sense they are often 'walking on eggshells'. What can often happen is that parents, in an attempt to support their child, invalidate their emotional experience by dismissing or minimizing how the situation was making their child feel. Parents attempting to solve the problem in this way will have a child respond as if they do not feel listened to or supported and this often causes the situation to escalate. Mental health nurses can help parents to understand that by validating their child's feelings through acknowledging that their feelings are genuine, and by understanding that this may be difficult for them, they will reduce the emotional intensity of their child's reaction. In this way, they can de-escalate the situation and continue the discussion, while offering support and advice regarding the cause of the initial outburst. Once the young person feels validated, the parent may be able to negotiate some form of compromise if a boundary has to be placed, such as when to be home from a party.

▼ Validation

For a continuation of the case study, see Box 16.4.

Box 16.4 Practice example

Sarah's clinician from the UCT can ask to meet with Sarah's mother separately to share with her some simple DBT techniques that will help validate Sarah's experience:

- When talking to Sarah, ensure Sarah's mother shows active listening skills by making eye contact with Sarah and staying focused.
- For Sarah's mother to be attentive to her own possible verbal and non-verbal reactions that Sarah could experience as invalidating.
- Sarah's mother to observe what Sarah is feeling in the moment and identify a word that describes that feeling.
- Sarah's mother to mirror, summarize, paraphrase, and reflect Sarah's feelings and experience back to her without judgement.
- Sarah's mother to be calm and show tolerance.

Reproduced from Rathus, J. H. and Miller, A. L. (2015). *DBT Skills Manual for Adolescents*. New York: Guilford Press.

Box 16.5 Practice example

For Sarah and her mother, spending positive time together could focus on Sarah's interests:

- TV shows on photography
- Accompanying Sarah to a place where she would like to take photographs
- Attend an exhibition on photography

- An activity they both enjoyed doing when Sarah was a child.

These activities will often be dependent on time and monies available to the parent but the important part is the that the parent carves out time and for the young person to be the parent's focus.

▼ Positive parenting strategies

In preparation for starting DBT when parents or carers attend services with a young person in crisis, they can start preparing by embracing some of the fundamentals and by starting to build a foundation to work on. They can do this by spending positive times together.

Spending positive times together

Often, as a child moves into adolescence, they spend more time independent of their parents. This can be part of normal behaviour and as a child moves into adulthood, they want to spend more time with their friends or concentrate on their studies so, for example, they may spend more time in their room. However, similarly to Sarah's story, when a family is going through a difficult time and communication has broken down between parent and child, there is often less time spent on ensuring positive times are spent together as each will often want to spend their time apart. Within this context, it is important for the mental health nurse to ensure that both the parent and young person understand the importance of spending time together and engage in activities they both enjoy (Box 16.5). Through this they can start to rebuild their relationship and have a firmer foundation when the next challenge arises that may test their relationship with one another.

A crisis plan can be developed by the mental health nurse with the young person and their family, and the family can help to implement the crisis plan following some psychoeducation from the nurse. An example of a crisis plan for Sarah is presented in Table 16.2.

▲ Conclusion

In this chapter we have given mental health nurses an understanding of the prevalence and causes of self-harm behaviours and completed suicide of young people in the UK. We have discussed the symptoms of BPD and the complexities of diagnosing young people with this health problem and have shared Linehan's behavioural patterns of BPD and the biosocial DBT theory. Then, through the use of a case study of Sarah, we showed mental health nurses how they can develop a crisis care plan by using a number of strategies from the DBT module which include how to validate and develop positive parenting.

✖ Tips from service users

1 The techniques do work. They sound simplistic and almost too easy but when you put them into practice, you will be amazed by the results.
2 Don't underestimate spending those 'positive times' with your child. It helps rebuild those ties that have become fractured and serves as a reserve for when the tough times come.
3 You are not alone. If you are able to attend 'Walking the middle path', meeting parents helps to realize that others need support as well and you can learn from one another.

W   Companion website

For extra resources on the topics covered in this chapter, visit the companion website at: www.oup.com/mhns

✚   References

Asarnow, J. R., Berk, M. S., Bedics, J., Adrian, M., Gallop, R., Cohen, J., Korslund, K., Hughes, J., Avina, C., Linehan, M. M., and McCauley, E. (2021). *Dialectical behaviour therapy for suicidal self-harming youth: emotion regulation, mechanisms, and mediators. Journal American Academic Child Adolescent Psychiatry 60(9), 1105–1115.*

Bellis, M. A., Hughes, K., Ford, K., Ramos Rodriguez, G., Sethi, D., and Passmore, J. (2019). *Life course health consequences and associated annual costs of adverse childhood experiences across Europe and North America: a systematic review and meta-analysis. Lancet Public Health 4(10), e517–e528.*

Brown, R. C. and Plener, P. L. (2017). *Non-suicidal self-injury in adolescence. Current Psychiatry Reports, 19(3), 20.*

Butera, C. (2014). *Brainstorm: the power and purpose of the teenage brain by Daniel J. Siegel M.D. International Journal of Adolescent Medicine and Health 26(3), 455.*

Chen, C. (2019). *Adverse childhood experiences and multidimensional perfectionism in young adults. Personality and Individual Differences 146, 53–57.*

Chen, W.-L. and Chun, C.-C. (2019). *Association between emotional dysregulation and distinct groups of non-suicidal self-injury in Taiwanese female adolescents. International Journal of Environmental Research and Public Health 16(18), 3361.*

Eyuboglu, M., Eyuboglu, D., Seval Caliskan, P., Oktar, D., Demirtas, Z., Arslantas, D., and Unsal, A. (2021). *Traditional school bullying and cyberbullying: prevalence, the effect on mental health problems and behaviour. Psychiatry Research 297, 113730.*

Fong, H.-F., Bennett, C. E., Mondestin, V., Scribano, P. V., Mollen, C., and Wood, J. N. (2021). *The impact of child sexual abuse discovery on caregivers and families:* a qualitative study. Journal of Interpersonal Violence 35(21–22), 4189–4215.

Hawton, K., Bergen, H., Kapur, N., Cooper, J., Steeg, S., Ness, J., and Waters, K. (2012). *Repetition of self-harm and suicide following self-harm in children and adolescents: findings from the Multicentre Study of Self-harm in England. Journal of Child Psychology and Psychiatry 53(12), 1212–1219.*

Linehan, M. M. (1993). *Cognitive Behavioural Treatment of Borderline Personality Disorder. New York: Guilford Press.*

Litvin, R., Trainor, G., and Dickinson, T. (2020). *Issues affecting trans⋆ young people: considerations for mental health nurses. Mental Health Practice 23(6), 14–21.*

Miller, A. L., Rathus, J. H., and Linehan, M. M. (2007). *Dialectical Behavior Therapy with Suicidal Adolescents. New York: Guilford Press.*

Neacsiu, A. D., Eberle, J. W., Kramer, R., Wiesmann, T., and Linehan, M. M. (2014). *Dialectical behavior therapy skills for transdiagnostic emotion dysregulation: a pilot randomized controlled trial. Behaviour Research and Therapy 59, 40–51.*

NHS Digital (2021). *Mental Health of Children and Young People in England 2021. Available at: https//digital.nhs.uk/data-and-infomration/publications/statistical/mental-health-of-children-and-young-people-in-england/2021-follow-up-to-the-2017-survey.*

Office for National Statistics (2020). *Mental Health of Children and Young People in the Pandemic. Available at: https://blog.ons.gov.uk. (Accessed: 25/05/2022).*

Patalay, P. and Fitzsimons, E. (2021). *Psychological distress, self-harm and attempted suicide in UK 17-year olds. British Journal of Psychiatry 219(2), 437–439.*

Peh, C. X., Shahwan, S., Fauziana, R., Mahesha, M., Sambasivam, R., Zhang, Y., How Ong, S., Chong, S. A., and Subrmaniam, M. (2017). *Emotion dysregulation as a mechanism linking child maltreatment exposure and self-harm behaviours in adolescents. Child Abuse & Neglect 67, 383–390.*

Public Health England (2016). *The Mental Health of children and Young People in England. Available at: https://assets.publishing.service.gov.uk/media/5a80c3e240f0b62305b8d06c/Mental_health_of_children_in_England.pdf*

Rathus, J. H. and Miller, A. L. (2015). *DBT Skills Manual for Adolescents. New York: Guilford Press.*

Williams, T., Stoianova, S., Sleap, V., Odd, D., Fleming, P. J., and Luyt, K. on behalf of the National Child Mortality Database (2021). *Child Review Data: Year Ending 31 March 2021. Bristol: National Child Mortality Database, University of Bristol.*

World Health Organization (1992). *The ICD-10 Classification of Mental and Behavioural Disorders. Geneva: World Health Organization.*

Young Minds (2018). *A New Era for Young People's Mental Health. Available at: https://www.youngminds.org.uk/media/5dilibjw/a-new-era-for-young-peoples-mental-health.pdf*

Key skills in working with children and young people

Annmarie Grealish   Gemma Trainor

Learning outcomes

By the end of this chapter, you should be able to:

1 Recognize the complexities of caring for children and young people's mental health

2 Discuss the effective communication skills with children and young people with mental health conditions

3 Identify key skills on how to talk to children and young people about their mental health

4 Apply patient-reported outcome measures for children and young people to explore, define, and clarify their condition(s) or problem(s).

▼ Introduction

This chapter aims to provide information on engagement, communication skills, and some practical suggestions that can make interactions with children and young people (CYP) more effective and efficient. The chapter is divided into two sections:

1 The first section provides information and practical suggestions on engagement and communication skills that enable you to talk to CYP about their mental health.

2 The second section describes assessment methods used in CYP's mental health and how the mental health nurse can help the child/young person to explore, define, and clarify their condition(s) or problem(s).

▼ Mental health of children and young people

Mental health problems are the most important single group of disorders in CYP aged 10–19 and contribute to almost half of all burden of disease in this age group (Gore et al., 2011; McGorry et al., 2013; Polanczyk et al., 2015). The World Health Organization (2021) found that 13% of young people globally aged 10–19 experience a mental health problem which is a critical point of biological, intellectual, and social development and called for the scaling up of efforts to promote improvements in mental well-being in young people. Young people's mental health is a key priority, and represents the main threat to the health, survival, future potential, and productivity of young people around the world (McGorry et al., 2022). Almost one in seven young people meet the diagnostic criteria for a mental health condition (Polanczyk et al., 2015) and 50% of all lifetime mental health disorders (classified by the *Diagnostic and Statistical Manual of Mental Disorders*, fourth edition) first emerge by 14 years and 75% by 24 years of age (Kessler et al., 2005). However, this landscape appears to have worsened since the start of the COVID-19 pandemic (Czeisler et al., 2020). NHS Digital (2020) found that one in six (16%) children aged between 5 and 16 years in England had a probable mental illness in 2020 which represents a 5% rise from one in nine children in 2017. This study was conducted in July 2020 during the COVID-19 pandemic when government-enacted nationwide or localized lockdowns were in force, which gave rise to increased cases of poor mental health in CYP. A recent report by Young Minds (2021) found that 80% of young people with mental health needs agreed that the COVID-19 pandemic had made their mental health worse and less than one in three received access to NHS care and treatment. The emotional legacy of COVID-19 gave rise to increased cases of mental health conditions in CYP such as panic disorders, general anxiety, and social anxiety disorders, which can often persist as long-term mental health problems into adulthood (Lehmann et al., 2021; Schmidt et al., 2021; Stevanovic et al., 2022).

Progression of mental health conditions in CYP is associated with higher costs to public services including health, social care, and criminal justice, creating a substantial global socioeconomic burden (McGorry et al., 2022; Pompili et al., 2012). Untreated mental health problems in CYP can have serious adverse effects on relationships, education, health, economic, and social outcomes and is related to higher levels of drug abuse, self-harm, and suicidal behaviour which can often persist into adulthood (McGorry et al., 2013; Pompili et al., 2012; Riegler et al., 2017). Considering that this is a vulnerable period for the onset of mental health problems, the importance of early detection and prompt access to professional treatment is vital. Mental health care systems are failing to identify and meet the growing demands for CYP's mental health needs; less than two-thirds of young people and their families access any professional help (Sadler et al., 2018; Scottish Parliament, 2018; Radez et al., 2021). It is estimated that 70% of CYP under the age of 19 with mental health problems have not had appropriate interventions at a sufficiently early age resulting in treatment only when they have become more complex or developed severe secondary disorders in adulthood (Birchwood et al., 2013; Gore et al., 2011; Reardon et al., 2017; Yap et al., 2013).

Despite commitment to improved access to mental health services for CYP, difficulties in accessing appropriate mental health facilities and provisions continue to persist and remain limited (Department of Health and NHS England, 2015; Ougrin et al., 2018; Patel et al., 2018). The UK *Future in Mind* report (Department of Health and NHS England, 2015) declared that this contributes to the pressure of escalating referrals, increased complexity, and rise in lengths of stay in inpatient care. Such was the level of need and concern, this report provided recommendations on how to improve mental health services for CYP and subsequently £1.5 billion of additional investment was provided over a 5-year period.

▼ Effective communication skills with children and young people with mental health conditions

Effective communication skills

When a child/young person experience a mental health problem, the mental health nurse is called upon to understand what happened to the person, how their strengths and resilience can be regained or improved, and how to support their recovery. Engagement permeates all aspects of nursing care. Engagement is considered a central activity and a high priority for nurses' clinical practice so that they can be competent in their holistic assessment and decision-making. Mental health nurses are expected to be competent in conducting a robust assessment so that they provide holistic and effective mental health care. Collecting relevant cues is an essential part of the assessment, as it is not possible to understand the person's problem(s) or condition(s) without this information. The therapeutic relationship has long been emphasized as a critical element of the assessment process and for treatment participation. It can help the nurse to better develop a detailed and shared understanding of the person's context, presenting problem(s) or condition(s), and can make interactions with CYP more effective and efficient.

Effective communication has been identified as an important indicator of quality of care as well as increasing patient satisfaction, adherence, and competency, and leading to a higher quality of life (Ditton-Phare et al., 2017; Flückiger et al., 2020; Lee et al., 2020; Papageorgiou et al., 2017). Communication skills are paramount to the therapeutic alliance (see Chapter 6), but this is often a factor neglected by healthcare professionals working with CYP (Hartley et al., 2022). Consequently, interpersonal and communication skills are one of the Nursing and Midwifery Council's (2018) core competencies with the goal for all nurses to communicate effectively using a wide range of strategies and interventions including the effective use of communication technologies.

Effective communication skills are paramount in providing high-quality care, as it allows the nurse to solicit the relevant mental health history to understand the person's concerns, generate a differential, build in-depth collaborative assessment, and then facilitate a discussion to engage the family in a shared decision-making process on the next steps in management. These communication skills include a combination of both verbal and non-verbal skills to help the nurse establish and sustain an effective working relationship with the person and allow the nurse the development of trust, and to obtain in-depth information on the person's experiences and presenting problem(s). It also stimulates the person's participation and collaboration, increases the reliability of the collected information, and makes the consultation more effective.

How to talk to children and young people about their mental health

This section describes some effective strategies that nurses can utilize to enable the child/young person to tell their story and explore their symptoms, emotion(s), or problem(s). An essential part of effective communication skills is to develop an understanding of the person's story (see case study in Box 17.1). Without good information it will not be possible to understand the person's problem(s), support the person to explore their experience, develop an understanding of their experience,

and develop strategies to enhance and maintain wellness. The best way to support the child/young person to tell their story and elicit information is making a 'human connection' (Sischy, 2006), asking 'careful' questions, and using psychotherapeutic skills, empathy, and reflective listening. It is also important for nurses to work constructively to engage parents or carers as a resource in the assessment and treatment of the child/young person (Brown, 2020). This chapter outlines some useful communication skills that are fundamental tenets of the therapeutic alliance, which is the strongest predictor of good treatment outcomes, no matter what intervention model or approach is utilized (Gergov et al., 2021; Hartley et al., 2022).

Specific interpersonal skills

The specific interpersonal skills in Table 17.1 need to be combined with the four-step model of relationship-building communication using the acronym PEARLS (Williamson, 2011), non-verbal-communication cues (Argyle, 1988) and awareness of these cues using the acronym SOLER (Egan, 1975), or SURETY (Stickley, 2011). It is paramount that an assessment interview should be conducted in a private room, with both the child/young person and the nurse comfortably seated in chairs of equal height, without being separated by a desk or table.

Box 17.1 Practice example: Tom

Tom is a 15-year-old boy who is living with generalized anxiety with some symptoms of low mood. Tom lives with his parents and brother Mark aged 12. Following his father's redundancy, the family had to move many miles away from home. Being away from their family and friends has placed strain on Tom who has found it difficult to cope and make new friends. Tom also misses his paternal grandfather who he spent a lot of time with—he found the talks they had helpful and supportive.

Since starting the new school, concerns have been raised by Tom's teachers that he has been struggling to settle in. They have reported that Tom seems to be quite tense in class and is often seen with what appears to be a worried expression on his face. They also noticed that Tom struggles to concentrate and appears to be very tired at times. However, his teachers' main concern is that Tom is often absent from class. He is

either late or asks on numerous occasions to use the toilet and/or to see the school nurse. Tom often complaints of stomach-ache, headache, and chest pain, while appearing to be quite breathless and sweaty.

Tom's mother admitted that it had gotten worse following the move, and that she struggles to get him into school. She said that he often has trouble sleeping, and lies in his bed for hours before finally going to sleep. When he finally falls asleep, he wakes up due to having a nightmare.

Consider the key engagement skills you would use to help Tom to talk about his mental health:

1 What kind of things might you want to know more about from Tom, his mother, and his brother?

2 Consider how you might map the elements of assessment process and the specific PROMs in Table 17.2.

Table 17.1 Four-step model of relationship-building communication

PEARLS	SOLER	SURETY
Partnership	**S**: Sit squarely to the person	**S**: Sit at an angle to the client
Empathy	**O**: Open posture, not crossing your arms or legs	**U**: Uncross legs and arms, shows openness
Acknowledgement		**R**: Relax, not too relaxed or too overconcerned
Respect	**L**: Lean slightly forward	**E**: Eye contact, not staring
Legitimization	**E**: Maintain Eye contact without staring.	**T**: Touch, appropriate use shows area is a safe zone
	R: Relax	**Y**: Your intuition, trust your own intuition

Source: data from Williamson (2011), Egan (1975), and Stickley (2011).

Talking to children and young people about their mental health

Open-ended questions

Using open broad questions, particularly in the early stage of the assessment, encourages the person to freely tell their story and aids connection and conversations. This gives the nurse time and space to listen and think about the child/young person's story, emotions, and problem(s), for example:

- How does that make you feel?
- Is something making you scared/sad?
- Can you tell me more …?
- May I ask why you think or believer that …?

Thinking about the 'six Ws' is also a useful framework for questioning (Figure 17.1)—**W**hat, **W**here, **W**hen, **W**hy, **W**ith, and **W**hom, allows the person to answer your questions in an open way.

Closed questions

Closed questions can discourage the person from talking, therefore, they should be used after the person's presenting

problem(s) has been explored and a good therapeutic alliance has been established. These are useful if skilfully used to investigate specific areas and to analyse symptoms in detail, as they imply a yes/no answer or a forced choice between two or more options, for example:

- Do you feel stressed about going home?
- Did you enjoy …?

Verbal and non-verbal cues

These can improve the therapeutic alliance with the child/young person. Games, vignettes, drawing, or using toys to act out emotions can help the child/young person to express feelings without words and teaches them to recognize other people's feelings, see Figure 17.2—the LinkyThinks 'How Do I Feel?' Wheel (https://www.linkythinks.com/). This wheel, with moving dials to help children pinpoint words and images that reflect their inner thoughts and outer behaviours, is an interactive, colourful emotions wheel, designed to help children process and communicate difficult feelings using words and images. Emotional literacy and self-awareness play an important role in supporting mental health. For children, both at home and at school, experiencing feelings for the first time can be confusing and difficult to explain, and typically children are encouraged to use language and terms that appeal to the understanding of a parent, teacher, or adult. The 'How Do I Feel?' Wheel gives CYP better agency over their mental health language, allowing them to communicate their feelings more on their own terms. Observing verbal and non-verbal cues also helps the nurse to pick up on the person's body language, facial expression, eye contact, tone of voice, and tune in to their possible meaning.

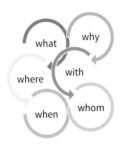

Figure 17.1 The 'six Ws' for open questions

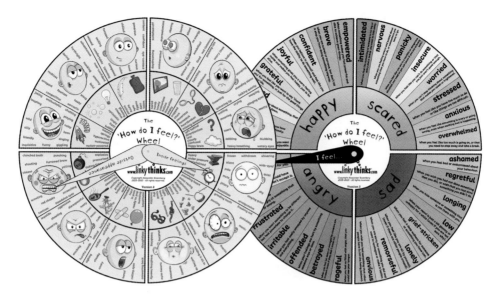

Figure 17.2   The LinkyThinks 'How Do I Feel?' Wheel

Listening (active, reflective)

Reflective listening helps to seek confirmation and determine the meaning of what you have heard. This reinforces the therapeutic alliance, for example:

- So, it sounds like you feel very angry about …
- I think I hear you saying you feel sad because of …
- I get a sense that …
- Help me to understand this, on the one hand you … and on the other hand …

Listening is more important than speaking especially when trying to give the child/young person the space and a voice to think about things that they may have not previously disclosed. Listen with your eyes and by listening attentively, this enables the person to complete statements without interruption and leaves space to think before answering or proceed after pausing. This can guide the person through their storytelling. Remember, there is little benefit in asking questions if you are unable to listen properly to the answers.

Passive listening (non-verbal responses)

Passive listening includes the appropriate use of silence and use of non-verbal and verbal facilitation. For example, nodding, use of eye contact, adopting an attentive posture, shaking your head, and facial expressions. Try not to interrupt, your role is to facilitate talk so the use of pauses, brief silence, and waiting time helps the person to express thoughts or feelings

that are occurring inside their mind, which can facilitate the person to tell you more.

Responding

Facilitating the child/young person's responses verbally and non-verbally indicates to the person that you are interested in what they are saying. For example, nodding your head, smiling, silence, or saying 'Ok', 'Uh-huh', 'Ah', 'I see', 'Go on', and 'What happened next?' Instead of offering solutions, help the child/young person to identify options. Solutions suggested or imposed by adults are often short term, resisted or agreed by the child/young person to maintain the therapeutic alliance or please the adult. Active listening will help the child/young person to find their own way, feel heard, understood, and supported, identify options, and decide on a course of actions. See Figure 17.3 for specific techniques for responding.

Reformulation

This strategy lies between data gathering and information giving. Reformulation is mostly related to the content expressed and combines elements of clarification, facilitation, and summarizing (Figure 17.3). Here you are adding something new or therapeutic messages, for example showing the linkage between events and emotions:

Child/young person: 'I am afraid … what happens if I can't breathe in the classroom or get another panic attack?'

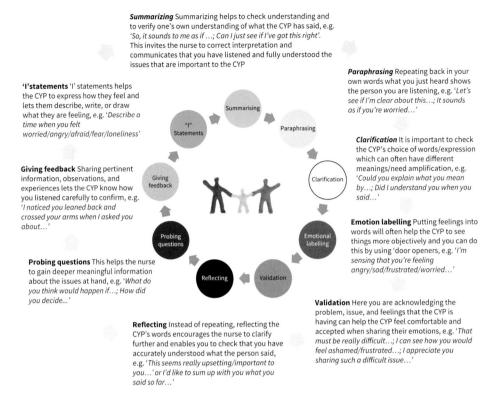

Summarizing Summarizing helps to check understanding and to verify one's own understanding of what the CYP has said, e.g. *'So, it sounds to me as if …; Can I just see if I've got this right'.* This invites the nurse to correct interpretation and communicates that you have listened and fully understood the issues that are important to the CYP

'I'statements 'I' statements helps the CYP to express how they feel and lets them describe, write, or draw what they are feeling, e.g. *'Describe a time when you felt worried/angry/afraid/fear/loneliness'*

Giving feedback Sharing pertinent information, observations, and experiences lets the CYP know how you listened carefully to confirm, e.g. *'I noticed you leaned back and crossed your arms when I asked you about…'*

Probing questions This helps the nurse to gain deeper meaningful information about the issues at hand, e.g. *'What do you think would happen if…; How did you decide…'*

Reflecting Instead of repeating, reflecting the CYP's words encourages the nurse to clarify further and enables you to check that you have accurately understood what the person said, e.g. *'This seems really upsetting/important to you…' or I'd like to sum up with you what you said so far…'*

Paraphrasing Repeating back in your own words what you just heard shows the person you are listening, e.g. *'Let's see if I'm clear about this…; It sounds as if you're worried…'*

Clarification It is important to check the CYP's choice of words/expression which can often have different meanings/need amplification, e.g. *'Could you explain what you mean by…; Did I understand you when you said…'*

Emotion labelling Putting feelings into words will often help the CYP to see things more objectively and you can do this by using 'door openers, e.g. *'I'm sensing that you're feeling angry/sad/frustrated/worried…'*

Validation Here you are acknowledging the problem, issue, and feelings that the CYP is having can help the CYP feel comfortable and accepted when sharing their emotions, e.g. *'That must be really difficult…; I can see how you would feel ashamed/frustrated…; I appreciate you sharing such a difficult issue…'*

Figure 17.3 Specific techniques for responding

Nurse: 'What you are telling me is that you are afraid that you might experience another panic attack in the classroom …'

Patient-reported outcome measures for children and young people

Patient-reported outcome measures (PROMs) were initially developed as standardized, validated questionnaires to monitor outcomes in clinical trials and research studies but are now used in routine clinical practice to assess the presence, severity, frequency, duration, and treatment outcomes for specific mental health conditions (Department of Health, 2011; Thapa Bajgain et al., 2023). The use of PROMs to review treatment progress in Child and Adolescent Mental Health Services (CAMHS) is an evidence-based intervention and are recommended by the Department of Health (2011). PROMs can help to explore, define, and clarify the child/young person's condition(s) or problem(s). There are calls to increase the use of PROMs in CAMHS as they can be used to measure effectiveness in healthcare delivery and place the child/young person at the centre of their healthcare (Dawson et al., 2010; Wolpert et al., 2012). Despite the recommendation by the CAMHS Outcome Research Consortium in 2006 to introduce routine

outcome monitoring into CAMHS (Ford et al., 2006), their use in CAMHS remains persistently low and neglected (Batty et al., 2013; Edbrooke-Childs et al., 2017; Morris et al., 2021).

PROMs can be used in CAMHS during the assessment phase, to monitor and review treatment progress and in the termination phase of treatment. PROMs can be used to help nurses understand the child/young person's reasons for attending CAMHS, their presenting problems, and their goals for treatment or intervention. These tools generate quantifiable measures of human experiences and can build up a picture of the presenting problems and concerns faced by the child/young person with mental health problems. The nurse in collaboration with the young person can then determine a problem formulation, which will determine a treatment or intervention regime. PROMs can also be used to review treatment progress and the child/young person's experience of care and services. This can help the nurse to monitor any change in symptoms and progress to determine whether further interventions are required, and to examine the closing stages of treatment or intervention. PROMs have the advantage of being relatively quick to deliver and review the characteristics and severity of the child/young person's thoughts, feelings, and actions. However, despite the large variety of assessment tools (Table 17.2), optimizing mental health is reliant, first and foremost, on the way that a child/young person's symptoms are assessed.

Table 17.2 Specific PROMs used in mental health assessment for children and young people

Subject	PROMs
General functioning	• The Children's Global Assessment Scale (C-GAS) • The Strengths and Difficulties Questionnaires (SDQ) • The Health of the Nation Outcome Scales for Children and Adolescents (HoNOSCA) • Behavior Assessment System for Children • Behavioural and Emotional Rating Scale
Depression	• Revised Children's Anxiety and Depression Scale (RCADS) • The Beck Youth Inventories (BYI) • Patient Health Questionnaire (PHQ-9)
Anxiety	• Revised Children's Anxiety and Depression Scale (RCADS19) • The Spence Children's Anxiety Scale (SCAS20) • Generalized Anxiety Disorder Assessment (GAD-7) • Liebowitz Social Anxiety Scale (LSAS) • The Social Anxiety Scale for Adolescents (SAS-A)
Psychosis	• The Prodromal Questionnaire—Brief (PQ-B) • Youth Psychosis At-Risk Questionnaire—Brief (YPARQ-B) • The Kiddie Version of the Positive and Negative Symptoms of Schizophrenia (K-PANSS) • Thought Control Questionnaire (TCQ)
Bipolar disorder	• The Young Mania Rating Scale (Y-MRS) • Mood and Feelings Questionnaire (MFQ)
Addiction	• Adolescent Relapse Coping Questionnaire • The Drug and Alcohol Problem (DAP) Quickscreen • The CRAFFT 2.1
Suicide risk	• Suicide Behaviors Questionnaire-Revised (SBQ-R) • Suicidal Ideation Questionnaire (SIQ)
Post-traumatic stress disorder and trauma	• Clinician-Administered PTSD Scale for DSM-5—Child/Adolescent Version (CAPS-CA-5) • Child Revised Impact of Events Scale (CRIES-8/CRIES-13)
Eating disorders	• Eating Disorder Examination Questionnaire (EDE-Q) • Eating Attitude Test (EAT12; EAT26) • Eating Disorder Inventory for Children (EDI-C) • The SCOFF questionnaire
Obsessive–compulsive disorder	• Child Yale-Brown Obsessive–Compulsive Scale (CY-BOCS) • The Obsessive–Compulsive Inventory—Children's Version (OCI-CV)

Link to the Child Outcomes Research Consortium (CORC) for data relating to mental health and well-being outcomes: https://www.corc.uk.net/about-corc/

▲ Conclusion

This chapter provides an overview of mental health difficulties of CYP and the key skills for nurses on how to talk to CYP about their mental health. This process is a combination of intuitive and effective communication skills, which requires open-mindedness, empathy, holism, and reflection on presuppositions. The process of how to talk to CYP about their mental health and to assess their mental health needs, requires, firstly, a foundation of specific and professional knowledge, and, secondly, shared decision-making as an underpinning value for the professional approach. A therapeutic validating relationship as well as specific communication skills with the young person are both essential.

✖ Tips from service users

1 Please let me explain what's happening in my own way and listen to what I am saying.
2 Provide me with a safe space to talk and be myself, please do not diagnose me, talk over me, or judge me without knowing the facts.
3 Do not pretend you know how I am feeling or worse still suggest your own coping strategies as something I should try.

W   Companion website

For extra resources on the topics covered in this chapter, visit the companion website at: www.oup.com/mhns

➕   References

Argyle, M. (1988). *Bodily Communication, 2nd ed.* Madison, CT: International Universities Press.

Batty, M. J., Moldavsky, M., Foroushani, P. S., Pass, S., Marriott, M., Sayal, K., and Chris, H. (2013). *Implementing routine outcome measures in child and adolescent mental health services: from present to future practice. Child and Adolescent Mental Health 18(2), 82–87.*

Birchwood, M. and Singh, S. P. (2013). *Mental health services for young people: matching the service to the need. British Journal of Psychiatry 202(Suppl. 54), s1–s2.*

Brown, J. (2020). *Engaging with parents in child and adolescent mental health services. Australian and New Zealand Journal of Family Therapy 41(2), 145–160.*

Czeisler, M. É., Lane, R. I., Petrosky, E., Wiley, J. F., Christensen, A., Njai, R., Weaver, M. D., Robbins, R., Facer-Childs, E. R., Barger, L. K., Czeisler, C. A.,

Howard, M. E., & Rajaratnam, S. (2020). *Mental health, substance use, and suicidal ideation during the COVID-19 Pandemic—United States, June 24–30, 2020. MMWR: Morbidity and Mortality Weekly Report 69(32), 1049–1057.*

Dawson, J., Doll, H., Fitzpatrick, R., Jenkinson, C., and Carr, A. J. (2010). *The routine use of patient reported outcome measures in healthcare settings. BMJ 340, c186.*

Department of Health (2011). *Talking Therapies: A Four-Year Plan of Action. London: Department of Health.*

Department of Health and NHS England. (2015). *Future in Mind: Promoting, Protecting and Improving our CYP's Mental Health and Wellbeing. Gov.uk. Available at: https://assets.publishing.service.gov.uk/government/uploads/system/uploads/attachment_data/file/414024/Childrens_Mental_Health.pdf*

Department of Health (2011). *Talking therapies: A four-year plan of action. London: Department of Health*

Ditton-Phare, P., Loughland, C., Duvivier, R., and Kelly, B. (2017). *Communication skills in the training of psychiatrists: a systematic review of current approaches. Australian and New Zealand Journal of Psychiatry 51(7), 675–692.*

Edbrooke-Childs, J., Barry, D., Mateos Rodriguez, I., Papageorgiou, D., Wolpert, M., and Schulz, J. (2017). *Patient reported outcome measures in child and adolescent mental health services: associations between clinician demographic characteristics, attitudes, and efficacy. Child and Adolescent Mental Health 22(1), 36–41.*

Egan, G. (1975). *The Skilled Helper: A Systematic Approach to Effective Helping. Pacific Grove, CA: Brooks/ Cole.*

Flückiger, C., Del Re, A. C., Wlodasch, D., Horvath, A., Solomonov, N., and Wampold, B. (2020). *Assessing the alliance-outcome association adjusted for patient characteristics and treatment processes: a meta-analytic summary of direct comparisons. Journal of Counseling Psychology 67(6), 706–711.*

Ford, T., Tingay, K., Wolpert, M., and CORC Steering Group (2006). *CORC's Survey of Routine Outcome Monitoring and National CAMHS Dataset Developments: A Response to Johnston and Gower. Child and Adolescent Mental Health 11(1), 50–52. https://doi.org/10.1111/ j.1475-3588.2005.00390.x*

Gergov, V., Marttunen, M., Lindberg, N., Lipsanen, J., and Lahti, J. (2021). *Therapeutic alliance: a comparison study between adolescent patients and their therapists. International Journal of Environmental Research and Public Health 18(21), 11238.*

Gore, F. M., Bloem, P. J., Patton, G. C., Ferguson, J., Jospeh, V., Coffey, C., Sawyer, S. M., and Mathers, C. D. (2011). *Global burden of disease in young people aged 10–24 years: a systematic analysis. Lancet 377(9783), 2093–2102.*

Hartley, S., Redmond, T., and Berry, K. (2022). *Therapeutic relationships within child and adolescent mental health inpatient services: a qualitative exploration of the experiences of young people, family members and nursing staff. PLoS One 17(1), e0262070.*

Kessler, R. C., Berglund, P., Demler, O., Jin, R., Merikangas, K. R., and Walters, E. E. (2005). *Lifetime prevalence and age-of-onset distributions of DSM-IV disorders in the National Comorbidity Survey Replication. Archives of General Psychiatry 62(6), 593–602.*

Lee, T., Cui, J., Rosario, H., Hilmara, D., Samuelson, K., Lin, E. C., Miller, V. A., and Lin, H. C. (2020). *Assessment of caregiver expectations of physician communication in a pediatric setting. BMC Health Services Research 20(1), 408.*

Lehmann, J., Lechner, V., and Scheithauer, H. (2021). *School closures during the COVID-19 pandemic: psychosocial outcomes in children—a systematic review. International Journal of Developmental Science 15(3–4), 85–111.*

McGorry, P. D., Bates, T., and Birchwood, M. (2013). *Designing youth mental health services for the 21st century: examples from Australia, Ireland and the UK. British Journal of Psychiatry 54, s30–s35.*

McGorry, P. D., Mei, C., Chanen, A., Hodges, C., Alvarez-Jimenez, M., and Killackey, E. (2022). *Designing and scaling up integrated youth mental health care. World Psychiatry: Official Journal of the World Psychiatric Association (WPA) 21(1), 61–76. https://doi.org/10.1002/ wps.20938*

Morris, A. C., Macdonald, A., Moghraby, O., Stringaris, A., Hayes, R. D., Simonoff, E., Ford, T., and Downs, J. M. (2021). *Sociodemographic factors associated with routine outcome monitoring: a historical cohort study of 28,382 young people accessing child and adolescent mental health services. Child and Adolescent Mental Health 26(1), 56–64.*

NHS Digital (2020). *Mental Health of CYP in England, 2020: Wave 1 Follow Up to the 2017 Survey. Available at: https://digital.nhs.uk/data-and-information/publicati ons/statistical/mental-health-of-children-and-young-people-in-england/2020-wave-1-follow-up*

Nursing and Midwifery Council (2018). *Future Nurse: Standards of Proficiency for Registered Nurses. Available at: https://www.nmc.org.uk/globalassets/sitedocume nts/standards-of-proficiency/nurses/future-nurse-profic iencies.pdf*

Ougrin, D., Corrigall, R., Poole, J., Zundel, T., Sarhane, M., Slater, V., Stahl, D., Reavey, P., Byford, S., Heslin, M., Ivens, J., Crommelin, M., Abdulla, Z., Hayes, D., Middleton, K., Nnadi, B., & Taylor, E. (2018). *Comparison of effectiveness and cost-effectiveness of an intensive community supported discharge service versus treatment as usual for adolescents with psychiatric emergencies: a randomised controlled trial. Lancet Psychiatry 5(6), 477–485.*

Papageorgiou, A., Loke, Y. K., and Fromage, M. (2017). *Communication skills training for mental health professionals working with people with severe mental illness. Cochrane Database of Systematic Reviews 6(6), CD010006.*

Patel, V., Saxena, S., Lund, C., Thornicroft, G., Baingana, F., Bolton, P., Chisholm, D., Collins, P. Y., Cooper, J. L., Eaton, J., Herrman, H., Herzallah, M. M., Huang, Y., Jordans, M. J. D., Kleinman, A., Medina-Mora, M. E., Morgan, E., Niaz, U., Omigbodun, O., . . . Unützer, J. (2018). *The Lancet Commission on global mental health and sustainable development. Lancet 392(10157), 1553–1598.*

Polanczyk, G. V., Salum, G. A., Sugaya, L. S., Caye, A., and Rohde, L. A. (2015). *Annual research review: a meta-analysis of the worldwide prevalence of mental disorders in children and adolescents. Journal of Child Psychology and Psychiatry and Allied Disciplines 56(3), 345–365.*

Pompili, M., Serafini, G., Innamorati, M., Biondi, M., Siracusano, A., Di Giannantonio, M., Giupponi, G., Amore, M., Lester, D., Girardi, P., and Möller-Leimkühler, A. M. (2012). *Substance abuse and suicide risk among adolescents. European Archives of Psychiatry and Clinical Neuroscience 262(6), 469–485.*

Radez, J., Reardon, T., Creswell, C., Lawrence, P. J., Evdoka-Burton, G., and Waite, P. (2021). *Why do children and adolescents (not) seek and access professional help for their mental health problems? A systematic review of quantitative and qualitative studies. European Child and Adolescent Psychiatry 30(2), 183–211.*

Reardon, T., Harvey, K., Baranowska, M., O'Brien, D., Smith, L., and Creswell, C. (2017). *What do parents perceive are the barriers and facilitators to accessing psychological treatment for mental health problems in children and adolescents? A systematic review of qualitative and quantitative studies. European Child and Adolescent Psychiatry 26(6), 623–647.*

Riegler, A., Völkl-Kernstock, S., Lesch, O., Walter, H., and Skala, K. (2017). *Attention deficit hyperactivity disorder and substance abuse: an investigation in young Austrian males. Journal of Affective Disorders 217, 60–65.*

Sadler, K., Vizard, T., Ford, T., Goodman, A., Goodman, R., and McManus, S. (2018) *Mental Health of CYP in England, 2017: Trends and Characteristics. Leeds: NHS Digital.*

Scottish Parliament (2018). *Public Audit and Post-legislative Scrutiny Committee. Available at: http://www.parliament.scot/parliamentarybusiness/report.aspx?r=11695&mode=pdf*

Schmidt, S. J., Barblan, L. P., Lory, I., and Landolt, M. A. (2021). *Age-related effects of the COVID-19 pandemic on mental health of children and adolescents. European Journal of Psychotraumatology 12(1), 1901407.*

Sischy, D. (2006). *Young People's Experiences of Relationships with Staff and Peers in Adolescent Inpatient Units. Doctoral thesis, University College London. Available at: https://discovery.ucl.ac.uk/id/eprint/1445090*

Stevanovic, D., Kabukcu Basay, B., Basay, O., Leskauskas, D., Nussbaum, L., and Zirakashvili, M. (2022). *COVID-19 pandemic-related aspects and predictors of emotional and behavioural symptoms in youth with pre-existing mental health conditions: results from Georgia, Lithuania, Romania, Serbia, and Turkey. Nordic Journal of Psychiatry 76(7), 515–522.*

Stickley, T. (2011). *From SOLER to SURETY for effective non-verbal communication. Nurse Education in Practice 11(6), 395–398.*

Thapa Bajgain, K., Amarbayan, M., Wittevrongel, K., McCabe, E., Naqvi, S. F., Tang, K., Aghajafari, F., Zwicker, J. D., and Santana, M. (2023). *Patient-reported outcome measures used to improve youth mental health services: a systematic review. Journal of Patient-Reported Outcomes 7(1), 14. https://doi.org/10.1186/s41687-023-00556-0*

Williamson, P. (2011). *A 4-step model of relationship-centered communication. In: A. Suchman, D. Sluyter, and P. Williamson, Eds., Leading Change in Healthcare: Transforming Organizations Using Complexity, Positive Psychology and Relationship Centered Care, pp. 311–318. Oxford: Radcliffe Publishing.*

Wolpert, M., Ford, T., Trustam, E., Law, D., Deighton, J., Flannery, H., and Fugard, A. (2012). *Patient reported outcomes in child and adolescent mental health services (CAMHS): use of idiographic and standardized measures. Journal of Mental Health 21(2), 165–173.*

World Health Organisation. (2021). *Adolescent mental health. Retrieved from https://www.who.int/news-room/fact-sheets/detail/adolescent-mental-health*

Yap, M. B., Reavley, N., and Jorm, A. F. (2013). *Where would young people seek help for mental disorders and what stops them? Findings from an Australian national survey. Journal of Affective Disorders 147(1–3), 255–261.*

Young Minds (2021). *Coronavirus: Impact on Young People with Mental Health Needs. Available at: https://www.youngminds.org.uk/media/esifqn3z/youngminds-coronavirus-report-jan-2021.pdf*

Key skills in working with people living with neurodevelopmental disorders

Jane Sedgwick-Müller

Learning outcomes

By the end of this chapter, you should be able to:

1 Interpret clinical and practical guidance for working with Attention Deficit Hyperactivity Disorder (ADHD) and Autism Spectrum Disorder (ASD)

2 Apply recommended screening tools to identify indicators of ADHD and ASD

3 Recognize when to refer service users with indicators of ADHD and ASD to specialist NHS services for further evaluation and treatment

4 Apply evidence-based knowledge and skills when working with ADHD and ASD

▼ Introduction

There are decades of research about childhood Attention Deficit Hyperactivity Disorder (ADHD) and Autism Spectrum Disorder (ASD) and well-established education, health, and social care services. This is not the same for adults where research and service provision is still in its infancy, owing to incorrect assumptions about neurodevelopmental disorders (NDDs) in childhood, such as ADHD and ASD, not persisting into adulthood. This is no longer the case because ADHD and ASD were reconceptualized as lifespan disorders in current versions of the *International Classification of Diseases*, 11th revision (ICD-11) (World Health Organization, 2019) and the *Diagnostic and Statistical Manual of Mental Disorders*, fifth edition, text revision (DSM-5-TR) (American Psychiatric Association, 2022), which are both used in the UK to diagnose NDDs. ADHD and ASD are the most prominent NDDs. Mental health nurses working in all contexts are likely to encounter service users with these disorders, and the knowledge and skills required to cater for their needs are discussed in this chapter.

▼ The evidence base: neurodevelopmental disorders versus neurodiversity

Developing skills for working with service users with ADHD and ASD begins by understanding the theory related to these disorders. NDDs arise from disturbances in the early maturation processes of neural architecture and connectivity, which causes neuroatypical expressions of thought, learning ability, memory, emotion, and self-control. NDDs are 'a group of conditions with an onset in the early developmental period, characterized by developmental deficits that produce

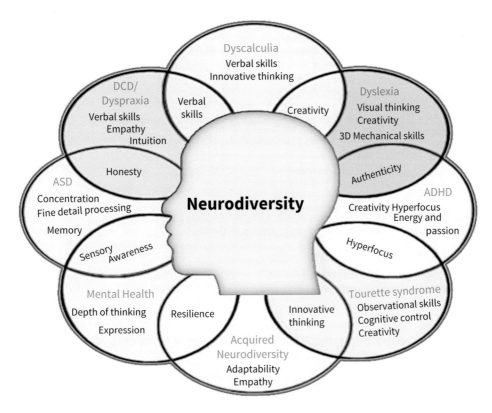

Figure 18.1 Model of neurodiversity: differences and overlapping strengths

Adapted with permission from Doyle, N. (2020). The world needs neurodiversity: unusual times call for unusual thinking, *Forbes*, 24 March, at: https://www.forbes.com/sites/drnancydoyle/2020/03/24/the-world-needs-neurodiversity-unusual-times-call-for-unusual-thinking/?sh=45fc5f556db2

impairments in personal, social, academic, or occupational functioning' (American Psychiatric Association, 2022; World Health Organization, 2019). NDDs are lifelong disabilities, whereas mental health disorders are more episodic. ADHD and ASD are the most common heritable NDDs with multifactorial genetic and environmental causes and heterogeneous clinical characteristics that make them 'spectrum disorders'. ADHD and ASD reflect lifelong traits; hence, one therapeutic aim is to advise on and support with environmental modifications. This approach embodies the 'neurodiversity model'.

Judy Singer coined the term 'neurodiversity' to describe neurological diversity and promote its recognition as 'difference' instead of 'disorder' (Singer, 1999). Service users can self-identify with terms like 'neurodivergent' or 'neuro*a*typical'. But the point is that neurodiversity opposes medical understandings of NDDs. By adopting the social model of disability, neurodiversity underscores systemic barriers like negative attitudes, prejudice, stigma, and exclusion (purposely or inadvertently) as more disabling than the actual/perceived 'disorder'. Mental health nurses need to know about neurodiversity and how the social model of disability relates to the Equality Act 2010, which mandates 'reasonable adjustments' for disabled people with conditions such as ADHD and ASD. The overlapping differences and strengths of neurodiversity are depicted in Figure 18.1 (Doyle, 2020). Mental health nurses also need to know how medical interventions like a correct diagnosis, medication, and psychosocial interventions (e.g. specialized cognitive behavioural therapy) can ease the burden of ADHD and ASD (National Institute for Health and Care Excellence (NICE), 2012, 2018).

▼ Attention Deficit Hyperactivity Disorder

ADHD begins in childhood and, in most cases, it persists into adulthood, where it has a prevalence estimate of 3-4%.

Impairing core symptoms of inattention and hyperactivity/ impulsivity characterize ADHD, but it can also coexist with

Table 18.1 Examples of conditions that can co-occur with Autism Spectrum Disorder and/or Attention Deficit Hyperactivity Disorder

Physical health	Mental health
• Gastrointestinal disorders	• Anxiety, depression, obsessive–compulsive disorder
• Metabolic disorders (e.g. diabetes mellitus)	• Patterns of disordered eating
• Allergies, eczema, asthma and respiratory tract infections	• Personality and post-trauma stress disorders
• Disrupted or poor patterns of sleep	• Addiction disorders
• Motor stereotypes (e.g. self-injurious behaviours)	• Gender dysphoria
• Epilepsy and intellectual disability	• Bipolar disorder, schizophrenia

Source: data from World Health Organization (2019). *International Classification of Diseases*, 11th ed. Geneva; and American Psychiatric Association (2022). *Diagnostic and Statistical Manual of Mental Disorders*, 5th ed., text rev. Washington, DC.

other NDDs and physical and mental health conditions listed in Table 18.1 (American Psychiatric Association, 2022; World Health Organization, 2019). ADHD is underdiagnosed in the UK, especially in females, who are at a greater risk of being misdiagnosed with mood, eating, or personality disorders (Young et al., 2020). The clinical picture of ADHD can be complicated by coexisting substance use or other disorders or by functional impairments that cause academic or occupational failure, antisocial behaviour, and imprisonment. However, the presentations and outcomes of ADHD are variable. There are also 'high-functioning' service users who may perceive their ADHD as a 'gift' with positive attributes that enable them to be creative thinkers, positive risk takers, and successful in life (Sedgwick et al., 2019).

Core skills for working with ADHD are 'identifying' indicators of the disorder, 'screening' for signs and symptoms, and making a 'referral' to primary or secondary specialist care. NICE (2018) guidance for treating and managing ADHD should be followed. The care pathway begins with being seen by a general practitioner (GP) or community mental health team, who can make a referral to an adult ADHD specialist clinic. A mental health nurse working in primary or secondary care, or a GP, might first administer for instance, the Adult ADHD Self-Report Scale (ASRSv1.1). The ASRSv1.1 is a widely used screening tool. A positive score is four or more of the six core indicators of ADHD on the scale, and this information can be added to the referral letter. Getting diagnosed with ADHD in adulthood can be a lengthy process due to significant waiting times to access specialist NHS services. **Specialist skills** are required to conduct a diagnostic assessment, prescribe medication, and deliver specific psychosocial therapies.

NICE (2018) guidance stipulates that **only** a healthcare professional (e.g. a mental health nurse, psychiatrist, or non-medical prescribing pharmacist) with specialist training and competency can conduct a diagnostic assessment for ADHD. This process involves gathering a detailed family, developmental, and clinical history, and conducting a mental state examination that includes an assessment of risk, other neurodevelopmental, substance use, and mental health disorders, and functional impairments, using, for example, the Weiss Functional Impairment Rating Scale—Self Report (WFRIS-S). The Diagnostic Interview for Adult ADHD (DIVA-5) is widely used to conduct a diagnostic assessment. ADHD is diagnosed when five or more in adults (or six or more in youth) of the 18 core symptoms of inattention and/or hyperactivity/impulsivity have been present for at least 6 months. Several symptoms must have an onset before the age of 12 years, not be better accounted for by another disorder and must cause functional impairments in at least two or more settings (e.g. education, work, home, or with friends or relatives). The diagnostic categories are ADHD **predominantly** 'inattentive' or 'hyperactive/impulsive' or 'combined'. Psychostimulant medicines such as methylphenidate or lisdexamfetamine are recommended as first-line treatment for ADHD in adults. A non-stimulant medicine like atomoxetine can also be prescribed if a stimulant produces a poor treatment response, or if the service user has coexisting problems with substance misuse, or presents with an elevated risk of non-medical use or diversion (Müller-Sedgwick and Sedgwick-Müller, 2020).

Prescribed stimulants are among the most effective medicines used in adult mental health and general medicine. Although they are good at treating ADHD, these medicines can also have side effects that tend to be dose related, mild, or transient. Side effects include headache, reduced appetite, nausea, palpitations, difficulties falling asleep, and dry mouth. Psychostimulants can also increase blood pressure and heart rate. Therefore, service users taking these medicines are assessed at baseline and monitored during treatment (NICE,

2018). For some service users, these side effects are undesirable, and they may decide to stop taking their medicine or only use it *pro re nata* (PRN; 'as needed'). Only a psychiatrist or trained non-medical prescriber (e.g. a mental health nurse or pharmacist) can prescribe psychostimulants, which are classified as controlled 'B' substances. Possessing psychostimulants without a prescription or illegal supply (and sharing) can attract a prison sentence, unlimited fine, or both (Misuse of Drugs Act 1971 (c.38): Schedule 2: Controlled Drugs). In some countries, stimulants are illegal, even when prescribed for personal use. Prescribing practitioners need to inform service users about this, advise them to contact a relevant embassy (or high commission) for country-specific advice, and carry a copy of their clinic letter or prescription when travelling outside of the UK. Psychostimulants alone can be effective for a subgroup of service users with ADHD, but in practice, persistent difficulties are often seen, and psychosocial interventions, including environmental modifications, help to address them (NICE, 2018). A mental health nurse can deliver most psychosocial interventions, although specialist types of therapy may require additional training. Psychosocial interventions are discussed in more detail in the section on 'Autism Spectrum Disorder and Attention Deficit Hyperactivity Disorder'.

▼ Autism spectrum disorder

ASD is a lifelong disorder that affects how individuals understand the world and relate to, and interact, with others. ASD has a prevalence of around 1%, although it is higher in males (2%) than in females (0.3%) (Baron-Cohen et al., 2009). ASD is characterized by pervasive difficulties across two domains: initiating and sustaining reciprocal social communication and interaction **and** a pattern of restricted, repetitive behaviours, interests, and activities. Autism usually presents by 2–3 years old. However, service users who are diagnosed in early childhood also tend to have more severe symptoms and impairments (American Psychiatric Association, 2022; World Health Organization, 2019). Autistic service users are more likely to experience poor educational outcomes, lower rates of employment, are less likely to live independently, be married, be in a long-term relationship, have at least one friend, and have elevated rates of physical and mental health problems (Lai et al., 2019). Autistic service users have reported difficulties with accessing appropriate health and social care services and, in some instances, have been subjected to alarming institutional abuse, such as that uncovered at 'Winterbourne View' (Department of Health, 2012). The Autism Act 2009 was introduced to increase awareness and mandate services for autistic adults. It provides Local Authorities and the NHS with minimum requirements for service delivery, awareness training for all staff, and specialist training for key staff such as GPs, community mental health teams, and social workers. Examples of recommendations in the NHS Long Term Plan (NHS England, 2019) are listed in Box 18.1.

Many service users, especially autistic females, tend to be diagnosed in adulthood. This may be due to poor recognition in childhood or to females presenting with fewer restricted/repetitive behaviours and/or 'social camouflaging' (using strategies 'to minimize the visibility of their autism in social situations') (Lai et al., 2019). Gender dysphoria (persistent distress that arises from a mismatch between sex assigned at birth and gender identity) is also over-represented in autistic females (Twist and de Graaf, 2019). Some autistic service users will not identify with their gender. Instead, they may self-identify with gender diverse terms such as 'non-binary, gender neutral or fluid, genderqueer, two-spirit, or bi-gender' and request that their gender term be used in clinical interactions, notes, and reports. Such requests should always be respected and implemented. Although autistic females, compared to autistic males and cisgender individuals, are more likely to be gender diverse, elevated rates of ASD, ADHD, and other mental health disorders are also reported among transgender

Box 18.1 Examples of recommendations

- Mandatory training for NHS staff (as per previous strategies).
- Introducing a 'digital flag' in a service user's record by 2023/2024 to ensure staff know that they have autism and put in place reasonable adjustments.
- Expanding the 'STOMP' project (Stopping the Over Medication of People with autism or a learning disability, or both).
- Where possible, helping autistic service users to access a personal health budget.
- Reducing levels of inpatient care for autistic service users.

Source: data from NHS England (2019). *NHS Long Term Plan*. https://www.longtermplan.nhs.uk/

individuals (Warrier et al., 2020). Risks of coexisting schizophrenia, self-harm, recurrent suicidal ideation, and death by suicide are elevated in autistic service users (Lai et al., 2019). However, some issues can be precipitated by sensory sensitivities, social communication, and emotional regulation difficulties. The use of 'interpersonal skills' is a core competency for mental health nurses, but these skills may need to be adjusted when interacting with autistic service users.

Presentations and outcomes in ASD are also variable. There are autistic service users who might never experience profound difficulties because they have robust protective factors like appropriate support from family, an academic institution, or work environment, or they are 'high functioning' and **savant** (i.e. remarkably talented in one or more domains such as music, maths, or technology). **Core skills** for working with people with ASD are 'identifying' indicators of the disorder, 'screening' for signs and symptoms, and making a 'referral' to primary or secondary specialist care. **Specialist skills** are required to conduct a diagnostic assessment and deliver specific behavioural therapies. NICE (2012) guidance for diagnosing and managing autism should be followed. The care pathway begins with a visit to a GP, or community mental health team, who can make a referral to a specialist neurodevelopmental service. A mental health nurse, or GP, may first administer for instance, the Autism-Spectrum Quotient (AQ-10) screening tool and a score of more than 6 out of 10 indicates that a referral for a specialist diagnostic assessment is appropriate.

NICE (2012) stipulates that a diagnostic assessment for ASD can only be conducted by a specially trained healthcare professional (e.g. a mental health nurse, clinical psychologist, or psychiatrist) and with multidisciplinary team input. The Autism Diagnostic Interview-Revised (ADI-R), Autism Diagnosis Observation Schedule, 2nd Edition (ADOS-2), and expert clinical judgement are the 'gold standard' for diagnosing ASD. The ADI-R is used to obtain a developmental history from an informant (e.g. a parent). Still, challenges can arise if informants refuse to participate, deny there were any issues, have passed away, or have no access to school reports. The ADOS-2 is a universally recognized tool for diagnosing ASD. It consists of activities and materials organized in four modules based on chronological age and language ability (preverbal

Box 18.2 Therapies not recommended for treating the core symptoms of Autism Spectrum Disorder

- Antipsychotics, anticonvulsants, antidepressants, cholinesterase inhibitors, oxytocin, secretin, or testosterone
- Exclusion diets (e.g. gluten- or casein-free and ketogenic diets)
- Vitamins, minerals and/or dietary supplements (e.g. vitamin B6 or iron)
- Chelation therapy/chelating agents
- Hyperbaric oxygen therapy.

Source: data from NICE (2012). Interventions for autism: 1.4.13–1.4.22. https://www.nice.org.uk/guidance/cg142/chapter/Recommendations#interventions-for-autism-2

to verbally fluent). Module four assesses verbally fluent older adolescents and adults (without an intellectual disability). It can take up to 1 hour to administer module four activities, which are designed to facilitate interactions between the assessor and service user. A protocol booklet provides structure and is used to make notes. A coding section at the end and a specified algorithm are used to formulate a score that produces one of three diagnostic classifications: **autism**, **autism spectrum**, or **non-spectrum**. The difference between autism and autism spectrum is severity. Autism has more pronounced and/or severe symptoms.

Unlike in ADHD, there are no medicines for treating ASD. However, medicines can be used to treat coexisting ADHD or other mental health disorders by following NICE guidance for the specific disorder. Examples of the other therapies not recommended for treating ASD are listed in Box 18.2. Mental health nurses may require training to deliver behavioural interventions that have a long history of use in ASD. For example, applied behaviour analysis (and interventions derived from it) has been extensively studied and is considered the most effective therapy for modifying behaviour that challenges or teaching autistic service users adaptive skills and behaviours (Matson et al., 2012).

▼ Autism Spectrum Disorder and Attention Deficit Hyperactivity Disorder

The DSM-5-TR and ICD-11, for the first time, allow for ASD and ADHD to be diagnosed concurrently. This makes sense because these disorders share several phenotypic similarities. Service users with ASD and ADHD tend to experience significant challenges when compared to service users with either disorder alone. It is often easier to diagnose more severe or straightforward cases of ASD and ADHD. Diagnostic challenges arise when symptoms are subtle, mild, hidden, or overshadowed by the physical or mental health comorbidities listed in Table 18.1 or when information to complete a developmental and/or clinical history is not readily available.

A multifaceted approach that combines the methods NICE recommends for each disorder is used in practice. Service users with ASD and ADHD must have a holistic, comprehensive, shared care plan that addresses their psychological, behavioural, educational, and/or occupational needs. The drive towards developing integrated 'neurodevelopmental services' is therefore welcome. This service model is likely to

Table 18.2 Example of how the ABC model was used in practice

Antecedent	Behaviour	Consequence
Describe the activity, situation, or event/s before the behaviour	**Describe exactly what the behaviour looked like**	**Describe the event/s that followed or results of the behaviour**
Daria was invited to lunch in the dining room. She came but had to wait in a queue to be served her food	When standing in the queue, Daria pulled the hair of the person standing in front of her and a scuffle broke out between them	Staff managed the scuffle by escorting Daria to the sensory room to de-escalate her stress
Daria was escorted by staff to the occupational therapy centre. There was a queue getting into the room	Daria barged past the person in front of her, hurting their arm in the process. Daria wanted to get into the room quickly to sit on her favourite seat	Daria was escorted back to the ward and into the sensory room to de-escalate her stress

Hypothesis: Daria can become aggressive towards other service users when standing behind them in a queue to get served food or to enter the occupational therapy centre. When these incidents occur, staff escort Daria to the sensory room to de-escalate the stress these incidents cause her. During her time in the sensory room Daria is alone, and no additional demands are placed on her

Testing the hypothesis:

Antecedent	Behaviour	Consequence
Describe the activity, situation, or event/s before the behaviour	**Describe exactly what the behaviour looked like**	**Describe the event/s that followed or results of the behaviour**
Daria was invited first into the dining room. There are no other people in the dining room and no queue. Daria was first to be served food	Daria sat on dining table and started to eat her meal	Other service users start coming into the dining room. Daria laughs at them standing in a queue. She finishes her meal quickly, leaves the dining room, and goes to sit alone in the TV room
Daria was escorted to the occupational therapy centre alone by nursing staff and there is no queue to get into room	Daria opens the door by herself, enters the room, and runs over to her favourite seat	Daria engages in artwork. She shows her picture to the therapist who comments that it is nice. Daria tears it up, throws it in the bin, and asks staff to take her back to the ward

be the most efficient and cost-effective way of catering to the needs of service users with ASD and ADHD.

Post-diagnosis, all service users with ASD and ADHD should be offered psychoeducation as a precursor to any intervention (NICE, 2012, 2018). Psychoeducation is a **core skill** for mental health nurses, who are well placed to deliver it on a one-to-one basis, in a group, and over time to reinforce messages. Even a one-off session can be helpful. Psychoeducation consists of giving information and having a discussion with service users about:

- the meaning and implications of having ASD and ADHD, including their similarities and differences

- practical options for treatment (medication and/or psychosocial interventions)

- advice about disclosure at work, college/university, or to family, friends, and peers

- advice about environmental modifications, including reasonable adjustments under the Equality Act 2010, Access to Work (https://www.gov.uk/access-to-work), or Disabled

Students Allowance (https://www.gov.uk/disabled-students-allowance-dsa).

After psychoeducation, other therapies like cognitive behavioural therapy, dialectical behaviour therapy, or coaching can be delivered with specialist training. Service users with ASD and ADHD may be or may become parents. In a few parents, their capacity to support a child/children may be questioned, especially if they are not being given appropriate support. If, at any time, social services need to be involved, all professionals involved in the case need to be aware of and understand the functional impairments that are caused by ASD and ADHD and offer the most appropriate support. Capacity and consent needs to be managed mindfully and sensitively, especially when there are differing views between the service user and their family members or caregivers. In some instances, it might be appropriate to refer the parties involved in any dispute(s) for 'family therapy', but with a therapist skilled in working with service users with NDDs.

▼ Pathological Demand Avoidance

Pathological Demand Avoidance (PDA) is one of the most controversial profiles in the neurodevelopmental literature. It describes a maladaptive response to everyday demands, low tolerance for uncertainty, and frustration that could be deemed 'controlling behaviour' (O'Nions et al., 2018). Some charities, organizations, service users, and health and social care professionals recognize PDA as a legitimate 'behaviour' on the autism spectrum. However, PDA is not listed in the ICD-11 or DSM-5-TR or clinical guidance, and research is not robust enough to inform nursing practice (O'Nions et al., 2018). PDA has been broadly associated with antisocial behaviours, delinquency, language disorder, epilepsy, ASD, and ADHD in a subset of service users with histories of a disrupted or traumatic childhood (Gillberg et al., 2015). 'Demand avoidance' can also be a rational choice a service user makes to maintain their autonomy. These caveats fuel controversies about whether PDA

is a well-defined syndrome. Practical implications can arise for mental health nurses when service users with ASD and ADHD self-identify with PDA. A way to give PDA clinical utility could be by viewing it as 'behaviour that challenges', which often is a secondary feature of ASD and ADHD. A core nursing skill is **case formulation**. Caregivers can be alerted to 'behaviour that challenges' by describing defining features in a case formulation, including how it may present or what function(s) it may serve. Describing 'demand avoidance' and 'emotional reactivity' as behaviours that challenge, including the impact they may have on daily functioning, can also be used to monitor and evaluate the effectiveness of care plans for managing them. Box 18.3 presents a practice example, and the functional assessment of behaviour and positive behaviour support (PBS) plan for the case is examined in more detail.

▼ What is a functional assessment?

A functional assessment is a process that systematically identifies factors that precipitate and maintain behaviour that challenges (or behaviour/s that is/are of concern). This process, depicted in Figure 18.2, begins by gathering information from 'direct observation' and 'key informants'. The behaviour being

observed must be clearly described, including the time and day it occurred, how often it occurred (**frequency**), how long it lasted (**duration**), potential triggers, the risks it posed to self and others (**severity**), and the consequences that followed. In the practice example, Daria's primary nurse implemented a

Box 18.3 Practice example: Daria

Daria is 24 years old. She has a family history of maternal personality disorder and paternal mild intellectual impairment She was taken into care at 6 months old and placed with different foster caregivers until she was adopted at 5 years old. As a child, Daria experienced speech, language, attention, and motor coordination difficulties, seizures, physical abuse, and neglect. At school, she had problems making friends, frequent temper tantrums, and bullied her peers. At 13 years old, she was transferred to a school for pupils with special education needs. She truanted from this school and was a victim of a traumatic rape at 15 years old. Complaints of physical and mental health problems, including recurring urinary tract infections, rectal bleeding, fluctuating weight, and self-harming behaviour marked Daria's teen years. At 17 years old, she was living in a hostel and was diagnosed with borderline personality disorder.

Daria had several admissions to an acute psychiatric ward. During her last admission, she was slapping, biting, kicking, verbally abusing staff and other service users, tearing off her clothes, threatening to get male staff 'fired', and, at times, using 'weapons' to attack staff (e.g. a broom, books, and chairs). She would spit out her prescribed medication (aripiprazole, 10 mg once daily; clonazepam, up to 2 mg PRN at night), once set a fire in her bedroom and swallowed dishwashing liquid. Her response to treatment and care was poor.

Daria was then transferred to a behaviour disorders assessment unit (BDAU) for a second opinion assessment. This resulted in her being re-diagnosed with autism, ADHD, and complex trauma. Her prescribed medication was continued, a functional assessment (see 'What is a functional assessment?') of her behaviour was conducted, and a PBS plan (Box 18.4) was formulated, regularly reviewed, and updated. Daria stayed on the BDAU for 8 months. She was then discharged into supported accommodation in the community, where she has lived for the past 14 months. She has a key worker and intermittent contact with a local neurodevelopmental service who also review her medication. Her recovery is progressing well, and Daria now has plans to complete her GCSEs at a local college. One day, she wants to be a librarian and have a family.

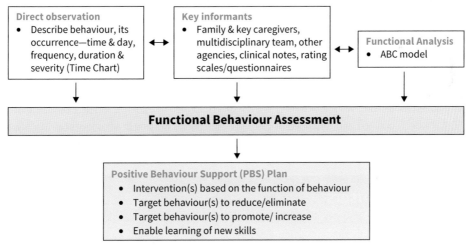

Figure 18.2 Example of the functional behaviour assessment process

plan to observe her behaviour over 7 days. The nursing staff allocated to care for Daria noted their observations on a 'time chart', which recorded the observed behaviour's date, time, frequency, duration, and severity. Daria's primary nurse used this information to complete a Functional Assessment Interview (FAI) questionnaire with her. After this, the ABC contingency model was used to conduct a more focused assessment. ABC is an acronym for **A**ntecedents (triggers for the behaviour), **B**ehaviour (actions observed), and **C**onsequences (events that occur immediately after the behaviour). In Table 18.2, an example of the ABC assessment completed by Daria's primary nurse shows how certain activities triggered her behaviour and the consequences. A simple formulation (or hypothesis) summarized why Daria's behaviours may be occurring. This hypothesis was tested, and the results were used to develop a PBS plan (Box 18.4).

Box 18.4 Positive behaviour support plan

Function of Daria's behaviour	Proactive strategies
Tangibles: • To be first to get served food in the dining room • To get her favourite seat in the occupational therapy centre	Nursing staff to: • invite Daria to dining room by herself so that she is first to be served food • escort Daria alone to the occupational therapy centre so that she is first to get through the door and sit on her favourite seat • if an incident of aggression towards staff or other patients occurs, escort Daria back to her bedroom for 1 hour time-out rather than to the sensory room

▼ What is a positive behaviour support plan?

A positive behaviour support (PBS) plan is an individualized care plan that combines person-centred values and a functional assessment. A PBS plan must provide clear and concise information for the mental health nursing team to deliver structured and consistent daily care and support, which aims to reduce the behaviour that challenges and optimize the service user's health, well-being, and quality of life. Mental health nurses can use strategies to modify the behaviour that challenges through environmental adaptations, active engagement, and support to manage anxiety or stress, such as time out in a sensory room (Department of Health and Social Care and Department of Education, 2021). The PBS plan shown in Box 18.4 is basic, but it should be frequently reviewed and updated with current information. Within different mental health settings, especially when service users have complex behavioural needs, a PBS plan may also detail strategies for primary and secondary prevention, reactive and risk management, and skills training.

▲ Conclusion

This chapter offers evidence-based advice and guidance for working with common NDDs and neurodiversity, from the perspective of a neuro*a*typical mental health nurse. The knowledge and skills required for working with service users with ADHD and ASD have been outlined and described. A case vignette was presented to demonstrate practical skills for conducting a functional assessment of behaviour and devising a PBS plan. Working with service users with ADHD and ASD can be challenging as well as rewarding. With knowledge and skills informed by evidence and NICE clinical guidance, mental health nurses working in all contexts can identify, assess, plan care, and effectively support service users with ADHD and ASD.

✖ Tips from service users

1 Be inclusive: give us opportunities to demonstrate our skills in ways that work for us, because we can do remarkable things.

2 Be mindful: when you do not listen to me you are simply refusing to see things from anything but a neurotypical frame of reference.

3 Cater for diverse needs: getting a 'correct' diagnosis, especially as a female, ensures the most appropriate care pathway can be followed.

W   Companion website

For extra resources on the topics covered in this chapter, visit the companion website at: www.oup.com/mhns

✚   References

American Psychiatric Association (2022). *Diagnostic and Statistical Manual of Mental Disorders, 5th ed., text rev. Washington, DC: American Psychiatric Association.*

Baron-Cohen, S., Scott, F. J., Allison, C., Williams, J., Bolton, P., Matthews, F. E., and Brayne, C. (2009). *Prevalence of autism-spectrum conditions: UK school-based population study. British Journal of Psychiatry 196(6), 500–519.Department of Health (2012). Transforming Care: A National Response to Winterbourne View Hospital. London: HM Government.*

Department of Health and Social Care, and Department of Education (2021). *The National Strategy for Autistic Children, Young People, and Adults: 2021–2026. London: HM Government.*

Doyle, N. (2020). *The world needs neurodiversity: unusual times call for unusual thinking. Forbes, 24 March. Available at:https://www.forbes.com/sites/drnancydoyle/2020/03/24/the-world-needs-neurodiversity-unusual-times-call-for-unusual-thinking/*

Gillberg, C., Gillberg, I. C., Thompson, L., Biskupsto, R., and Billstedt, E. (2015). *Extreme ('pathological') demand avoidance in autism: a general population study in the Faroe Islands. European Child and Adolescent Psychiatry 24(8), 979–984.*

Lai, M., Kassee, C., Besney, R., Bonato, S., Hull, L., Mandy, W., Szatmari, P., and Ameis, S. H. (2019). *Prevalence of co-occurring mental health diagnosis in the autism population: a systematic review and meta-analysis. Lancet Psychiatry 6(10), 819–829.*

Matson, J. L., Turygin, N. C., Beighley, J., Rieske, R., Tureck, K., and Matson, M. L. (2012).*Applied behavior analysis in autism spectrum disorders: recent developments, strengths, and pitfalls. Research in Autism Spectrum Disorders 6(1), 144–150.*

Müller-Sedgwick, U. and Sedgwick-Müller, J. A. (2020). *Drugs to treat attention deficit hyperactivity disorder. In: P. M. Haddad and D. J. Nutt, Eds., Seminars in Clinical Psychopharmacology, pp. 392–432. Cambridge: Cambridge University Press.*

National Institute for Health and Care Excellence (2012). *Autism Spectrum Disorder in Adults: Diagnosis and Management. Clinical guideline [CG142]. Available at: https://www.nice.org.uk/guidance/cg142*

National Institute for Health and Care Excellence (2018).*Attention Deficit Hyperactivity Disorder: Diagnosis and Management. NICE guideline [NG87]. Available at: https://www.nice.org.uk/guidance/ng87*

NHS England (2019). *NHS Long Term Plan. Available at: https://www.longtermplan.nhs.uk/*

O'Nions, E., Viding, E., Floyd, C., Quinlan, E., Pidgeon, C., Gould, J., and Happé, F. (2018). *Dimensions of difficulty in children reported to have an autism spectrum diagnosis and features of extreme/'pathological' demand avoidance. Child and Adolescent Mental Health 23(3), 220–227.*

Sedgwick, J. A., Merwood, A., and Asherson, P. (2019). *The positive aspects of attention deficit hyperactivity disorder: a qualitative investigation of successful adults with ADHD. Attention Deficit and Hyperactivity Disorders 11(3), 241–253.*

Singer J. (1999). *'Why can't you be normal for once in your life?' From a 'problem with no name' to a new category of disability. In: M. Corker and S. French, Eds., Disability Discourse, pp. 59–67. Buckingham: Open University Press.*

Twist, J. and de Graaf, N. M. (2019). *Gender diversity and non-binary presentations in young people attending*

the UK's National Gender Identity Development Service. Clinical Child Psychology and Psychiatry 24(2), 277–290.

Warrier, V., Greenberg, D. M., Weir, E., Buckingham, C., Smith, P., Lai, M., Allison, C., and Baron-Cohen, S. (2020). Elevated rates of autism, other neurodevelopmental and psychiatric diagnoses, and autistic traits in transgender and gender-diverse individuals. Nature Communications 11(1), 3959.

World Health Organization (2019). International Classification of Diseases, 11th ed. Geneva: World Health Organization.

Young, S., Adamo, N., Ásgeirsdóttir, B. B., Branney, P., Beckett, M., Colley, W., Cubbin, S., Deeley, Q., Farrag, E., Gudjonsson, G., Hill, P., Hollingdale, J., Kilic, O., Lloyd, T., Mason, P., Paliokosta, E., Perecheria, S., Sedgwick, J., Skirrow, C., ... Woodhouse E. (2020). Females with ADHD: an expert consensus statement taking a lifespan approach providing guidance for the identification and treatment of attention-deficit/hyperactivity disorder in girls and women. BMC Psychiatry 20(404), 1–27.

(19) Medicines management

Mark Pearson   **Alan Pringle**

Learning outcomes

By the end of this chapter, you should be able to:

1 Outline the nature of, and some of the influences on, non-adherence with medication

2 Describe a range of evidence-based interventions for collaborative approaches to engage with service users to discuss all aspects of medication management

3 Outline general principles and skills for communication with service users and carers that encourage service user and carer involvement in shared decision-making around the subject of medication.

▼ Medication management

Mental health nurses play an essential role in the administration and management of medicines. Medicines are potent treatments that can be life-changing for service users but can also present significant risks and nurses have a key role in both the safe administration of medication and in the monitoring for effects and side effects of any medication taken. In the 2018 document *Future Nurse: Standards of Proficiency for Registered Nurses*, the NMC states that all registered nurses must understand the principles of safe and effective administration of medicines and demonstrate proficiency in this area. All nurses should be aware that individual NHS trusts, private healthcare providers, and third-sector organizations that are involved in medication administration will each have local policies that govern the management of medicines in their own specific areas that need to be adhered to. In every episode of medication administration, irrelevant of the setting, service user safety is paramount at all times. Errors in the administration of any medication should be reported immediately to appropriate senior members of staff so that immediate action can be taken.

When service users require assistance in adhering to medication regimens, the use of compliance aids such as weekly dosing or Dosette boxes may be used. These boxes should ideally be dispensed and sealed by a pharmacist but where a pharmacist is unable to dispense the medications in a compliance aid, a nurse may do so. Compliance aids are intended for use by individuals who recognize the need for treatment but have problems in either remembering to take their medication or in identifying which medication should be taken at a specific time. Other aids to compliance can include alarms and smartphone apps.

While the practical skills of medication management are important, effective medication management is more than just the completion of a set of mechanical tasks. The management of medication should be facilitated by effective communication with service users and carers that encourages a collaborative working relationship and focuses on four key areas: safety, impact on symptoms, side effects, and service user satisfaction. Where more complex reasons for non-adherence are found, a variety of psychosocial approaches may be helpful and the remainder of this chapter focuses on engaging with people for whom non-adherence with long-term medicines is a part of their health behaviour.

▼ Non-adherence with long-term treatment

Choosing not to take medication, or ceasing to take medication that was previously accepted, is usually referred to as non-compliance or non-adherence and is a recurring phenomenon in mental health care (Lin et al., 2022). Brown and Grey (2015) have reported that up to 75% of mental health patients will completely stop medication within 18 months of treatment commencing and they go on to suggest that this is important because non-adherence is the most powerful predictor of relapse. A mean non-adherence rate of 41% has been reported among those diagnosed with schizophrenia (Bradley and Green, 2018). For other medications, the non-adherence rates can be 30% for antidepressants, and up to 56% for mood stabilizers (Sudak and Ayub, 2017). A recent systematic review by Semahegn et al. (2020) proposed several determinant factors which influence medication adherence for people prescribed psychiatric medications including sociodemographic factors, substance misuse, perceived stigma, and cost.

The language used in this area can sometimes have an impact on the actions of people involved. The words compliance or adherence can be perceived as power-related terms that have the potential to imply that service users should do as they are told by professionals and are not able to make choices themselves. Bradley and Green (2018) report some service users stating that prescribing decision-making is not inclusive and that they have had feelings of being disempowered by prescribers who have made decisions **for** them and not **with** them.

It should be considered whether these terms 'compliance' or 'adherence' should therefore be replaced by others in discussions. As an alternative to the word adherence, the word 'concordance' is a term being used increasingly in the literature. The implication of the word concordance is that a joint process takes place between service user and service provider that involves discussing and managing treatment. In this process the discussion is the important thing and even if a service user chooses to not take the medication in the end, the process of having the discussion can still be viewed as concordant. This process of discussion and inclusion that De Las Cuevas (2011) describes as 'shared decision-making' has been found to be a reliable way to increase adherence to prescriptions (Lin et al., 2022).

▼ Influences on non-adherence/non-concordance

Non-adherence to long-term treatment can have significant consequences for service users. There is clear evidence to suggest that stopping medicines in conditions that are episodic or enduring can place service users at a higher risk of relapse than those who continue taking treatment as prescribed (Bradley and Green, 2018; Brown and Grey, 2015; Hadler et al., 2020).

Some of the reasons that people do not adhere to medication regimens can include the service user's perspective of the medication they are consuming. People who are non-adherent have more negative attitudes about medication itself than those who are adherent (De Las Cuevas, 2011). The complementary view that positive beliefs and attitudes towards medicines help compliance levels is presented by Richardson et al. (2013) and Greene et al. (2018) who suggested that positive patient beliefs and attitudes towards medicines 'have usually been found to be a sound variable in forecasting compliance'.

Some other factors thought to determine adherence levels are related to how much control an individual feels they have over their lives and their condition; to how much service users see medication as something that limits their freedom to think, feel, or behave; and to their beliefs about how well they might cope without taking medication (De Las Cuevas et al., 2017).

In some cases, characteristics of the medication itself can influence adherence (Levy et al., 2018). An example of this could be a service user's experience of, or knowledge of, side effects of the medication. If the side effects create a noticeable difference in the quality of life for a service user, for example, weight gain, lethargy or loss of libido, some service users might choose not to take medicines simply because of this. However, some research suggests that if service users have a knowledge of side effects and can recognize them for what they are, they may still choose to accept this for the sake of mental wellness (El-Mallakh and Findlay, 2015).

▼ Interventions to enhance adherence/concordance

Research into medication adherence can be complicated. One example of this can be that the sampling of service users who agree to take part in research might be more likely to be adherent than service users who do not participate. It could be argued that if this is the case, the samples used in trials may not represent the spectrum of service users seen in everyday clinical practice. In mental health settings, although several conditions have been addressed, a large proportion of research into medication non-adherence has focused on service users with psychosis.

Educational interventions aim to provide information to service users about both their condition and their medication. Group and individual service user education has been evaluated and results suggest that although giving information improves service users' understanding of their illness and medication, it does not necessarily improve adherence rates. Levy et al. (2018) suggest that how the education is administered may have some effect on its impact. Live web-based educational interventions that became more common during the COVID-19 pandemic appear to perform as well as in-person education and were the most potent method for education, whereas educational mailings and pamphlets appear to offer minimal benefit.

Face-to-face family interventions involving psychoeducation have been shown to improve rates of adherence. El-Mallakh and Findlay (2015) and Kopelowicz et al. (2012) both describe programmes that trained family members to be involved with medication regimens significantly increased compliance.

Behavioural interventions try to help service users tailor their treatment to suit their daily routines. For example, encouraging service users to take medication at a set time of day, such as before they go to bed to minimize sedation, or similarly taking medication with other routine behaviours (e.g. when leaving the house in the morning or after brushing their teeth).

Research to enhance adherence has examined cognitive behavioural approaches and interventions in this area. These interventions focus on enabling the practitioner to work collaboratively with service users to explore their beliefs about illness and treatment using cognitive behavioural therapy techniques. Miller and Rollnick (2013) describe how cognitive behavioural therapy is often used in conjunction with motivational interviewing, to resolve ambivalence about taking medications, to address perceptions about the importance of taking medications, and to examine confidence in the ability to adhere to a medication regimen. Studies using this process by Grey et al. (2006) and Cavezza (2013) showed positive outcomes.

Medication management approaches should try to help people to maximize the effectiveness of their medication. The aim is not to force people to take medication, but to work collaboratively with service users to enable them to make informed choices that maximize health. When clinicians work in this concordant way, service users are more involved in the process, more satisfied with treatment, and therefore less likely to stop taking medication.

The suggested approaches aimed at maintaining concordance would be appropriate in both community and inpatient settings. It is acknowledged that it can be difficult to maintain collaboration when service users refuse treatment and are compelled to take medication under mental health legislation. In these situations, the health care professional has a duty of care to enforce treatment to maintain the health and safety of the service user and others. This duty of care at times takes priority over individual rights to autonomy and choice, and health care professionals should focus on maintaining engagement with the service user and encouraging shared decision-making where possible even in these challenging circumstances.

The opportunity to engage in meaningful dialogue with health care professionals can provide a space for some of these subjective experiences to be explored and mental health nurses can play an important role in providing opportunities for greater dialogue with service users in relation to their medications (Pearson et al., 2021).

▼ Assessing and managing side effects

There is potential for all medications to cause side effects; however, the tolerability of side effects is often reported by service users as a significant reason for discontinuing their medication (McCann et al., 2008; Wong et al., 2011). Psychiatric medications perhaps require greater scrutiny due to their broad side effects profiles and the complex subjective experiences which might arise for those taking these medications (Flore et al., 2019). While some of the potential side effects might be mild and transient, others might be profoundly distressing and even fatal, therefore, identification and management of side effects is important in ensuring medication safety and optimization.

Between 50% and 70% of people prescribed antipsychotic medications will experience some form of side effect (Arana, 2000), these include extrapyramidal side effects, sedation, and metabolic disorders (Miller et al., 2008; Morrison et al., 2015). For those taking antidepressants, the rates of experienced side effects are similar (Anagha et al., 2021; Cascade et al., 2009) and most commonly include gastrointestinal disturbances, weight gain, and sexual side effects (Gartlehner et al., 2008). However, the potential for side effects is higher within certain vulnerable populations such as older people and those with underlying physical health conditions (Tveito et al., 2016).

Mental health nurses may have variable knowledge of side effects (Begum et al., 2020) despite often being the primary contact in administering the medication. This limited knowledge may result in medication errors but also limit the ability of the nurse to engage in meaningful conversations with service users about their medication and adequately assess their side effects (Begum et al., 2020). Assessment tools have the potential to support the identification of side effects, but these are often underused within clinical practice (Stomski et al., 2016). Examples of these tools include the Akathisia rating scale (Barnes, 1989) and the Glasgow antipsychotic rating scale (Waddell and Taylor, 2008). These tools have the potential to support identification and dialogue in relation to side effects. However, different tools can vary in their validity and reliability (Stomski et al., 2015).

Based on the 'ten commandments of wise medicines management' (Mutsatsa, 2016, p. 241), the following key points are suggested as foundational principles in supporting the effective assessment and management of side effects:

- Ensure the service user is well informed about the medication from the time of first prescription.

- Provide effective safety netting advice (Silverston, 2014) to service users to ensure that they are aware of potential side effects and how to proceed should these side effects arise. This process should also involve agreeing a timescale for the prescription to be reviewed.

- Ensure that people are taking the medication correctly.

- Always consider the service user's viewpoint, as this is critical.

▼ Assessing and managing withdrawal

As previously discussed, many people will discontinue their medications for a variety of reasons. However, the period of time during which the person discontinues and withdraws from their medication can be very difficult, potentially resulting in increased distress and both physical and emotional withdrawal symptoms (Watts et al., 2021). Importantly, although discontinuation syndrome is a discrete phenomenon, these withdrawal symptoms can also be misunderstood as a relapse of the original mental health problem (Horowitz and Taylor, 2019; Moncrieff, 2006).

In recent years, there has been increasing recognition of the significant impact of withdrawing from antidepressants, particularly selective serotonin reuptake inhibitors. Withdrawal effects might be increasingly likely for those who are prescribed high doses of medications or multiple medications (Read and Williams, 2018). The onset of symptoms is linked to the half-life of the medication; medications such as venlafaxine or paroxetine are known to have a shorter half-life and therefore result in potentially more severe and immediate withdrawal effects (Henssler et al., 2019).

The Maudsley prescribing guidelines (Taylor et al., 2021) suggest the following key points when supporting people to withdraw from antidepressant medication:

- Avoid abruptly stopping medication—medication should be tapered off gradually. All relevant professionals, including the prescriber of the medicine, should be informed of the plan to withdraw the medication so that a reducing regimen can be agreed with the service user.

- Consider prolonged tapering for people at increased risk—people who have been taking antidepressants for over 8 weeks, people who have been taking high doses of medications, or people who are also taking other medications such as antipsychotics may need to be tapered off these medications at a slower pace.

- If the discontinuation symptoms are severe, and the service user is in agreement, it may be helpful to reintroduce the antidepressant or an alternative with a longer half-life. The tapering can then continue under increased monitoring.

- Alternative short-term medications, such as benzodiazepines, may be helpful in alleviating some withdrawal effects such as increased anxiety or insomnia.

Similar principles underpin the process of withdrawing from antipsychotic medications. The tapering down of medication is advised as abrupt stopping of antipsychotics is more likely to result in significant withdrawal effect or relapse (Huhn et al., 2021). Importantly, when reducing antipsychotic medication there is also the potential for psychosis to re-emerge. There is debate as to whether this is a re-emergence of the original psychotic condition or a psychosis resulting from the withdrawal of the medication which itself has physiologically changed the brain, known as supersensitivity psychosis (Chouinard et al., 2017; Moncrieff, 2006). However, regardless of this debate, it is important that those withdrawing from the medication are informed of the potential risks and supported robustly and compassionately throughout this process.

▼ Motivation and ambivalence

The term ambivalence refers to a state of mixed feeling or contradictory ideas; the experience of, for example, both simultaneously wanting and not wanting something (Weisbrode, 2012). Ambivalence, if unresolved, may represent a significant obstacle to change (Wagner, 2013). In relation to medication, an individual may be interested in taking medications as they feel that these may improve their mental health, while also simultaneously be worried about side effects, potential stigma or other issues associated with medication.

Motivational interviewing can be described as a way of structuring conversations, so that 'people talk themselves into change, based on their own values and interests' (Miller and Rollnick, 2013, p. 4). This is a collaborative process, as the goal is not to convince the person to take medications but is rather to explore their feelings, and potential ambivalence, in relation to medicines, an outcome of which could lead to resolved ambivalence, greater motivation, and increased concordance (Inwanna et al., 2022).

Miller and Rollnick (2013) use the acronym OARS to describe the foundational skills in any motivation interviewing intervention:

- **O**—Open questions. Using open questions when starting a discussion about medication has the potential to invite greater discussion and dialogue around the issue.

- **A**—Affirming. This process of affirmation is focused on highlighting the good and the positive. In this process of affirming, the nurse is able to prevent a conversation which purely focuses on the potential difficulties or deficits of a person, but also emphasizes their strengths, abilities, and resources.

- **R**—Reflecting. Offering reflections during a conversation can be more helpful than continuing with a series of questions as reflections can provide both the nurse and the service user with the chance to consider what has been said during the interaction.

- **S**—Summaries. Summaries may also function as reflections in that they function to collect everything that has been said in the interaction. Summaries can be important in any interaction as they allow the service user to reflect on what has been discussed. Summaries can also support the transition of the conversation to different areas or topics.

The overall process of motivational interviewing is targeted towards supporting people to articulate their reasons for changing, by increasing the frequency of this 'change talk' and offering people the opportunity to explore this in a compassionate and reciprocal environment. The goal is to strengthen the intention to change (Rosengren, 2018).

▼ Problem-solving

Problem-solving approaches are psychosocial interventions aimed at supporting people to cope with stressors in order to lessen the impact on mental and physical health (Nezu et al., 2012). While this approach, as with motivational interviewing, is not solely related to medication management, it can offer potential tools which nurses can use to support meaningful conversations in relation to medications. A structured problem-solving approach can be used to identify solutions and behavioural strategies that can be integrated into solutions to make taking medication easier for service users.

A potential structure to a problem solving intervention, based on the framework by Falloon (2000) consists of six steps:

Step 1   What is the problem statement?:

- What is the problem (use the service user's own words)?
- Where/when does it occur?
- What makes it worse or better?
- What are the consequences of the problem?
- How does the person feel about the consequences?

Step 2   List all solutions:

- Encourage the service user to think about as many solutions as possible (these may not all be appropriate) and make a list of all generated solutions.
- If helpful and appropriate, the nurse can help to make suggestions.
- Do not discuss whether these are good or bad, no judgements should be made about the possible solutions at this point.

Step 3   Explore the main advantages and disadvantages of all suggested solutions:

- Evaluate/choose solution.
- Explore what would be good and not-so-good about each solution.
- In light of this information, ask the service user to choose the solution that they think is most likely to be effective.

Step 4   Action plan (needs to be detailed):

- List the steps needed to put their plan into action.
- What do they need to do?

- Consider utilizing the SMART acronym:

   Specific

   Measurable

   Achievable

   Realistic

   Time limited.

- Who else may be able to help them?
- Might anything get in the way?
- How might they get round potential obstacles?

Step 5   Implement solution:

- Follow the action plan over the agreed period.
- Ask the service user to make a mental or physical note about progress.

Step 6   Evaluation:

- Reflect on all the efforts that has been made, even if the initial plan has not been fully completed—the evaluation is not a matter of success or failure but an opportunity to reflect on how the person has experienced the action plan.
- Ask the service user to score how successful the solution was out of ten (this encourages recognition of partial success).
- If not solved, explore why.
- If solved, explore what has been learnt?
- Consider if the service users want to tackle another problem on the list?

▼ Ethical and philosophical issues

Although medication management remains a ubiquitous element of mental health nursing practice (Duxbury et al., 2010; White et al., 2018) this is perhaps one of the areas of practice most rife with ethical and philosophical dilemmas. These ethical issues become heightened when considering the frequency in which medicines might be administered to an individual against their will, under restraint, and representing a form of coercive control. This process of forced administration may very well fall within the legal remit of the Mental Health Act (1983/2007), and in many situations may well be ethically and morally justifiable. However, the development of a reflective, critical, and curious position towards these ethical, moral, and philosophical issues has

the potential to enhance nursing practice and prevent the proliferation of ineffective or inappropriate treatments (Day and McKeown, 2018).

Developments within psychopharmacology have had a remarkable impact on practices within mental health services; however, the notion that the application of these developments within clinical practice is a value-neutral, objective science is erroneous (Singh and Singh, 2016). Even considering the fundamental question of 'Who should be prescribed medication?' is complex within mental health care. There are treatment guidelines to guide the diagnostic and prescriptive process such as those published in the UK by the National Institute for Health and Care Excellence (e.g. 2009, 2014). However, Kramer (1994)

Box 19.1 Practice example: Peter

Peter is a 34-year-old man who was diagnosed with a psychotic disorder as a teenager and who has had four admissions to hospital since then. On each admission, Peter had features of paranoia and felt that there was a conspiracy to inject substances into his bloodstream to control his thinking and his personality.

Peter has been free from such thoughts and ideas since commencing on clozapine as a medication 11 months ago. You are Peter's community psychiatric nurse and when planning your next visit Peter has requested that you discuss some specific topics on your next time together.

Peter says he has looked at a lot of online and social media postings about clozapine and is confused. Some say it is a good drug and works, some say it is a terrible drug whose side effects are worse than its benefits and one Instagram post calls it the most dangerous drug ever. He has tried reading the drug information leaflet in the box but says he doesn't really understand what it says.

Peter says he feels he never really got a choice of whether to start the drug or not as his family and medical professionals all told him he needed to take it and now wonders if he made a mistake in saying yes. He says that because he is what he describes as an 'informal patient' he might say no to any more doses.

Peter suggests that another concern he has about the drug is that he has joined an online dating forum and every picture of him is one in which he looks fat. He says he has been told that antipsychotic drugs 'put stones of weight on people that can never be shifted' and wants to know if this is true.

Consider the following questions:

1 How might you prepare for your meeting with Peter and how might you try to structure the interaction?

2 What are the key messages you would want Peter to take away from your meeting together?

3 How might you try to check if these messages have been heard and understood?

---

proposes the prescription of psychiatric medication may represent a form of cosmetic psychopharmacology, and that as psychiatric medications become increasing prevalent within society 'we have to decide how comfortable we are with using chemicals to modify personality' (p. 15).

Beauchamp and Childress (2009) propose the four pillars of biomedical ethics which remain omnipresent in health care discourse (Page, 2012):

- Non-maleficence: the obligation and duty to do no harm
- Beneficence: to work in a way which is believed to be in the best interests of the service user
- Autonomy: respect the decision-making capacity of others and supporting others to make informed choices
- Justice: ensure that all service users in similar positions are treated in a similar manner and have access to similar resources.

These pillars can serve as useful tools in supporting reflection on practice and the ethical and moral implications of decisions in relation to medications. While there may be no easy answers to some of these ethical or moral issues, being aware of, and reflecting upon, these issues can prevent complacency and the passive acceptance of unethical practice.

See Box 19.1 for a practice example.

▲ Conclusion

Medication management remains a large component of the nursing role, especially within acute inpatient environments. Moreover, regardless of setting it is likely that mental health nurses have a unique role to play in ensuring the safe and effective management of medications. Individual may choose to take or not to take a medication for a variety of reasons and therefore it is essential that mental health nurses are equipped with the skills and knowledge to effectively facilitate dialogues with people in relation to their medications. This chapter has provided some examples of evidence-based interventions which may be helpful in facilitating these dialogues and highlighted some of the crucial practical and ethical elements of medications management which should always be considered.

✖ **Tips from service users**

1 Always tell the mental health nurse you are working with if you don't feel that you have been fully involved in decisions about your medicines.
2 Ask questions and discuss any concerns you might have in relation to medication—these may be in relation to the medicine itself or associated issues such as difficulties in accessing prescriptions.

3 Try to avoid poor-quality evidence sources in relation to medications. Some sources of information, especially online, can contain incorrect and potentially dangerous information.

W   Companion website

For extra resources on the topics covered in this chapter, visit the companion website at: www.oup.com/mhns

✚   References

Anagha, K., Shihabudheen, P., and Uvais, N. (2021). *Side effect profiles of selective serotonin reuptake inhibitors: a cross-sectional study in a naturalistic setting. The Primary Care Companion for CNS Disorders 23(4), 35561.*

Arana, G. W. (2000). *An overview of side effects caused by typical antipsychotics. Journal of Clinical Psychiatry 61(4), 5–13.*

Barnes, T. R. (1989). *A rating scale for drug-induced akathisia. British Journal of Psychiatry 154, 672–676.*

Beauchamp, T. L. and Childress, J. F. (2009). *Principles of Biomedical Ethics, 6th ed. New York: Oxford University Press.*

Begum, F., Mutsatsa, S., Gul, N., Thomas, B., and Flood, C. (2020). *Antipsychotic medication side effects knowledge amongst registered mental health nurses in England: a national survey. Journal of Psychiatric and Mental Health Nursing 27(5), 521–532.*

Bradley, E. and Green, D. (2018). *Involved, inputting or informing: 'shared' decision making in adult mental health care. Health Expectations 21(1), 192–200.*

Brown, E. and Gray, R. (2015). *Tackling medication non-adherence in severe mental illness: where are we going*

wrong? Journal of Psychiatric and Mental Health Nursing 22(3), 192–198.

Cascade, E., Kalali, A. H., and Kennedy, S. H. (2009). *Real-world data on SSRI antidepressant side effects. Psychiatry 6(2), 16–18.*

Cavezza, C. (2013). *A consumer-centred intervention to enhance antipsychotic medication adherence. InPsych 35(2), 18–19.*

Chouinard, G., Samaha, A. N., Chouinard, V. A., Peretti, C. S., Kanahara, N., Takase, M., and Iyo, M. (2017). *Antipsychotic-induced dopamine supersensitivity psychosis: pharmacology, criteria, and therapy. Psychotherapy and Psychosomatics 86(4), 189–219.*

Day, J. and McKeown, M. (2018). *Psychopharmacology for mental health nurses. In: K. Wright and M. McKeown, Eds., Essentials of Mental Health Nursing, pp. 507–523. London: SAGE.*

De Las Cuevas, C. (2011). *Compliance, adherence and concordance in medicine taking of psychiatric patients. Current Clinical Pharmacology 6(2), 71–73.*

De Las Cuevas, C., de Leon, J., Peñate, W., and Betancort, M. (2017). *Factors influencing adherence to psychopharmacological medications in psychiatric* patients: a structural equation modeling approach. *Patient Preference and Adherence 11, 681–690.*

Duxbury, J. A., Wright, K., Bradley, D., and Barnes, P. (2010). *Administration of medication in the acute mental health ward: perspective of nurses and patients. International Journal of Mental Health Nursing 19(1), 53–61.*

El-Mallakh, P. and Findlay, J. (2015). *Strategies to improve medication adherence in patients with schizophrenia: the role of support services. Neuropsychiatric Disease and Treatment 11, 1077–1090.*

Falloon, I. R. H. (2000). *Problem solving as a core strategy in the prevention of schizophrenia and other mental disorders. Australian and New Zealand Journal of Psychiatry 34(Suppl. 2), S185–S190.*

Flore, J., Kokanović, R., Callard, F., Broom, A., and Duff, C. (2019). *Unravelling subjectivity, embodied experience and (taking) psychotropic medication. Social Science & Medicine 230, 66–73.*

Gartlehner, G., Thieda, P., Hansen, R. A., Gaynes, B. N., Deveaugh-Geiss, A., Krebs, E. E., and Lohr, K. N. (2008). *Comparative risk for harms of second generation antidepressants. Drug Safety 31(10), 851–865.*

Glantz, A., Örmon, K., and Sandström, B. (2019). *'How do we use the time?'—an observational study measuring the task time distribution of nurses in psychiatric care. Practical Issues in Geriatrics 18, 67.*

Greene, M., Yan, T., Chang, E., Hartry, A., Touya, M., and Broder M. S. (2018). *Medication adherence and discontinuation of long-acting injectable versus oral antipsychotics in patients with schizophrenia or bipolar disorder. Journal of Medical Economics 21(2), 127–134.*

Gray, R., Leese, M., and Bindman, J. (2006). *Adherence therapy for people with schizophrenia. European multicentre randomised controlled trial. British Journal of Psychiatry 189, 508–514.*

Hadler, A., Sutton, S., and Osterberg, L. (2020). *Working with people with mental health difficulties to improve adherence to medication. In: A. Hadler, S. Sutton, and L. Osterberg, Eds., The Wiley Handbook of Healthcare Treatment Engagement: Theory, Research, and Clinical Practice, pp. 430–454. London: Wiley.*

Henssler, J., Heinz, A., Brandt, L., and Bschor, T. (2019). *Antidepressant withdrawal and rebound phenomena. Deutsches Ärzteblatt International 116(20), 355–361.*

Horowitz, M. A. and Taylor, D. (2019). *Tapering of SSRI treatment to mitigate withdrawal symptoms. Lancet Psychiatry 6(6), 538–546.*

Huhn, M., Leucht, C., Rothe, P., Dold, M., Heres, S., Bornschein, S., Schneider-Axmann, T., Hasan, A., and Leucht, S. (2021). *Reducing antipsychotic drugs in stable patients with chronic schizophrenia or schizoaffective disorder: a randomized controlled pilot trial. European Archives of Psychiatry and Clinical Neuroscience 271(2), 293–302.*

Inwanna, S., Duangchan, C., and Matthews, A. K. (2022). *Effectiveness of interventions to promote medication adherence in schizophrenic populations in Thailand: a systematic review. International Journal of Environmental Research and Public Health 19(5), 2887.*

Kopelowicz, A., Zarate, R., Wallace, C. J., Liberman, R. P., Lopez, S. R., and Mintz, J. (2012). *The ability of multifamily groups to improve treatment adherence in Mexican Americans with schizophrenia. Archives of General Psychiatry 69(3), 265–273.*

Kramer, P. D. (1994). *Listening to Prozac. New York: Penguin Books.*

Levy, A. E., Huang, C., Huang, A., and Michael Ho, P. (2018). *Recent approaches to improve medication adherence in patients with coronary heart disease: progress towards a learning healthcare system. Current Atherosclerosis Reports 20(1), 5.*

Lin, Y.-Y., Yen, W.-J., Hou, W.-L., Liao, W., and Lin, M. (2022). *Mental health nurses' tacit knowledge of strategies for improving medication adherence for schizophrenia: a qualitative study. Healthcare 10(3), 492.*

McCann, T., Boardman, G., Clark, E., and Lu, S. (2008). *Risk profiles for non-adherence to antipsychotic medications. Journal of Psychiatric and Mental Health Nursing 15(8), 622–629.*

Miller, D. D., Caroff, S. N., Davis, S. M., Rosenheck, R. A., McEvoy, J. P., Saltz, B. L., Riggio, S., Chakos, M. H., Swartz, M. S., Keefe, R. S., Stroup, T. S., Lieberman, J. A., and Clinical Antipsychotic Trials of Intervention Effectiveness (CATIE) Investigators (2008). *Extrapyramidal side-effects of antipsychotics in a randomised trial. British Journal of Psychiatry 193(4), 279–288.*

Miller, W. R. and Rollnick, S. (2013). *Motivational Interviewing: Helping People Change, 3rd ed. New York: Guilford Press.*

Moncrieff, J. (2006). *Does antipsychotic withdrawal provoke psychosis? Review of the literature on rapid onset psychosis (supersensitivity psychosis) and withdrawal-related relapse. Acta Psychiatrica Scandinavica 114(1), 3–13.*

Morrison, P., Meehan, T., and Stomski, N. J. (2015). *Living with antipsychotic medication side-effects: the experience of Australian mental health consumers. International Journal of Mental Health Nursing 24(3), 253–261.*

Mutsatsa, S. (2016). *Medicines Management in Mental Health Nursing. London: Learning Matters.*

National Institute for Health and Care Excellence (2009). *Depression in Adults: Recognition and Management. Clinical guideline [CG90]. Available at: https://www.nice.org.uk/guidance/cg90*

National Institute for Health and Care Excellence (2014). *Psychosis and Schizophrenia in Adults: Prevention and Management. Clinical guideline [CG178]. Available at: https://www.nice.org.uk/guidance/cg178*

Nezu, A. M., Nezu, C. M., and D'Zurilla, T. (2012). *Problem-Solving Therapy: A Treatment Manual. New York: Springer.*

Nursing and Midwifery Council (2018). *Future Nurse: Standards of Proficiency for Registered Nurses. Available at: https://www.nmc.org.uk/globalassets/sitedocuments/education-standards/future-nurse-proficiencies.pdf*

Page, K. (2012). *The four principles: can they be measured and do they predict ethical decision making? BMC Medical Ethics 13, 10.*

Pearson, M., Sibson, T., and Carter, T. (2021). *A qualitative study of service users' experiences of mental health nurses' knowledge and skills in relation to medication Journal of Psychiatric and Mental Health Nursing 28(4), 682–691.*

Read, J. and Williams, J. (2018). *Adverse effects of antidepressants reported by a large international cohort: emotional blunting, suicidality, and withdrawal effects. Current Drug Safety 13(3), 176–186.*

Richardson, M., McCabe, R., and Priebe, S. (2013). *Are attitudes towards medication adherence associated with medication adherence behaviours among patients with psychosis? A systematic review and meta analysis. Social Psychiatry and Psychiatric Epidemiology 48(4), 649–657.*

Rosengren, D. B. (2018). *Building Motivational Interviewing Skills: A Practitioner Workbook, 2nd ed. New York: Guilford Press.*

Semahegn, A., Torpey, K., Manu, A., Assefa, N., Tesfaye, G., and Ankomah, A. (2020). *Psychotropic medication non-adherence and its associated factors among patients with major psychiatric disorders: a systematic review and meta-analysis. Systematic Reviews 9(1), 17.*

Silverston, P. (2014). *Effective safety-netting in prescribing practice. Nurse Prescribing 12(7), 349–352.*

Singh, A. R. and Singh, S. A. (2016). *Bioethical and other philosophical considerations in positive psychiatry. Mens Sana Monographs 14(1), 46.*

Stomski, N. J., Morrison, P., and Meyer, A. (2015). *Antipsychotic medication side effect assessment tools: a systematic review. Australian & New Zealand Journal of Psychiatry 50(5), 399–409.*

Stomski, N. J., Morrison, P., and Meehan, T. (2016). *Mental health nurses' views about antipsychotic medication side effects. Journal of Psychiatric and Mental Health Nursing 23(6-7), 369–377. https://doi.org/https://doi.org/10.1111/jpm.12314*

Sudak, D. and Ayub, S. (2017). *Psychotherapeutic strategies to enhance medication adherence. Psychiatric Times 34(9), 22–23.*

Taylor, D. M., Barns, R. E., and Young, A. H. (2021). *The Maudsley Guidelines in Psychiatry, 14th ed. Hoboken, NJ: John Wiley & Sons.*

Tveito, M., Correll, C. U., Bramness, J. G., Engedal, K., Lorentzen, B., Refsum, H., and Høiseth, G. (2016). *Correlates of major medication side effects interfering with daily performance: results from a cross-sectional cohort study of older psychiatric patients. International Psychogeriatrics 28(2), 331–340.*

Waddell, L. and Taylor, M. (2008). *A new self-rating scale for detecting atypical or second-generation antipsychotic side effects. Journal of Psychopharmacology 22(3), 238–243.*

Wagner, C. C. and Ingersoll, K. S. (2013). *Motivational Interviewing in Groups. New York: Guilford Press.*

Watts, M., Murphy, E., Keogh, B., Downes, C., Doyle, L., and Higgins, A. (2021). *Deciding to discontinue prescribed psychotropic medication: a qualitative study of service users' experiences. International Journal of Mental Health Nursing 30(Suppl. 1), 1395–1406.*

Weisbrode, K. (2012). *On Ambivalence: The Problems and Pleasures of Having it Both Ways. Cambridge, MA: MIT Press.*

White, S., Goodman, J., and Behan, L. (2018). *Nurses' use of appropriate needle sizes when administering intramuscular injections. Journal of Continuing Education in Nursing 49(11), 519–525.*

Wong, M., Chen, E., Lui, S., and Tso, S. (2011). *Medication adherence and subjective weight perception in patients with first-episode psychotic disorder. Clinical Schizophrenia and Related Psychoses 5(3), 135–141.*

(20) Law and practice

Richard Griffith

Learning outcomes

By the end of this chapter, you will be able to:

1 State the principles of the Mental Health Act 1983
2 Describe the requirements for compulsory admission

3 Evaluate the safeguards designed to protect patients undergoing treatment for a mental disorder
4 Discuss the arrangements for the rehabilitation and after-care of patients detained for treatment.

▼ Introduction

The position of the patient with mental health problems is now more legalized than ever before (Brown, 2016; Unsworth, 1987). In addition to the provisions of the Mental Health Act 1983, a strong body of case law has developed that informs your practice on issues of liberty, autonomy, and respect.

▼ The Mental Health Act 1983

In England and Wales, mental healthcare is regulated through the provisions of the Mental Health Act 1983 (Legislation. gov.uk, 1983) as amended by the Mental Health Act 2007 (Legislation.gov.uk, 2007). It is accompanied by a code of practice that provides guidance on the application of the provisions of the Act in practice.

The fundamental aim of the 1983 Act is to strengthen the rights of patients made subject to its compulsory powers. This is achieved through five key principles that all have a liberal thrust.

Increased recourse to review of detention

Detention in hospital has been limited by time since the Lunacy Act 1890. Detained patients have a right to appeal against detention through the Mental Health Review Tribunal, which considers whether the criteria for detention continue to be met.

To ensure that all detained patients have their case independently reviewed, hospital managers now have a duty to refer a case to the Mental Health Review Tribunal where the patient has not appealed and remains detained in hospital for 6 months following their admission (Mental Health Act 1983, section 68).

Hospital managers are also empowered to conduct their own reviews of detention and order discharge where three or more agree that the detention conditions are not met (Mental Health Act 1983, section 23). Hospital managers can only discharge a patient if three or more of them agree the detention conditions are no longer met (*R (Tagoe-Thompson) v Central and North West London Mental Health NHS Trust* [2002]).

Enhanced civil and social status

This principle was advocated mainly on therapeutic rather than legal grounds. One way the law was able to implement this principle was through the right to vote. Informal inpatients were given the right to vote by allowing them to register their entitlement using a previous address (Representation of the People Act 1983).

Detained patients did not gain the right to vote until an amendment to the House of Lords Reform Act 2001 granted it subject to the patient's capacity to decide on who to vote for.

Ideology of entitlement

This principle promoted the concept of access to services as a legal right. Patients who have been detained for treatment are entitled to aftercare services as a right.

There is a duty on the health and social services to continue to provide aftercare until it appears to them that the patient is no longer in need of that service (Mental Health Act 1983, section 117). The duty is owed to individual patients who cannot be charged for the aftercare services (*R (Stennett)* v *Manchester City Council* [2002]).

Least restrictive alternative

Any use of formal powers under the 1983 Act must be the least restrictive means of meeting the needs of the patient.

The approved mental health professional (AMHP) has a duty to ensure that the person is actively resisting admission to hospital and that compulsory admission is the most appropriate method of dealing with the case.

The AMHP must also certify that the detention order used is the least restrictive method of meeting the needs of the patient.

Multidisciplinary review of medical decisions

When formal admission under the Mental Health Act 1983 is considered, this falls to the AMHP whose role is to ensure that the person appears to be suffering from a mental disorder that warrants compulsory confinement. This initial safeguard ensures that people who do not have a mental disorder or those who do not actively resist admission are not improperly detained.

Further multidisciplinary reviews of medical decisions occur under part 4 of the 1983 Act, which provides safeguards concerning consent to treatment in certain cases. For example, patients who are subject to the consent to treatment provisions have a legal right to be supported through the treatment process by an independent mental capacity advocate (Mental Health Act 1983, section 130A).

▼ Scope of the Mental Health Act 1983

Part 1, section 1 of the Mental Health Act 1983 makes it clear that the Act shall have effect with respect to 'the reception, care and treatment of mentally disordered patients, the management of their property and other related matters'. From the outset, it is clear that the 1983 Act only applies to people who suffer from a mental disorder.

Definition of mental disorder

Mental disorder is the legal term used by the 1983 Act to establish who can be made subject to its provisions. It is defined as 'any disorder or disability of the mind' (Mental Health Act 1983, section 1(2)).

As the definition is very broad, two safeguards are included to narrow the scope of the 1983 Act. A person with a learning disability cannot be compulsorily admitted for treatment or guardianship unless their disability is associated with abnormally aggressive or seriously irresponsible conduct (Mental Health Act 1983, section 1(2A)). Furthermore, dependence alone on alcohol or drugs cannot be considered a mental disorder for the purpose of the Act (Mental Health Act 1983, section 1(3)).

In *St George's Healthcare NHS Trust* v *S* [1998], a pregnant woman with pre-eclampsia was detained under section 2 of the Mental Health Act 1983 when she refused hospital treatment for this life-threatening physical condition. The court held that her detention was unlawful because she did not have a mental disorder and the 1983 Act cannot be used to detain someone just because their thinking seemed unusual, irrational, or contrary to public opinion. The Mental Health Act 1983 can only be used to justify detention for mental disorder.

▼ Principles of compulsory detention

The process of detention aims to ensure that the only people made subject to the compulsory provisions of the 1983 Act are those who:

- are or appear to be suffering from a mental disorder, and
- are actively resisting admission to hospital.

In all other cases, informal admission under the provisions of section 131 of the Mental Health Act 1983 is more appropriate.

Deprivation of liberty

Compulsory detention means that a person is deprived of their liberty. Detention on the grounds that a person is suffering from a mental health problem is not in itself unlawful. If it is carried out in accordance with the law, it will comply with the European Convention on Human Rights (Council of Europe, 1950). In *Winterwerp* v *The Netherlands* [1979], the law requires that (unless it is an emergency):

- the person is reliably shown by objective medical evidence to be suffering from a mental disorder, and
- the disorder is of a nature or degree that warrants continued compulsory confinement.

✖ Activity 1. Evidence-based practice and research

Detention conditions
Look at the requirements for detention for each of the powers detailed in sections 2, 3, and 4 of the Mental Health Act 1983. Do the requirements meet the conditions specified by the European Court of Human Rights in *Winterwerp* v *The Netherlands* [1979], previously listed?

▼ Compulsory admission

The detention process is a division of responsibility between three key people:

- the AMHP
- a registered medical practitioner
- the patient's nearest relative.

The doctor(s) and the AMHP must see the person face to face. Assessments for detention under the Mental Health Act 1983 cannot be done remotely (*Devon Partnership NHS Trust* v *Secretary of State for Health and Social Care & Others* [2021]).

Approved mental health professionals

AMHPs include nurses and social workers who have been approved by the local authority as having appropriate competence in dealing with people who have a mental disorder (Mental Health Act 1983, section 114).

The AMHP generally makes the application for detention once they are satisfied that the person is suffering from a mental disorder and is actively resisting admission to hospital and has a duty to conduct a suitable interview with the person before making the application. The AMHP provides a safeguard against the misuse of detention powers and cannot be directed by their local authority or employer to apply for a person's detention.

Registered medical practitioners

Reliable, objective medical evidence is a fundamental requirement of lawful detention and an application for detention must be founded upon two medical recommendations (one in an emergency). One doctor must also be a clinician recognized as being competent in the diagnosis of mental disorder. This requirement meets the need for objective medical evidence under human rights law (Mental Health Act 1983, section 12).

The medical recommendation must indicate that the person is suffering from a mental disorder of a nature or degree that warrants continued compulsory confinement. The degree of the disorder is its current severity. The nature of the disorder is its prognosis and the person's past history, including previous admissions and compliance with treatment. Only one of these criteria needs to be satisfied to meet the requirements for detention (*R* v *Mental Health Review Tribunal for South Thames Region Ex p. Smith* [1998]).

The nearest relative

The nearest relative is a statutory friend allocated to a detained patient. The person is drawn from a hierarchy of relatives set out under section 26 of the 1983 Act, with the person in the highest category becoming the nearest relative unless someone lower down the list:

- ordinarily resides with the patient, or
- cares for the patient.

Where there are two or more people in the same category, the older person will be the nearest relative (*Dewen* v *Barnet Healthcare Trust & Barnet London Borough Council* [2000]).

The hierarchy of nearest relative under section 26 of the Mental Health Act 1983 is:

- husband, wife, or civil partner
- son or daughter
- mother or father
- brother or sister
- grandparent
- grandchild

- uncle or aunt
- nephew or niece
- a person who is not a relative, but with whom the patient has been living for not less than 5 years.

The purpose of the nearest relative is to provide a statutory friend for the detained patient, and that person has the power to:

- make applications to admit a person under compulsion; where the AMHPs make the application they have to take reasonable steps to inform the nearest relative about an application, and are required to have regard to any wishes expressed by the nearest relative
- veto an application for treatment (section 3) and guardianship (section 7)
- be given information by the hospital managers about the patient's detention and discharge unless the patient objects
- discharge their relative from detention by giving 72 hours' notice to an authorized person at the hospital; the discharge can be barred by the responsible clinician and a further application cannot be made for 6 months; the nearest relative then has 28 days to make an application to a Mental Health Review Tribunal for discharge
- apply to the tribunal for discharge in respect of a patient detained by a criminal court under section 37 of the Act
- have the right to be involved in any consideration as to the aftercare needs of a patient unless the patient objects
- make a formal complaint to the hospital managers and the Mental Health Act Commission.

A nearest relative may be removed by the county court if they act unreasonably or are otherwise unsuitable. The patient, another relative, a person living with the patient, or an AMHP can apply to have a nearest relative removed and replaced by the court (Mental Health Act 1983, section 29(2)).

Detention

The properly completed Mental Health Act 1983 forms are sufficient authority to detain the patient and convey them to the named hospital. Once in hospital the managers have a duty, usually delegated to a registered nurse, to inform the patient of the conditions of detention and their right to appeal or complain (Mental Health Act 1983, section 132).

Under the civil detention provisions, a person can be detained either for assessment or for treatment (Mental

Health Act 1983, sections 2, 3, and 4). Where a person is detained for treatment, appropriate medical treatment must be available. This is defined as medical treatment appropriate to the patient's case, taking into account the nature and degree of the mental disorder and other circumstances of his or her case.

Informal admission

A person can enter hospital for assessment and treatment of their mental disorder without the need to be detained. Since 1959, formal admission to hospital has been reserved for those who actively resist admission, whether or not that person has the mental capacity to refuse admission. Informal admission is used for those who consent, those who are incapable of deciding on admission, and those who come into hospital informally rather than be detained (Mental Health Act 1983, section 131).

A 16- or 17-year-old child must consent themselves to admission on an informal basis. Where that child refuses admission on an informal basis, the decision cannot be made by a person with parental responsibility (Mental Health Act 1983, section 131(2)).

Holding powers

Informal patients who wish to leave hospital against medical advice can be made subject to the holding powers under section 5 of the 1983 Act. The approved clinician or their nominated deputy may hold a patient for up to 72 hours to allow for an assessment to be made with a view to their detention under section 2 or section 3. Where the immediate attendance of an approved clinician cannot be secured, a nurse of the prescribed class may hold the person for up to 6 hours or until the clinician arrives on the ward.

For the purposes of the power to detain a patient in hospital for a maximum of 6 hours under section 5(4) of the Mental Health Act 1983, a nurse of the prescribed class is a first- or second-level registered nurse whose registration includes an entry indicating that the nurse's field of practice is either mental health or learning disabilities nursing (Mental Health (Nurses) (England) Order 2008 (SI 2008/1207)).

▼ Consent to treatment

Compulsory admission and treatment under the Mental Health Act 1983 are dealt with separately. Detention under the Act does not necessarily mean compulsory treatment. Section 56 of the Act specifically excludes most of the emergency provisions and holding powers from the consent to treatment provisions, including patients detained by virtue of:

- an emergency application (section 4)
- holding powers under sections 5(2) or (4)
- remand to hospital for a report on their mental condition (section 35)
- a detention by the police (section 135 or 136)
- a detention in a place of safety (section 37(4) or 45A(5)).

They also do not apply to a patient who is:

- conditionally discharged and not recalled to hospital (section 42, 73, or 74)
- a community patient and not recalled to hospital (section 17A), or
- subject to guardianship (section 7).

The approved clinician

The care of a detained mental health patient is supervised by an approved clinician who is called the patient's responsible clinician. This person is not necessarily a consultant psychiatrist. Amendments introduced by the Mental Health Act 2007 have extended the professionals who can be appointed as approved clinicians to include consultant clinical psychologists, consultant nurses, and occupational therapists.

The approved clinician will supervise the patient's treatment, grant leave, and, where necessary, renew a detention order or discharge the patient from hospital (Mental Health Act 1983, sections 20 and 145).

Even though the provisions of the Mental Health Act 1983 allow for compulsory treatment without consent under section 63 of the 1983 Act, it is essential that care and treatment are given in a climate of consent with respect for the rights and dignity of the patient. The European Convention on Human Rights (1950) places a negative obligation—a duty not to breach a patient's human rights—on mental health nurses. Treatment for mental disorder can engage rights under article 3: the right to be free from torture, inhuman and degrading treatment, and article 8: the right to respect for private and family life, which includes respect for personal autonomy and dignity (*R (on the application of PS) v RMO (DR G) and SOAD (DR W)* [2003]).

Treatment under the provisions of the Mental Health Act 1983 is defined as nursing, psychological intervention, and specialist mental health habilitation, rehabilitation, and care, the purpose of which is to alleviate or prevent a worsening of the disorder or its symptoms (Mental Health Act 1983, sections 145(1) and (4)). This recognizes a treatment as a whole approach to mental disorder and allows for the treatment of a wide range of symptoms, including physical symptoms that occur as a result of a mental disorder (*B v Croydon Health Authority* [1995]).

Safeguards

Some treatment under the 1983 Act may only be given where provisions safeguarding patients have been met. There are three categories of safeguard:

*   Treatments that require consent and a second opinion, including psychosurgery: these require both the consent of the patient and an agreeable second opinion from a doctor appointed by the Mental Health Act Commission (Mental Health Act 1983, section 57).

*   Treatments that require consent or a second opinion, including the giving of medication for mental disorder beyond 3 months from when it was first administered: these require either the consent of the patient or an agreeable second opinion from an appointed doctor (Mental Health Act 1983, section 58).

In the case of electroconvulsive therapy (ECT):

*   treatment cannot be given without the consent of a capable patient

*   treatment cannot be given without agreement from an appointed doctor where the person is incapable.

The second-opinion appointed doctor will not be entitled to authorize ECT for an incapable patient where:

*   there is a valid and applicable advance decision refusing ECT

*   an attorney with authority under a lasting power of attorney refuses consent

*   a deputy with authority refuses consent.

(Mental Health Act 1983, section 58A).

The nurse as consultee

When asked to sanction treatment for a patient, second-opinion appointed doctors must consult with two people, one a nurse and one who cannot be a doctor or a nurse, about the patient's condition.

✖ Activity 2. Reflection

The nurse's role as consultee
Imagine that you are to act as consultee for a patient whose treatment is being considered by a second-opinion appointed doctor. Note down the topics you are likely to discuss with the doctor before they decide on the suitability of treatment for the patient.

The nurse will need direct knowledge of the person's history and condition, and be in a position to comment on the issues affecting the patient including:

*   the proposed treatment and the patient's ability to consent to it

*   other treatment options

*   the way in which the decision to treat was arrived at

*   the facts of the case, progress, etc.

*   the view of the patient's relatives on the proposed treatment

*   the implications of imposing treatment upon a non-consenting patient

*   the reasons for the patient's refusal of treatment

*   any other matter relating to the patient's care on which the consultee wishes to comment.

Patients who initially consent to treatment may withdraw that consent. Treatment would have to cease unless it could be justified as urgent as set out in section 62.

▼ Independent Mental Health Advocacy service

An Independent Mental Health Advocacy service was established under the 1983 Act by an amendment introduced by the Mental Health Act 2007.

There is a duty to instruct an independent mental health advocate (IMHA) where a patient is a qualifying patient. A patient is a qualifying patient if they are:

- detained under the Mental Health Act (other than sections 4, 5(2), 5(4), 135 or 136)
- subject to guardianship, or
- a community patient, or
- discussing with a registered medical practitioner or approved clinician the possibility of being given treatment under section 57, or
- under 18 and not detained and discussing with a doctor or approved clinician the possibility of being given ECT.

The role of the IMHA is to help obtain information about and improve the patient's understanding of:

- the provisions of this Act
- any conditions or restrictions to which he or she is subject
- what (if any) medical treatment is given, proposed, or discussed
- why it is given, proposed, or discussed
- the authority under which it is, or would be, given
- the requirements of this Act which apply to giving the treatment to him or her.

To fulfil their role the IMHA may:

- visit and interview the patient in private
- visit and interview the person professionally concerned with his or her medical treatment
- require the production of and inspect any records relating to his or her detention or treatment or aftercare service and records held by a local social services authority which relate to him or her.

▼ Rehabilitation and aftercare

Leave of absence

Testing a patient's response to treatment by allowing controlled periods away from hospital is an important element of the rehabilitation process. A responsible clinician may grant a detained patient a leave of absence from hospital. The leave may be subject to any conditions the approved clinician considers necessary (Mental Health Act 1983, section 17). The period of leave is at the responsible clinician's discretion and can range from hours to weeks, or longer if the persons treatment continues to include a significant hospital based component (*DB* v *Betsi Cadwaladr UHB* [2021]). The use of extended leave as a fallback because community treatment order is deemed unsuitable is not acceptable. A patient may be recalled to hospital if they do not fulfil the conditions set out when the leave was granted, without the need to undergo a new detention application.

Community treatment orders

Where long-term leave of over 7 days is contemplated, the responsible clinician must consider the use of a community treatment order. This order allows an approved clinician to test the rehabilitation of a patient detained for treatment by discharging the patient subject to their being recalled to hospital if they do not continue with treatment in the community.

A patient subject to a community treatment order is known and referred to in mental health law as a **community patient**. A community patient cannot be made to take treatment by force in the community. Where compulsory treatment is deemed necessary, recall to hospital would be necessary.

The responsible clinician may make a community treatment order for a patient detained under the Mental Health Act 1983 for treatment under sections 3, 47, and 48 of the 1983 Act if they are satisfied that the following criteria are met and an AMHP agrees that a community treatment order is appropriate for that patient:

- The patient must need medical treatment for their mental disorder for their own health or safety, or for the protection of others.
- It must be possible for the patient to receive the treatment they need without having to be in hospital.
- The patient may be recalled to hospital for treatment should this become necessary.

- Appropriate medical treatment for the patient must be available while living in the community.

- The responsible clinician must state the conditions of the order that have been agreed with the AMHP.

- Where the patient does not comply with the conditions, this can be taken into account when considering a recall to hospital.

- The responsible clinician may also recall a community patient to hospital if:

  - they require medical treatment in hospital for mental disorder, and

  - there would be a risk of harm to the health or safety of the patient or to other persons if they were not recalled to hospital for that purpose.

Aftercare

Patients detained for treatment under the Mental Health Act 1983 have a right to aftercare under section 117 of the Act. It is the duty of the health and social services to provide any aftercare services they consider necessary for the patient. As aftercare is a right, the services provided cannot be charged for. The provision of aftercare must continue as long as the health and social services consider the patient requires it. The decision to end aftercare services must be a joint one (*R v Ealing District Health Authority Ex p Fox* [1993]).

Guardianship

Under the Mental Health Act 1983, section 7, guardianship provides an alternative to detention for compulsory treatment by requiring a person with a mental disorder to:

- live at an address specified by the guardian

- provide access to people named by the guardian, such as a doctor, nurse, or social worker

- attend any place the guardian may specify for medical treatment, occupation, education, or training.

No treatment may be given to the patient without consent. Guardianship is administered by the local social services authority. They will name a social worker as guardian or accept a person known to the patient, such as a relative who is suitable and willing to act in the role.

▼ Proposals for reform of the Mental Health Act 1983

The Westminster Government published a draft Bill on the reform of the Mental Health Act 1983 in the summer of 2022 (Department of Health and Social Care and Ministry of Justice, 2022). The draft Bill set out initial Government proposals for implementing the recommendations of the Wessely review of mental health law (Department of Health and Social Care, 2018), that sought to answer why:

- detentions under the 1983 Act had risen some 40% since 2007

- a disproportionate number of people from black and minority ethnic groups are detained under the Act, with black people four times more likely than white people to be detained

- the processes for detention care and treatment have more in common with Victorian era laws than a modern mental health care system.

The draft Bill takes forward the recommendations of the review and suggests how the guiding principles emerging from the review might be implemented in law to ensure:

- choice and autonomy—ensuring service users' views and choices are respected

- least restriction—ensuring the Mental Health Act powers are used in the least restrictive way

- therapeutic benefit—ensuring patients are supported to get better, so they can be discharged from the Mental Health Act

- the person as an individual—ensuring patients are viewed and treated as individuals.

A draft Bill is a form of consultation document and allows for further discussion and amendment by select committees in Parliament before a final Bill is presented to parliament and the process of enacting the reforms begins. Despite the Government receiving the report into the review of the Mental Health Act 1983 and publishing a white paper and draft bill on modernizing mental health law in England and Wales, a final decision on what a twenty-first-century mental health law will provide for is still not clear. It is a little disquieting that the draft Bill currently proposes amending the Mental Health Act 1983 rather than introducing a new Act for the twenty-first century. Given that the 1983 Act was amended in 1995 and again in 2007, with further legislation regulating its implementation and principles in Wales in 2010, it is still not considered fit for purpose in the twenty-first century.

▲ Conclusion

- Mental healthcare is regulated through the provisions of the Mental Health Act 1983 as amended by the Mental Health Act 2007.
- Only people who are suffering from a mental disorder and who actively resist admission to hospital are considered for compulsory detention under the Mental Health Act 1983.
- Detained patients must be informed of the conditions of detention and their right to appeal or complain once in hospital; managers usually delegate this duty to a registered nurse.
- Some treatment under the Mental Health Act 1983 may only be given where provisions safeguarding patients have been met.
- The requirements of the Mental Health Act 1983 and its code of practice must be followed to ensure that patients are cared for with respect and with due regard for their fundamental rights and freedoms.

✖ Tips from service users

1 The Mental Health Act 1983 codes of practice set out how dignified and compassionate mental health care should be delivered including under conditions of detention. Always inform your practice by reference to the codes.

2 Always work in a climate of consent when you have the authority to give compulsory treatment. Consent has two purposes, a legal purpose as a defence against unlawful touching and a clinical purpose. Effective mental health nursing requires cooperation from the service user and this is best achieved by explaining the care and treatment you are proposing to the services user so they can give permission for and cooperate with the delivery of their nursing care.

3 Remember that mental health units have a positive operational obligation under the European Convention on Human Rights to protect service users from harm. You must take reasonable operational measures to protect service users including those who want to harm themselves or take their own life.

W   Companion website

For extra resources on the topics covered in this chapter, visit the companion website at: www.oup.com/mhns

✚   References

B v Croydon Health Authority [1995] 2 WLR 294.

Brown, J. (2016). *The changing purpose of mental health law: from medicalism to legalism to new legalism. International Journal of Law and Psychiatry 47, 1–9.*

Council of Europe (1950). *European Convention on Fundamental Human Rights and Freedoms.* Rome: Council of Europe.

DB v Betsi Cadwaladr UHB [2021] UKUT 53 (AAC).

Department of Health and Social Care (2018). *Modernising the Mental Health Act: Increasing Choice Reducing Compulsion. Chair Sir Simon Wessley. Available at: https://assets.publishing.service.gov.uk/government/ uploads/system/uploads/attachment_data/file/778897/ Modernising_the_Mental_Health_Act_-_increasing_choi ce__reducing_compulsion.pdf*

Department of Health and Social Care and Ministry of Justice (2022). *Draft Mental Health Bill. CP699. Available at: https://assets.publishing.service.gov.uk/government/ uploads/system/uploads/attachment_data/file/1093 555/draft-mental-health-bill-web-accessible.pdf*

Devon Partnership NHS Trust v Secretary of State for Health and Social Care & Others [2021] EWHC 101 (admin).

Dewen v Barnet Healthcare Trust & Barnet London Borough Council [2000] 2 FLR 848.

Legislation.gov.uk (1983). *Mental Health Act 1983. Available at: https://www.legislation.gov.uk/ukpga/ 1983/20/contents*

Legislation.gov.uk (2007). *Mental Health Act 2007. Available at: https://www.legislation.gov.uk/ukpga/ 2007/12/contents*

R (Stennett) v Manchester City Council [2002] UKHL 34.

R (Tagoe-Thompson) v Central and North West London Mental Health NHS Trust [2002] EWHC 2803. *Admin.*

R v Ealing District Health Authority Ex p Fox [1993] 1 WLR 373.

R v Mental Health Review Tribunal for South Thames Region Ex p. Smith [1998] EGCS 55. CA.

St George's Healthcare NHS Trust v S [1998] 3 WLR 936. CA.

Unsworth, C. (1987). *The Politics of Mental Health Legislation. Oxford: Clarendon Press.*

Winterwerp v The Netherlands [1979] 6301/73 ECHR 4.

Considering and responding to risk when working with people living with mental health problems

Dan Warrender   Chris Young

▼ Introduction

Risk is defined as a chance of losing something of value (Fischhoff and Kadvany, 2011), which may contribute to a degree of harm. Often considered narrowly, usually in terms of violence to self or others, risk has greater complexity when we begin to consider the subjectivity of human experience, the different things which we each value, and that some may be valued more than others. In the case of mental health (MH) nursing, the human beings of note are nurses, service users and the people close to them, and the wider nursing and multidisciplinary teams who may contribute to decision-making around risk. We would encourage the reader to keep in mind not only what MH professionals would say is of value, but also a curiosity about what others may value.

Risk cannot be completely eliminated, only changed. As we address one risk, we may create another, and harm may be caused to service users through professional responses. Take a moment to review some important dimensions of risk which are detailed here, and reflect on how they relate to MH nursing practice:

Important aspects of risk (Fischhoff and Kadvany, 2011):

- Risk is a chance of losing something of value, and people may value different things

- Risk can appear in many forms

- It may involve one event or repeated events

- It may be imposed on a person or arise from their own actions

- It can have immediate or delayed effects

- It may impact a person directly or indirectly

- Impacts may be material or psychological

- Outcomes may be certain or uncertain.

Reflection point: think about some things which you value more than others.

This chapter will critically discuss approaches to risk, and promote collaboration and sharing risk with service users as far as possible. Given this is a skills book, we would suggest that the key skills when working with risk are self-awareness, empathy, critical thinking, and relational competence.

▼ Evidence base

Given that risk assessment is a prominent feature of MH nursing, the evidence base is surprisingly poor, with little evidence supporting effectiveness in predicting and reducing risk of harm to self or others (Wand, 2012). In an explicit example, a national inquiry cited that of 1,538 deaths by suicide in individuals in the UK who had been in contact with MH services in the previous 12 months, '88% were judged to be at low or no immediate risk of suicide by clinicians at their final service contact' (National Confidential Inquiry into Suicide and Safety in Mental Health, 2018, p. 5).

Moreover, the same inquiry noted clinicians' views critiquing the use of risk assessment tools (National Confidential Inquiry into Suicide and Safety in Mental Health, 2018, p. 14):

- Compared to full clinical case records, it is not easy to find relevant information.
- Tools can be lengthy and time consuming to complete.
- Tables and tick boxes are not always read by staff.
- Information may not always be accessible if updated incorrectly.

- Difficult to input information and track back, leading to details being lost.
- The use of tools may prevent staff from using experience and clinical judgement and provide false reassurance.

Perhaps contributing to this predictive impotence of risk assessment, Ahmed et al. (2021) found that shared decision-making is not a concept commonly used in MH services, noting studies have shown service users not directly involved in the risk assessment process, and sometimes even unaware that one has taken place. This approach is unlikely to be conducive to good care. Deering et al. (2019) found that from the perspective of service users, beneficial risk management practice includes good interpersonal relationships with staff, clear communication around decisions, and participation in their care. While the purpose of any risk assessment and response should be to understand how we can help, it has been associated with causing harm to service users (Deering et al., 2019).

▼ Iatrogenic harm

It is important to be aware that risk does not just exist within the service user, and also comes from measures used by MH nurses to manage risk. It is common for MH practitioners to see themselves as heroes. Imagine firefighters coming to the rescue, pulling victims from the flames of their inner turmoil just in the nick of time. Who cares about a bit of water damage if you have just saved someone's life?

Iatrogenic harm, like water damage, is defined as 'inadvertent' injury caused to service users by well-meaning care. It is trauma often seen as both accidental and incidental as we administer interventions in controlled environments for what we believe to be the good of service users.

But consider the often-detrimental effects of that input. Let us not call them side effects, because that minimizes the actual harm done to thousands of people by the less desirable foibles inherent in the system. Take any psychotropic medication—the short-, medium-, and long-term undesired effects of taking them are well

documented, from erectile dysfunction to type 2 diabetes, from suicidal ideation to dissociation, and yet we often minimize them, leaving them undiscussed with the traumatized service user we see before us. Similarly, much of the coercion and control we use on our service users breaches human rights (see the companion website for an online activity), and can retraumatize them, triggering many of the events that led to their 'mental illness' in the first place by repeating them.

The cognitive dissonance generated by a caring system that causes harm is often too much for us to take. After all, we are the good guys—the firefighters—we have come to the rescue … have we not? We know objectively what is best for our service users … do we not? When we use interventions that we know may cause harm to our service users, even in the most challenging environments, even with the best of intentions, we can no longer claim this is 'inadvertent' iatrogenic harm.

▼ Assessing risk through relational practice

Given risk assessment tools cannot effectively predict nor assure level of risk, we suggest that the best way to assess risk is through empathic, genuine, and curious conversations. Attending to the principles of establishing good therapeutic relationships is essential, as without trust and compassion, a service user is unlikely to share their inner world. Given the complexity of human beings, there is no clear 'how-to' in addressing risk. Rather, there are a series of things to think about to ensure we help and avoid harm. As with all approaches, models, and tools, they are of limited benefit without attending to the context of the human relationships in which they occur.

We suggest the following principles form the bedrock from which any assessment and response should take place. We have coined these ingredients the Goldilocks 'just right' response.

Goldilocks 'just right' response

- **Person centred**—with empathy towards the service user, as they are seen and treated as a unique person rather than a stereotype or diagnosis.
- **Relational**—with communication and engagement from MH nurses demonstrating the necessary skills, techniques, and considerations involved in establishing genuine, hopeful, and trusting therapeutic relationships.

- **Collaborative**—with a transparent decision-making process, which seeks to share risk with the service user, fully involves them as the expert of their own experience and needs, and as per the triangle of care should involve family and supportive people if helpful to the service user. Collaboration should also extend, where appropriate, to integrating and coordinating communication between relevant agencies and care providers who may be involved in the service user's care.
- **Mentalizing**—with attention paid to the mental states of all people involved, particularly the underlying distress experienced by service users which contributes to risk, and any distress resulting from measures used to contain risk. Mentalizing involves both an acute self-awareness of nurse's mental states as well as an explicit empathy for service users. This awareness of our own and others' mental states considers the motivations behind decisions and behaviours.
- **Least restrictive**—where any measure taken to contain risk must allow the service user as much freedom as possible while keeping them safe, is reviewed regularly, with full autonomy and freedom given back to the service user as soon as possible.
- **Reflective**—through clinical supervision or formal reflection, MH nurses should actively reflect on decisions taken, ensuring that the service users' needs are being met while avoiding iatrogenic harm

▼ Case vignette

The vignette in Box 21.1 is a true story (pseudonym used). We would encourage readers to read this and keep this person in mind as you explore the models which follow. You may also find it useful to refer to Chapter 23, which explores suicide and self-harm in more detail.

Given the extreme but not rare occurrence illustrated with Abeo in Box 21.1, it is understandable that when working with risk, nurses can become overwhelmed with anxiety and critical thinking can become redundant. The following two models, the triangle of risk (Figure 21.1) and the action/consequences model (Table 21.1), are presented as aids to considering risk.

The triangle of risk (T. Dickinson, personal communication, 2021) is a model to aid risk assessment, composed of three

elements of risk which, akin to the triangle of fire, when present in combination may increase the likelihood of adverse outcomes:

- **Method—a way of doing something**. For example, a person who is motivated to self-harm and their chosen method is a razorblade. A method may relate to an action which would cause harm, and importantly, there may be a variety of methods which need to be considered. Methods may be specific objects, part of the environment, or even at times the person's own body. Identifying potential methods is important in terms of reducing the risk of harm, as intervention may then address the means and ability to utilize these methods. While methods are an important consideration, unless a person's ability or motivation to act is addressed, one method of harm can quickly be replaced by another.

Box 21.1 Practice example: Abeo

Abeo was in her twenties when she completed suicide while under 15-minute observations in the psychiatric hospital where she had been detained. This was the devastating conclusion to her short life that was marred by abuse, neglect, and invalidation by those charged with her care.

In her late teens she was given the label of borderline personality disorder after a childhood of sexual abuse by her step-father because she was displaying a number of 'symptoms' including suicidal ideation and behaviour, self-harm, and dissociation.

Over a period of 10 years, Abeo was given a variety of diagnoses and medications from antidepressants to antipsychotics and sedatives by a steady procession of psychiatrists who, as a rule, saw her once before moving on in their rotation.

At no point in that time was she offered any non-medical treatments such as psychotherapy or access to a therapeutic community.

She was detained on numerous occasions, being regularly told by a wide range of staff including MH nurses, that she was manipulative and attention seeking and that her problems were 'behavioural' and/or incurable.

In her early twenties, she was given a 2-year prison sentence for trespass after attempting to take her own life on a railway line. She was released into the community after 6 months on the condition that she wore an electronic tag and attended weekly meetings with a criminal justice social worker, where she was told to change her undefined 'offending behaviours'.

Once her sentence was complete, she was placed on a waiting list for a placement at a therapeutic community. Just before she got to the top of the list, a psychiatrist redefined her condition as antisocial personality disorder, making her ineligible for that service.

Abeo completed suicide shortly after that.

- **Means—the ability to do something**. For example, a person has a method of harming themselves such as self-harm with a razorblade, and they have access to razorblades. If a method is identified, assessment needs to consider the means in terms of ability to act using that method. Means may require to be addressed in terms of removal of objects or implements which could harm, though as methods may be environmental or even the person themselves, the means may include access to certain places, or time spent alone.

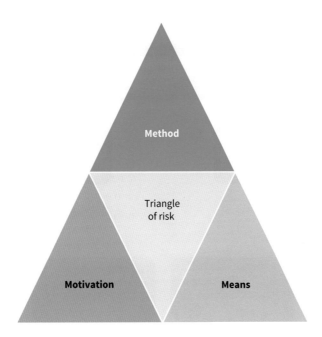

Figure 21.1 The triangle of risk

Table 21.1 The action/consequences model

| Actions | Potential consequences | | | | |
	Benefits	Dangers	Short term	Long term	Interpretation of motive
Containing risk	Service user safety	Retraumatization Disempowerment	Service user safety MH nurse comfort	MH nurse comfort Creating dependence Alienation Evolution of risk	Care and compassion Punitive control
Tolerating risk	Service user autonomy	Retraumatization Invalidation MH nurse complacency Significant and lasting harm	Short-term risk MH nurse anxiety	MH nurse anxiety Opportunity for service user to develop own coping mechanisms	Neglect Trust and freedom

Adapted from Warrender, D. (2018). Borderline personality disorder and the ethics of risk management: the action/consequences model. *Nursing Ethics* 25(7), 918–927.

- **Motivation—the drive to act**. For example, a person is motivated to die by suicide due to feelings of hopelessness and emotional distress. While with fire if we remove one ingredient from the triangle the fire disappears, risk in human beings is more complex. We can remove both means and method, but the person may still be in distress, and attention needs to be drawn to an iatrogenic circle; the fact that

removing means and method may involve restricting a person's freedom and human rights, which may cause further distress, thus contributing to the motivation to act on risk (Figure 21.2).

While safety is important, it is not wellness. Consideration needs to be given to the fuel—any mental states, distress, or experiences which may contribute to the motivation for

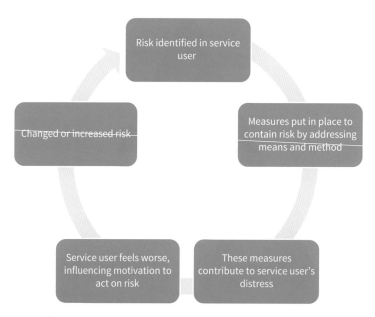

Figure 21.2 Iatrogenic cycle of containing risk

service users acting in risky ways. Arguably, addressing motivation is most important, as without motivation to act on risk, method and means become inconsequential. Overlooking motivation is often noted as a failing of MH care, with nurses often responding to behaviour without exploring underlying distress.

▼ The action/consequences model

Having assessed risk, the MH nurse must make decisions regarding appropriate intervention. The action/consequences model (Warrender, 2018), updated here (Table 21.1), explores potential consequences based on the actions of containing and tolerating risk.

Actions

Actions are what nurses do. Containing risk is any action which places barriers in between the person and their ability to act in a way which may put them or others at risk of harm. Containment may be physical, chemical, or legal, and examples may range between hospital admission, use of medication, the Mental Health Act, and physical restraints. Conversely, tolerating risk at its most extreme sees a service user having full autonomy, though with no input from services (and they may be frustrated with the term service user, when they do not access any services). Tolerating risk is preferred to the term 'positive risk taking', as it could be strongly argued that many risks are anything but positive. Between these two extremes of action exists a spectrum whereby risk can be contained or tolerated to various degrees.

Potential consequences

MH care has been criticized as either excluding people from care or becoming so risk averse that people spend lengthy spells in hospital against their will. Whether we contain or tolerate risk, there are consequences to these actions or omissions. There may be ethical consequences of beneficence (doing good), but also maleficence (doing harm). One of the first principles of healthcare is to do no harm, thus it is essential that careful consideration is given to the potential for iatrogenic harm, which can present itself in various ways. The potential consequences of each action are taken here in turn, and presented as potentials rather than certainties, and things to think about rather than a 'how-to' guide.

▼ The potential consequences of containing risk

Benefits and dangers

The obvious benefit of containing risk is that service users may be kept safe; however, the way in which this is done needs careful consideration. As some risk management practices can remove human rights and are restrictive and coercive by nature, they may become iatrogenic harm through retraumatizing people and echoing their previous experiences of adversity, or even becoming an index trauma themselves. In these instances, nurses should ask themselves, 'Does our approach to safety **feel safe** for the service user?'

Restrictive practice may disempower people from using their own coping mechanisms, for example, being on locked hospital wards unable to exercise, or more controversially, people who use self-harm as a coping mechanism being prevented from doing so. While we would never actively encourage self-harm, careful thought does need to be given to removing a service user's usual coping mechanism, without acknowledging the distress this may cause or replacing it with something of equal value.

Short term and long term

In the short term, a service user may be safe from the assessed risk of harm, and the degree of comfort nurses themselves may experience due to this may be a driver of decisions. Containing risk in the long term, however, becomes much more complex. As a crisis intervention has been defined as that which ensures safety and recovery and lasts no longer than 1 month (Borschmann et al., 2012), containing risk beyond this point may be considered long term.

If a service user has been contained for a period of time, stepping away from that may be daunting. A feeling of understandable attachment and dependence may occur, unless risk is shared, and transition to increasing self-efficacy and autonomy is gently managed.

Alienation may occur where containing risk becomes what has been described as a 'state of nervous paternalism' (Wand, 2012, p. 6), with distressed service users and anxious nurses experiencing a breakdown in relationships. Good relational practice and critical reflection is essential to minimize the likelihood of this occurring.

Risk can never be completely eliminated, only changed. If a service user is contained in the long term with increasing restriction, risk will simply evolve. Using an analogy, if you hold a piece of jelly in your hand, close your hand, and try to contain it more and more, no matter how hard you press, it will gradually flow outside your hand and through your fingers. In the same way, if a person is distressed and contained more and more, removal of means and method may simply force a person to reconsider means and method. Containing risk in of itself is not treatment, and therapeutic responses need to address underlying distress.

▼ The potential consequences of tolerating risk

Benefits and dangers

The obvious benefit of tolerating risk is that this approach embodies the least restrictive response, with no infringement on a service user's rights or liberty. The dangers of this approach arise when risk is overlooked, minimized, or communication deviates from the Goldilocks 'just right' response.

As many service users have experienced trauma, neglect, and adversity, they may experience a retraumatization through invalidation if they are communicating needs which are not listened to, or not deemed serious enough to meet the threshold for service provision by gatekeepers. For people who have experienced neglect in their lives, it may reinforce low self-worth and steal hope.

The most significant danger when tolerating risk is complacency, when serious risk is overlooked, possibly resulting in significant and lasting harm such as death through suicide. Complacency may occur around service users who have presented to services in repeated crises, perhaps surviving attempted suicide several times. There may be the naïve assumption that as they have previously not met with significant and lasting harm, that this will always be the case. As mortal beings, it only takes one falsifier for this theory to be shattered. People can and do die.

Short term and long term

In the short term, tolerating risk is most likely to cause an acute professional anxiety. While this is understandable, particularly given potential for significant and lasting harm, decisions made should be about the needs of service users rather than alleviating the anxiety of MH nurses. As more risk is tolerated and a service user remains safe, the anxiety may dissipate. However, given the unpredictability of human beings and risk, a level of anxiety may continue long term. The goal is not to ignore or overcome anxiety, but to acknowledge it and its impact on clinical decisions.

As tolerating risk is least restrictive, it is the best place from which a service user can be independent and potentially develop their own coping mechanisms. An important caveat, however, is that tolerating risk should never be seen as a reason to do nothing, as this development will not occur by magic, and may be unlikely without effective support. This calls into question some clinical practice which sees some people as 'too unstable' for longer-term interventions. Tolerating risk may mean not containing risk, though useful therapeutic responses and interventions still need to be provided.

▼ Interpretation of motive

The interpretation of motive behind actions and decisions on risk is incredibly important, given the human relationships in which these occur. Decisions are seen by service users, their loved ones and families, colleagues, managers, the organization, professional bodies such as the Nursing and Midwifery Council, the media, and wider society. Given this context, nurses might have concerns not only of how they justify their decisions, but of how those decisions may be perceived by all of the aforementioned parties. The best interest of service users is paramount and doing good rather than looking good to anyone else. One recognized phenomenon is 'defensive psychiatry', where decisions are made for fear of litigation, and based on risk to MH professional rather than service user.

The potential for misinterpreting decisions requires excellent relational practice and transparency around decision-making, talking to service users with empathy, and sharing why we have made the decisions we have. One may imagine how containing risk may appear caring and compassionate, rescuing someone from harm. However, not all containment is experienced as caring and compassionate, and may be understood as punitive control. Likewise, tolerating risk may either be perceived as neglect, not taking service users seriously and

not caring, or perceived as evidence of trust, empowerment, hope and belief in the service users' strengths. The perceptual consequences of these actions may influence the trajectory of care.

In concluding the model, it is essential to re-emphasize the importance of critical thinking, and the skill of not only acting but effectively communicating that action's intent. To have any hope of building and maintaining a therapeutic alliance we must do good, aim to avoid harm, communicate decisions with empathy, and be willing to say a genuine sorry when we get it wrong.

▼ Maintaining values in social systems and challenging poor practice

Obedience is not synonymous with morality. The risks of professional conformity, obedience, and bystander apathy are significant in MH care. As social animals, no matter how independently minded we would like to think we are, the desire to fit in can be incredibly powerful (see the companion website for an online activity). Studies on conformity, obedience, and bystander apathy have frequently shown humans will act contrary to their knowledge, beliefs, and values to be accepted as part of the larger group (Mermillod et al., 2015).

This risk is greatest when we enter new and unfamiliar environments—for example, if we are newly qualified and/or working for an organization for the first time. This can be particularly challenging when we encounter prejudice and discrimination in our working environment. Thompson (1997) describes prejudice occurring at three levels:

- **The personal**—an individual member of staff may hold, voice, and act on views that clearly discriminate against service users or groups of service users.
- **The cultural**—the organization may allow this member of staff, and others like them, to continue discriminatory behaviour unchallenged and unsanctioned—perhaps seen as a bit of fun, or banter. This can apply to wards, hospitals, services, and professional groups.
- **The structural**—our society still negatively discriminates against people with mental illness and distress.

This becomes apparent when we think about our collective acceptance of poor support and services and negative attitudes towards this vulnerable group. Our governments, media, education, criminal justice, welfare benefit, and employment systems can all contribute to the stigma experienced by people with mental ill-health.

Reflection point: think about how some of your values may be different to colleagues you have worked with.

It is worth exploring the systems your organization has in place to challenge any prejudices and considering how you may feel when challenging these attitudes. The interplay between the personal, cultural, and structural environments can make any kind of awareness raising or whistle-blowing difficult, especially when pernicious guidelines and policies can make the whistle-blower the problem.

As an individual, as part of a team or organization, and as a member of society, it is not enough to be non-discriminatory. We need to be anti-discriminatory, questioning, and challenging prejudice wherever we encounter it.

> If you are neutral in situations of injustice, you have chosen the side of the oppressor.
>
> Archbishop Desmond Tutu

▲ Conclusion

Risk does not exist solely in the presenting problems of service users and working with risk requires critical thinking which

may be guided by models, but necessarily requires the foundations of the Goldilocks 'just right' response. It is essential that we consider the life story service users have experienced before arriving at the point of risk assessment, and not only the actions we take when considering risk but also how we communicate intent. Just as importantly, it is crucial that we consider the risks we bring to the situation, and the ways in which well-intended 'care' can harm service users, before we embark on a journey of what we deem to be best for them.

✖ Tips from service users

1 Working with risk might be your day-to-day job, but please remember this is a significant life experience for me.
2 Please remember I'm a person with a story and a past, and I might have good reasons for not trusting the MH care system.
3 Risk doesn't just come from the things I do, and you need to think about what you and other professionals do too.

W   Companion website

For extra resources on the topics covered in this chapter, visit the companion website at: www.oup.com/mhns

---

✚   References

Ahmed, N., Barlow, S., Reynolds, L., Drey, N., Begum, F., Tuudah, E., and Simpson, A. (2021). *Mental health professionals' perceived barriers and enablers to shared decision making in risk assessment and risk management: a qualitative systematic review. BMC Psychiatry 21(1)*, 594.

Borschmann, R., Henderson, C., Hogg, J., Phillips, R., and Moran, P. (2012). *Crisis interventions for people with borderline personality disorder. Cochrane Database of Systematic Reviews 6, CD009353.*

Deering, K., Pawson, C., Summers, N., and Williams, J. (2019). *Patient perspectives of helpful risk management practices within mental health services. A mixed studies systematic review of primary research. Journal of Psychiatric and Mental Health Nursing 26(5–6), 185–197.*

Fischhoff, B. and Kadvany, J. (2011). *Risk: A Very Short Introduction. Oxford: Oxford University Press.*

Mermillod, M., Marchand, V., Lepage, J., Begue, L., and Dambrun, M. (2015). *Destructive obedience without pressure: beyond the limits of the agentic state. Social Psychology 46(6), 345–351.*

National Confidential Inquiry into Suicide and Safety in Mental Health (2018). *The Assessment of Clinical Risk in Mental Health Services. Manchester: The University of Manchester. Available at: https://www.research.man chester.ac.uk/portal/files/77517990/REPORT_The_ assessment_of_clinical_risk_in_mental_health_servi ces.pdf*

Thompson, N. (1997). *Anti-Discriminatory Practice, 2nd ed. Basingstoke: Macmillan.*

Wand, T. (2012). *Investigating the evidence for the effectiveness of risk assessment in mental health care. Issues in Mental Health Nursing 33(1), 2–7.*

Warrender, D. (2018). *Borderline personality disorder and the ethics of risk management: the action/ consequences model. Nursing Ethics 25(7), 918–927.*

22 Practising safe and effective observation

Mark J. Baker
Susan Sookoo

Haseem Usman

Learning outcomes

By the end of this chapter, you should be able to:

1 Describe the current evidence and best practice guidance regarding observation

2 Define the concept of restrictive practice

3 Apply the core skills and competencies required to observe service users 'at risk' in an effective and supportive way

4 Explain the potential benefits and limitations of conducting observation at different levels of intensity.

▼ Introduction

This chapter addresses the core skill of observation. It can be confusing for everyone (nurses, service users, carers) that there is no universal term used to describe the procedure of observation. Instead, the procedure is known by various terms in different places and countries. Here is a list of some of the terms you may encounter in your reading and practice: nursing observation; formal observation; close observation; special observation; maximum observation; continuous or constant observation or supervision; suicide watch or precaution; 15-minute, timed, or intermittent checks; specialing; one-to-one nursing; within eyesight; and within arm's length. In this chapter, for purposes of consistency, the simple term of 'observation' is used.

The main purpose of observation is to keep service users safe when they are acutely mentally unwell. It is a commonly used intervention for service users 'at risk' of harming themselves or others, or at risk of being harmed by others. The procedure of observation should be performed according to prescribed 'levels' of observation, which vary in intensity according to the degree of assessed risk. Service users assessed to be at greatest risk of harming themselves or others are nursed on continuous observation, with service users never being left alone by nurses, and with the nurse often within 'arm's reach' of the service user.

The Chief Nursing Officer's Review of Mental Health Nursing (Department of Health (DoH), 2006) identified risk and risk management as a key area requiring good practice guidance, with the aim of improving outcomes for service users; a position recently echoed in the NHS Long Term Plan (NHS England, 2019). Regarding the practice of observation, the Chief Nursing Officer's review specified that mental health nurses are required to 'demonstrate an understanding of the benefits and limitations of the use of levels of observation to maximise therapeutic effect on in-patient units' (DoH, 2006, p. 29). Callagan et al. (2012) note the Chief Nursing Officer's review prompted direct and indirect positive changes in the practice of observation in mental health.

Observation is designed to be a therapeutic intervention, yet it is acknowledged that there are benefits, limitations, and challenges involved. The challenge for nurses who conduct observation is to maintain the safety of service users who are at 'high-risk', while providing person-centred care.

▼ The evidence base

National guidelines exist to govern the practice of observations in mental health contexts, such as the Standing Nursing and Midwifery Advisory Committee (DoH, 1999); National Institute for Health and Care Excellence (NICE) guidelines: *Violence and Aggression: Short-Term Management in Mental Health, and Community Settings* (2015), *Violent and Aggressive Behaviours in People with Mental Health Problems* (2017), and *Self-harm: Assessment, Management and Preventing Recurrence* (2022); *Mental Health Act 1983: Code of Practice* (DoH, 2015); and the *Mental Health Act 1983* (as amended) (Legislation.gov.uk, 1983). Policy evidence is also available, such as the *Mental Capacity (Amendment) Act 2019: Liberty Protection Safeguards* (Department of Health and Social Care, 2020), and *Positive and Proactive Care: Reducing the Need for Restrictive Interventions* (DoH, 2014). In addition, local trust policies may be relevant across various clinical contexts, such as observation and engagement, management of violence and aggression, positive behaviour management, and seclusion.

Despite a range of policy and guidance documents there is very little evidence regarding the efficacy and impact of observation (Chu, 2016). There are various policies and good practice documents regarding observation, at international, national, and local levels. Research indicates mixed findings about the effectiveness of observation in preventing people from self-harming (Reen et al., 2020; Slemon et al., 2017). Some surveys report fewer suicides when patients are being observed (Flynn et al., 2017) while other studies report no relationship (Stewart et al., 2009). Harmful effects associated with observation have also been reported (Stewart et al., 2012). These varying views reflect how therapeutic, effective, and 'safe' observation really is. In this section, the main principles of observation are described and the current evidence base discussed.

What is observation?

Observation is a commonly used mental health nursing intervention for service users who are assessed to be at risk of harming themselves or others, or at risk of being harmed or exploited by others (Bowers and Park, 2001; Reen et al., 2020). Observation is widely defined as: 'regarding the service user attentively while minimising the extent to which they feel that they are under surveillance' (DoH, 1999, p. 2). More recently, NICE (2015) broadened this definition: 'minimally restrictive intervention of varying intensity in which a member of the healthcare staff observes and maintains contact with a service user to ensure the service user's safety and the safety of others'. Observation involves the allocation of one staff healthcare worker, usually from the nursing team—which may sometimes involve two or more healthcare workers—to one service user for a prescribed length of time to provide intensive care. As highlighted by the definition of observation, a great challenge for nurses who conduct observation is to maintain service users' safety while minimizing restrictive practice, that is, the custodial nature of the intervention (Chu, 2016; Reen et al., 2020).

Observation can be used as an intervention in several different situations and is commonly used for service users who are:

- suicidal or actively interested in harming themselves
- aggressive and who pose a danger to staff or other service users
- vulnerable
- likely to abscond
- sexually disinhibited (Bowers, 2014; Slemon et al., 2017).

Observation and suicide

The purpose of observing service users who are suicidal or at risk of self-harm is to keep service users safe, and to also support service users in feeling safe. Indeed, research that asked service users about observation demonstrated that the interpersonal aspect of observation is important, with supportive interactions with staff enhancing service users' feelings of safety and hope (Barnicot et al., 2017, Jones et al., 2000; Reen et al., 2020). However, an influential report by the National Confidential Inquiry into Suicide and Homicide by People with Mental Illness (2006) has shown that a minority of service users do not remain safe in hospital, even when they are being observed closely. This study found that out of all suicides in England and Wales during that period, 27% (6,367 individuals) were current or recent mental health inpatients. Some 856 of these individuals had committed suicide while in hospital, and of these 185 (22% of all inpatient suicides) were at the time under observation, with 18 (3%) of these cases reported to be under the most intensive one-to-one observation when the suicide occurred. Although these figures may seem relatively small, it demonstrates that observation is not 100% effective in preventing inpatient suicides. In fact, some research highlights that service users do not always remain safe in hospital despite being under observation (Flynn et al., 2017).

Observation and disturbed/violent behaviour

Service user disturbed/violent behaviour occurs for several reasons and nurses are often at the forefront of managing this behaviour (Morrison, 1990a, 1990b) with observation as a primary intervention in the recognition, prevention, and therapeutic management of violence (NICE, 2015). NICE (2015) guidance recommends the use of observation as a least restrictive intervention for the short-term management of violence and aggressive behaviour in mental health and other settings. A key evolution of these guidelines has been to reduce the use of restrictive interventions with a focus on therapeutic engagement that is person-centred in reducing the risk of violence and aggression.

Observation levels

Central to all observation policies is the prescribed 'level' of observation. NICE (2015) recommends staff working in inpatient mental health wards consider using the following definitions for levels of observation, unless a locally agreed policy states otherwise, that is, within an individual hospital or health care service:

- **Low-level intermittent observation**: the baseline level of observation in a specified psychiatric setting. The frequency of observation is once every 30 to 60 minutes.

- **High-level intermittent observation**: usually used if a service user is at risk of becoming violent or aggressive but does not represent an immediate risk. The frequency of observation is once every 15 to 30 minutes. Or arbitrarily timed checked (e.g. four checks within the hour).

- **Continuous observation**: usually used when a service user presents an immediate threat and needs to be kept within eyesight or at arm's length of a designated one-to-one nurse, with immediate access to other members of staff if needed.

- **Multiprofessional continuous observation**: usually used when a service user is at the highest risk of harming themselves or others and needs to be kept within eyesight of two or three staff members and at arm's length of at least one staff member.

Observation and restrictive practice

The practice of observation has been labelled as a custodial task, rather than a therapeutic intervention (Cutcliffe and Barker, 2002; Dodds and Bowles, 2001). Stevenson and Cutcliffe (2006) described observation as 'the regulatory function of the "gaze" of professional codes and government policy in relation to restricting professional practices' (p. 713), while Cutcliffe and Barker (2002) note that observation originally served the function of providing feedback to a doctor about a service user's status. No matter the function or purpose, observation can be viewed as a restrictive intervention.

Restrictive interventions are defined in *Positive and Proactive Care: Reducing the Need for Restrictive Interventions* (DoH, 2014, p. 14) as:

> deliberate acts on the part of other person(s) that restrict an individual's movement, liberty, and/or freedom to act independently in order to:
> - take immediate control of a dangerous situation where there is a real possibility of harm to the person or others if no action is undertaken; and
> - end or reduce significantly the danger to the person or others; and
> - contain or limit the person's freedom for no longer than is necessary.

Positive and Proactive Care was in response to investigations about the abuses at Winterbourne View and the findings of MIND (2013) and as such focuses on reducing the need for physical interventions. However, the definition of restrictive interventions certainly fits the practice of, in particular, constant observation. The DoH (2015) identifies enhanced observation (along with physical and mechanical restraint, rapid tranquillization, seclusion, and long-term segregation) as a restrictive intervention. Similarly, the Safewards model of conflict and containment (Bowers et al., 2014) includes aggression, self-harm, suicide, absconding, substance/alcohol use, and medication refusal as conflict behaviours and special observation as a containment measure.

Observation, particularly continuous observation, is a restrictive practice, and policy and research emphasize an imperative to reduce the need for restrictive practice. The *Mental Health Act 1983: Code of Practice* (DoH, 2015) explicitly states that 'there may be times when enhanced levels of observation are required for the short-term management of behavioural disturbance or during periods of distress to prevent suicide or serious self-harm' (2015, para. 26.30) adding that any restrictive intervention should only be used in a way that respects human rights. In practice, the use of observation is not isolated, but occurs in the context of a complex decision-making process (Barnicot et al., 2017) which is in turn influenced by the 'ecology' (Bowers et al., 2008), or culture, of the service. Restrictive interventions should only ever be used as a last resort and then for the shortest time possible, and services should provide a culture in which people's needs are met and their quality of life enhanced. The pertinent issues are using observation in a way that respects human rights, while also finding ways to reduce the need for observation as an intervention.

The statutory framework which directs the use of observations is set out in the *Mental Health Act 1983: Code of Practice* (DoH, 2015) and indicates observation should be caring rather than custodial. New NICE (2022) guidelines extend our understanding about the practice of observation and suggest the use of therapeutic risk taking: 'a process that aims to empower people who self-harm to make decisions about their own safety and to take risks to enable recovery'. The process of taking risks should be based on joint decision-making between the service user and the multidisciplinary team (for further discussion on risk assessment, see Chapter 21) and involve collaborative care planning (NICE, 2022) (for further discussion on collaborative care planning, see Chapter 10). A qualitative study by Barnicot et al. (2017) reported that factors which enable good practice are short-term use of observation as part of a risk-taking approach, collaborative decision-making with the service user, and supportive team working. MacKay et al.

(2005) explain that the balance between control and caring is achieved through a staff philosophy of 'least restrictive intervention and in the best interests of the patient' (p. 469). In practice, least restrictive interventions may involve using different levels of observation. For example, lower levels of self-harm have been associated with use of intermittent observations rather than constant observation, which was in the service user's best interests (Bowers et al., 2008).

Observation is much more than 'just watching' (MacKay et al., 2005) or 'sitting and staring' at the service user (Altschul and McGovern, 1985) but is a complex, caring intervention which can engender hope (Cutcliffe and Barker, 2002). Its use as a restrictive intervention should be minimal and attention should be paid to the factors underlying self-harm and safety. Janner (2007, p. 76) highlights that research 'repeatedly demonstrates that providing a stimulating, therapeutic environment, and crucially one where service users feel listened to by staff, is not a distraction from ensuring safety. On the contrary, it is a prerequisite'. Altschul and McGovern (1985) argue that nurses can provide a stimulating and therapeutic environment for service users under constant observation by offering to play board and/or card games, reading aloud, and actively listening to them. They posit the importance of the nurse remaining vigilant and not becoming so absorbed in any work that they will not notice the service user's every move and point out that the effect of constant observation is often that 'the [service user] observes the staff more efficiently than nurses are able to observe the [service user] (Altschul and McGovern, 1985, p. 167).

▼ Observation in practice

We have considered the evidence for observation and the principles underlying its use. In this section we will apply these

to a practice example (Box 22.1). This section applies the principles of the *Mental Health Act 1983: Code of Practice* (DoH,

Box 22.1 Practice example: illustrating observation in practice

You are a mental health nurse and you have worked on the same acute ward for 2 years since qualifying. You arrive at 07:00 to start a 12-hour shift. The other nurse who should be on the shift with you has called in sick, so an agency nurse has been booked who has not worked on the ward before. There are also two support workers—one a regular member of staff, one who is doing a bank shift. The night staff give a handover for each of the 16 service users on the ward. One, Aisha, has set a fire in her room during the night. She was assessed by the duty doctor and nurse in charge and said that she wanted

to commit suicide by inhaling the smoke from the fire. Aisha had been admitted 24 hours previously due to low mood and has been withdrawn, staying in her room, for most of this time. Since admission she has drunk tea but not joined patients for meals. Her mother has phoned several times since Aisha's admission to ask how she is. Suicide risk was assessed as high and constant observations were started at 03:00. You are in charge of coordinating the shift so you must make sure a rota is done for constant observations of the service user, delegate care of the other 15 service users, and allocate staff tasks.

Table 22.1 Application of the Mental Health Act 1983: Code of Practice to the practice example

Mental Health Act 1983: Code of Practice (DoH, 2015) guidance	Observation in practice
Para. 26.33 Provider policies should cover the use of enhanced observation and include: • which staff (profession and grade) are best placed to carry out enhanced, constant, observation and under what circumstances it might be appropriate to delegate this duty to another member of the team • how the selection of a staff member to undertake enhanced observation should take account of the individual's characteristics and circumstances (including factors such as ethnicity, sexual identity, age, and gender)	• There are four staff on the shift who can carry out observations. As nurse in charge, the rota for observations will need to allow for each staff member to have a break • As some of the staff are not permanent, you will need to make sure they are aware of local observation policies • You will need to discuss with Aisha her wishes about who will carry out observations and liaise with a manager if these wishes cannot be met by the staff on the shift
Para. 26.33 (cont.) • how enhanced observation can be undertaken in a way which minimizes the likelihood of individuals perceiving the intervention to be coercive	• Service users and their carers should be involved in the planning and delivery of person-centred care (NICE, 2015). A major complaint among service users who experience observation is the lack of information provided about why they need to be observed and by whom (Jones et al., 2000; Staniszewska et al., 2019). Service users report feeling more supported when the observer is known and actively engages with them (Barnicot et al., 2017). Engagement is key to fostering a therapeutic relationship and experience (McAllister et al., 2021) • It is imperative that every effort is made to involve Aisha and her mother in the decision-making process regarding observation, and you must ensure that the procedure and the reasons for its implementation are explained clearly and documented
Para. 26.33 (cont.) • how observation can be carried out in a way that respects the individual's privacy as far as practicable and minimizes any distress. In particular, provider policies should outline how an individual's dignity can be maximized without compromising safety when individuals are in a state of undress, such as when using the toilet, bathing, showering, dressing, etc.	• The care plan that accompanies any period of observation should involve Aisha. When appropriate, each handover from one observer to another and each evaluation of the care plan should also include Aisha • You will need to discuss the care plan with Aisha and the multidisciplinary team to decide on what to do when Aisha is using the toilet etc. • You will also need to plan for staffing issues such as ethnicity, sexual identity, age, and sex when deciding who should carry out observations when Aisha is in a state of undress

(*continued*)

Table 22.1 Continued

Mental Health Act 1983: Code of Practice (DoH, 2015) guidance	Observation in practice
	• With Aisha's permission, an explanation of the plan of care, including the rationale for observation, should also be provided to her mother. Her feedback on the care plan should be considered, as her knowledge and experience of Aisha may help to explain her presentation and inform the choice of appropriate therapeutic interventions
Para. 26.30 Enhanced, or constant, observation is a therapeutic intervention with the aim of reducing the factors which contribute to increased risk and promoting recovery. It should focus on engaging the person therapeutically and enabling them to address their difficulties constructively (e.g. through sitting, chatting, encouraging/supporting people to participate in activities, to relax, to talk about any concerns, etc.)	• Each member of staff carrying out observations will need to engage with Aisha, adapting to her needs at the time • This may include sitting silently with her, talking about her mood, and carrying out activities like eating or playing board games • Staff members should not use their phone or read magazines/newspapers when observing Aisha, even if she does not want to engage with them, as this may signal to Aisha that they are preoccupied with other tasks, when their sole task should be to ensure her safety and therapeutically engage with her
Para. 26.34 Staff should balance the potentially distressing effect on the individual of increased levels of observation, particularly if these are proposed for many hours or days, against the identified risk of self-injury or behavioural disturbance. Levels of observation and risk should be regularly reviewed, and a record made of decisions agreed in relation to increasing or decreasing the observation	• You will need to plan for the next review of Aisha's observations and discuss with her the criteria for reducing the level of observations • You will need to coordinate the multidisciplinary team for this review which includes Aisha and her mother

Source: data from Department of Health (2015). *Mental Health Act 1983: Code of Practice*. London: The Stationery Office.

2015) guidance for enhanced, constant, observation to a practice example to illustrate its use (Table 22.1).

▲ Conclusion

This chapter has described the core skills and competencies required to observe service users 'at risk' on acute inpatient mental health wards. There is some emerging evidence, but rigorous evaluative research is required to assess the effectiveness of observation and to guide effective practice. This chapter has referred a great deal to the existing written guidance on observation, specifically the revised NICE (2015) guidance.

Observing a service user who is deeply distressed and potentially suicidal or aggressive is one of the most difficult and demanding roles to undertake for a nurse. It involves the challenge of maintaining the safety of service users, while minimizing the custodial nature of the intervention. As highlighted by Duffy (1995) and Barnicot et al. (2017), conducting observation reveals the inherent tension around service user-focused care, because the aim of 'keeping someone safe' may in reality mean having to stop a service user from doing something they are intent on doing, for example, attempting to harm themselves in some way, attempting to abscond, or behaving aggressively towards others. However, service users tell us from their experience of being observed that, when observation is conducted by nurses who engage with them in a supportive way, therapeutic benefits can include feeling cared for, protected, safer, and more optimistic. This is what mental health nurses should strive to achieve in their practice of observation.

✖ Tips from service users

1   Ask service users about their experience of being under observation.
2   Ask service users, and carers, how they would like to be involved in planning their care with observation.
3   Read policy, guidance, and journal articles keeps you up to date with current evidence.
4   Develop an understanding of observation and the levels in your area of employment. Read local policy and practice guidelines.

W   Companion website

For extra resources on the topics covered in this chapter, visit the companion website at: www.oup.com/mhns

✚   References

Altschul, A. and McGovern, M. (1985). *Psychiatric Nursing, 6th ed. London: Bailliere Tindall.*

Barnicot, K., Insua-Summerhayes, B., Plummer, E., Hart, A., Barker, C., and Priebe, S. (2017). *Staff and patient experiences of decision-making about continuous observation in psychiatric hospitals. Social Psychiatry and Psychiatric Epidemiology 52(4), 473–483.*

Bowers, L. (2014). *Safewards: a new model of conflict and containment on psychiatric wards. Journal of Psychiatric and Mental Health Nursing 21(6), 499–508.*

Bowers, L. and Park, A. (2001). *Special observation in the care of psychiatric inpatients: a literature review. Issues in Mental Health Nursing 22(8), 769–86.*

Bowers, L., Whittington, R., Nolan, P., Parkin, D., Curtis, S., Bhui, K., Hackney, D., Allan, T., and Simpson, A. (2008). *Relationship between service ecology, special observation, and self-harm during acute in-patient care: City-128 study. British Journal of Psychiatry 193(5), 395–401.*

Callagan, P., Repper, J., Clifton, A., Stacey, G., and Carter, T. (2012). *Evaluation of the Chief Nursing Officer's review of mental health nursing in England: findings from case studies in mental health trusts. Psychiatric and Mental Health Nursing 19(5), 455–465.*

Chu, S. (2016). *Special observations in the care of psychiatric inpatients: a review of the literature and*

developments in practice. *ARC Journal of Psychiatry 1(1), 21–31.*

Cutcliffe, J. and Barker, P. (2002). *Considering the care of the suicidal client and the case for 'engagement and inspiring hope' or 'observations'. Journal of Psychiatric and Mental Health Nursing 9(5), 611–621.*

Department of Health (1999). *Practice Guidance: Safe and Supportive Observation of Patients at Risk. Mental Health Nursing—Addressing Acute Concerns. London: The Stationery Office.*

Department of Health (2006). *Best Practice Competencies and Capabilities for Pre-Registration Mental Health Nurses in England. The Chief Nursing Officer's Review of Mental Health Nursing. London: The Stationery Office.*

Department of Health (2014). *Positive and Proactive Care: Reducing the Need for Restrictive Interventions. London: The Stationery Office.*

Department of Health (2015). *Mental Health Act 1983: Code of Practice. London: The Stationery Office.*

Department of Health and Social Care (2020). *Mental Capacity (Amendment) Act 2019: Liberty Protection Safeguards. Available at: https://www.gov.uk/governm ent/collections/mental-capacity-amendment-act-2019-liberty-protection-safeguards-lps*

Dodds, P. and Bowles, N. (2001). *Dismantling formal observation and refocusing nursing activity in acute inpatient psychiatry: a case study. Journal of Psychiatric and Mental Health Nursing 8, 183–188.*

Duffy, D. (1995). *Out of the shadows: a study of the special observation of suicidal psychiatric in-patients. Journal of Advanced Nursing 21(5), 944–950.*

Flynn, S., Nyathi, T., Tham, S. G., Williams, A., Windfuhr, K., Karpur, N., Appleby, L., and Shaw, J. (2017). *Suicide by mental health in-patients under observation. Psychological Medicine 47(13), 2238–2245.*

Janner, M. (2007). *From the inside out: Star Wards–lessons from within acute in-patient wards. Journal of Psychiatric Intensive Care 3(2), 75–78.*

Jones J., Lowe, T., and Ward, M. (2000). *Inpatients' experiences of nursing observation on an acute psychiatric unit: a pilot study. Mental Health Care 4(4), 125–129.*

Legislation.gov.uk (1983). *Mental Health Act 1983. Available at: https://www.legislation.gov.uk/ukpga/ 1983/20/contents*

MacKay, I., Paterson, B., and Cassells, C. (2005). *Constant or special observations of inpatients presenting a risk of aggression or violence: nurses' perceptions of the rules of engagement. Journal of Psychiatric and Mental Health Nursing 12(4), 464–471.*

McAllister, S., Simpson, A., Tsianakas, V., and Robert, G. (2021). *'What matters to me': a multi-mixed method qualitative study exploring service users', carers' and clinicians' needs and experiences of therapeutic engagement on acute mental health wards. International Journal of Mental Health Nursing 30(3), 703–714.*

MIND (2013). *Mental Health Crisis Care: Physical Restraint in Crisis: A Report on Physical Restraint in Hospital Settings in England. London: MIND.*

Morrison, E. F. (1990a). *A typology of violent psychiatric patients in a public hospital. Scholarly Inquiry for Nursing Practice 4(1), 65–82.*

Morrison, E. F. (1990b). *The tradition of toughness: a study of nonprofessional nursing care in psychiatric settings. Journal of Nursing Scholarship 22(1), 32–38.*

National Confidential Inquiry into Suicide and Homicide by People with Mental Illness (2006). *Avoidable Deaths: Five Year Report of the National Confidential Inquiry into Suicide and Homicide by People with Mental Illness. Manchester: University of Manchester.*

National Institute for Health and Care Excellence (2015). *Violence and Aggression: Short-Term Management in Mental Health, Health and Community Settings. NICE guideline [NG10]. Available at: https:// www.nice.org.uk/guidance/ng10*

National Institute for Health and Care Excellence (2017). *Violent and Aggressive Behaviours in People with Mental Health Problems. Quality standard [QS154]. Available at: https://www.nice.org.uk/guidance/qs154*

National Institute for Health and Care Excellence (2022). *Self-harm: Assessment, Management and Preventing Recurrence. NICE guideline [NG225]. Available at: https://www.nice.org.uk/guidance/ng225*

NHS England (2019). *The NHS Long Term Plan. Available at: https://www.longtermplan.nhs.uk/wp-content/uplo ads/2019/08/nhs-long-term-plan-version-1.2.pdf*

Reen, G. K., Bailey, J., Maughan, D. L., and Vincent, C. (2020). *Systematic review of interventions to improve constant observation on adult inpatient psychiatric* wards. *International Journal of Mental Health Nursing 29(3), 372–386.*

Slemon, A., Jenkins, E., and Bungay, V. (2017). *Safety in psychiatric inpatient care: the impact of risk management culture on mental health nursing practice. Nursing Inquiry 24(4), e12199.*

Staniszewska, S., Mockford, C., Chadburn, G., Fenton, S., Bhui, K., Larkin, M., Newton, E., Crepaz-Keay, D., Griffiths, F., and Welch, S. (2019). *Experiences of in-patient mental health services: systematic review. British Journal of Psychiatry 214(6), 329–338.*

Stevenson, C. and Cutcliffe, J. (2006). *Problematizing special observation in psychiatry: Foucault, archaeology, genealogy, discourse, and power/knowledge. Journal of Psychiatric and Mental Health Nursing 13(6), 713–721.*

Stewart, D., Bowers, L., and Ross, J. (2012). *Managing risk and conflict behaviours in acute psychiatry: the dual role of constant special observation. Journal of Advanced Nursing 68(6), 1340–1348.*

Stewart, D., Bowers, L., and Warburton, F. (2009). *Constant special observation and self-harm on acute psychiatric wards: a longitudinal analysis. General Hospital Psychiatry 31 (6), 523–530.*

23 The recognition and therapeutic management of self-harm and suicide prevention

Rachel Lees
Keith Waters

Andy Willis

Learning outcomes

By the end of this chapter, you should be able to:

1 Recognize the impact of suicide and self-harm on individuals, families, the community, and healthcare professionals, and appreciate the importance of looking after ourselves

2 Outline the importance of compassion and language and an individualized approach when working with people who are experiencing suicidality

3 Explain the importance of engagement and collaboration with service users, carers, and other supporters of the individual when working with someone experiencing suicidality, which may include self-harm

4 Identify components essential in the practice of assessment, risk formulation, and care planning (including safety planning) to promote safety concerning self-harm and suicide.

▼ Introduction

Suicide prevention, and effective responses to suicidality and self-harm, are essential for healthcare, public health, and society. Evidence and policy relating to suicide prevention and self-harm continue to emerge. Risk assessment and reducing access to means to self-harm or suicide have long been important aspects of prevention. There is an increasing understanding of the importance of compassion, validation, and exploring the meaning of self-harm and suicide for the individual. The importance of collaboration and involvement with people who have lived experience (service users and those around them) in delivering individualized care and developing services and policy is increasingly recognized.

▼ The impact of suicide and self-harm, and looking after ourselves

A person experiencing suicidality may do so for various reasons and in response to many different factors. Feelings of hopelessness, distress, and overwhelmedness can be common. Self-harm and suicide can impact families and carers too, and there is increasing recognition of the impact that suicide bereavement has across society, including for healthcare professionals exposed to suicide through their roles (McDonnell et al., 2022). As many as 135 people may be affected to some degree by every person who dies by suicide (Cerel et al., 2019).

Anyone can be affected by suicidality. Healthcare professionals' experiences can affect their responses to service users who may already be experiencing mental health crises, suicidality, and distress. Healthcare professionals must be aware of their views, attitudes, and assumptions and reflect on these. It can be common for healthcare professionals to experience anxiety and also to experience feelings of guilt and bereavement when someone they have cared for dies by suicide. It is critical to consider staff health and well-being concerning this, which may include:

- reflection and being aware of our feelings and responses
- being prepared for conversations about suicidality and self-harm
- peer support, clinical supervision, and training
- staff health and well-being resources, self-care, and safety planning
- postvention (an organized response in the aftermath of a suicide) and post-incident support.

▼ Suicide and self-harm

Suicide and self-harm are significant public health and social issues and intensely individual experiences. Self-harm is often about coping and responding to distress, and the final function may not be to die. It is not the case that everyone who self-harms will experience suicidal ideation or intent, nor will everyone who dies by suicide have a history of self-harm. However, self-harm is a significant risk factor for suicide. Any relationship between self-harm and suicide needs to be explored during assessment. Individuals who self-harm are more likely to die by suicide in the 12 months after an episode of self-harm than those who do not (Geulayov et al., 2019). Feelings of suicidality and hope can change between self-harm episodes (Townsend et al., 2016). It should not be assumed that because someone may have self-harmed previously without suicidal ideation or intent that these may not be present at other times. The principles in this chapter apply to both self-harm and suicidality.

More than 700,000 people die by suicide yearly (World Health Organization, 2021). It is difficult to present an accurate picture of the extent of suicide and self-harm, as it can be challenging to identify suicide with certainty after the event and data can be generated only for reported episodes of self-harm. Therefore, suicide and self-harm are likely to be underreported. Self-harm is frequently encountered in mental health services. The National Confidential Inquiry into Suicide and Safety in Mental Health (NCISH) collects information on all suicides in the UK. NCISH make recommendations to improve patient safety in mental health settings and reduce patient suicide rates (Figure 23.1).

Models attempting to understand the psychology of suicidality commonly recognize feelings of hopelessness, entrapment, thwarted belongingness, and overwhelming distress. Some models also attempt to explain the transitions from ideation to action (Connor and Kirtley, 2018). Self-harm may be a response to distress and overwhelming feelings and a person's effort to cope and respond to these. Having thoughts of suicide and self-harm can be distressing and anxiety-provoking. Possible reasons for self-harm include:

- expressing or coping with emotional distress and overwhelming feelings
- trying to feel in control
- a way of punishing themselves
- relieving distress and tension
- intrusive thoughts
- for self-soothing or care (from self or others) following self-harm.

These reasons may change over time, as can suicidality and the effect that self-harm creates for the individual.

There can often be feelings of conflict or ambivalence rather than a definitive presence or absence of suicide intent. The opportunity to explore one's feelings therapeutically and collaboratively can aid in understanding the factors and circumstances leading to this.

> I often struggled with a dangerous internal yin and yang dialogue of knowing I needed to be somewhere safe from myself yet deceived during risk assessments to avoid at all costs an inpatient admission.

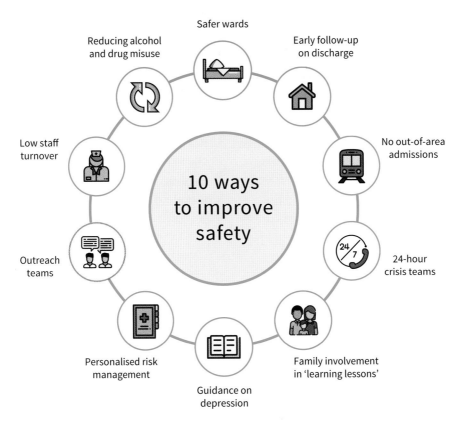

Figure 23.1 The National Confidential Inquiry into Suicide and Safety in Mental Health recommendations to improve patient safety in mental health settings and reduce patient suicide rates

Reproduced with permission from National Confidential Inquiry into Suicide and Safety in Mental Health (NCISH) (2022). *Annual Report: UK patient and general population data, 2009–2019, and real-time surveillance data*. The University of Manchester, p. 7. Available at: https://documents.manchester.ac.uk/display.aspx?DocID=60521. Copyright © [2023] Healthcare Quality Improvement Partnership.

▼ Skills for responding to self-harm and suicidality

Competency frameworks (National Collaborating Centre for Mental Health, 2018a, 2018b) identify activities that are needed to support people, including:

- early recognition of signs of self-harm and suicidality

- responding appropriately with empathy, professional curiosity, and non-judgemental responses

- assessing risk using interviews and other assessment measures

- the ability to judge when urgent action is needed and how to access this

- knowing how to complete a formal risk assessment, how to document this, and when this needs to be updated

- recognizing other sources of help

- knowing how to intervene to help service users manage risk and safety.

- appreciating normal personal reactions, developing self-awareness, and appropriate self-care.

Every service user should be treated with compassion, respect, and dignity. Negative experiences of services can impede further attempts to seek treatment, support, or specialist care. Attitudes to suicide and self-harm have changed over time, but stigma, myths, and misconceptions remain. Cultural, societal, and religious beliefs can also impact individuals' understanding of suicide and self-harm and contribute to these further.

Language is essential for conveying attitudes and values. Phrases such as 'committed suicide' have historically negative connotations from when suicide was considered a sin or a crime. More respectful language, such as 'died by suicide', should be used instead. Language and terminology implying judgements can prevent conversations about suicide and self-harm from continuing. Listening, validating, and using the same language the individual uses can make a meaningful difference, both for the quality of therapeutic relationships and for avoiding assumptions and misunderstandings. The impact of negative attitudes and unconscious judgements on clinical decisions and care must be avoided (Dickinson and Hurley, 2012).

Providing a validating response which promotes engagement and rapport is essential. Service users identify one-to-one time, collaboration, being listened to, and establishing trust as essential for ensuring that compassionate conversations about suicidality and self-harm take place. Indeed, Bruch and Bond (1998) argue that a good therapeutic relationship is more valuable than technique.

> During times of extreme personal crisis with my mind scrambled with intense and disturbing thoughts, I was still able to detect those who had compassion for me and those who seemed to be just going through the motions of a tick box exercise.

▼ Asking about suicide and self-harm

> Asking me about suicidal thoughts never put these ideas into my head because those thoughts were already there. When asked the right way, these sorts of questions showed care and a genuine interest in me remaining alive.

It is important to expect that anyone may experience suicidality and to believe someone when they say they feel suicidal, including when this is communicated in a manner which feels unexpected or incongruent. The UK's first mental health nurse pioneer, Annie Altschul, argued that 'all expressions of suicidal thoughts and every gesture the patient makes to take their life should receive [the nurse's] full attention' (Altschul and McGovern, 1985, p. 161). It is important to ask direct and open questions and allow the individual time to think, answer and process their responses. There may be a 'gut feeling' which needs to be explored further through assessment and by demonstrating professional curiosity.

Many terms can be used to refer to different aspects of suicidality, and individuals will describe their own experiences differently. For clinicians, the most crucial focus is to explore and understand these experiences for the individual and determine the factors impacting suicidality, however this may be defined (Kapur and Goldney, 2019). Trauma-informed care recognizes the high prevalence of trauma, the effects of traumatic experiences, and the potential for trauma to occur within care (Sweeney et al., 2018). Trauma-informed care involves a shift from asking, 'What is wrong with you?' to asking, 'What happened to you?' The importance of trauma-informed care is especially significant when considering the impact of trauma and the prevalence of trauma for many (but not all) who self-harm.

'Are you having suicidal thoughts?', 'Have you been having thoughts of ending your life?', and 'Can you tell me more about that?' are questions that might be asked (further examples are included in the online activities associated with this chapter on the companion website).

There are often stages of revelation throughout the assessment, as suicidality is explored. More may also be revealed by what is not said or implied than by what someone says explicitly. For example, someone unable to identify reasons to live or future plans may indicate hopelessness more than an expression of hopelessness. It is also important to note that asking or prompting someone to make assurances for their safety can provide false assurance.

> I saw someone talking compassionately about suicide with me as representing good care. It never gave me ideas because, in my lived experience, suicidal ideation or thoughts of planning were already present or absent.

▼ Psychosocial assessment, risk assessment, and formulation

A psychosocial assessment is a comprehensive assessment including an evaluation of the person's needs and risks that is designed to identify personal psychological and environmental (social) factors to:

- engage people and develop a collaborative therapeutic relationship
- develop a shared understanding of self-harm and suicidality
- ensure that needed care is received
- give the individual and their family members or carers information about their condition and diagnosis
- explore historical (static), changeable (dynamic), and current (contextual) factors, future factors, and protective or mitigating factors (National Institute for Health and Care Excellence (NICE), 2022).

Risk assessment and formulation must be based on individual risk. Risk assessment should not be a checklist and treatment decisions should not be determined by a score (NICE, 2022).

Risk is dynamic, and the assessment of risk is an ongoing process. This is also true for people who may have self-harmed on several occasions. Every episode of self-harm should be considered in the current context for the person, as risks and intent can vary and change. For a more detailed exploration of risk and risk assessment within mental health nursing, please see Chapter 21.

▼ A suggested structure

A Prepare and establish rapport, asking questions such as 'What has brought you here?' and 'Can you tell me about what has been happening for you?' Demonstrate compassion and professional curiosity.

B Take a personal and social history, including a history of suicidal behaviour, family history of suicide and mental health difficulties, withdrawal, and isolation (note strengths, coping, reasons for living, and any other resources that someone may mention).

C Explore the service user's current situation and the previous 24 hours to this event (self-harm, suicide attempt, or high intensity of suicidal feelings). Develop a shared understanding of the build-up to the current situation.

D Investigate suicidal thoughts, explore their reasons for living, thoughts to harm themselves, warning signs, and plans. Explore suicidal intent, planning, and any steps taken towards this, including any research and access to methods to self-harm.

✖ Tip

If someone appears to be struggling to articulate what they are experiencing, it can sometimes be helpful to share broad statements and ask if any of those feelings resonate (or not) with the person before following up with further open questions.

Every interaction and assessment can be therapeutic, and there is an opportunity for any assessment to be an intervention. It may be the first time someone has had the opportunity to share their distress, and discuss, explore, and reframe their experience. The impact of compassion and validation, and opportunities for hope to be promoted, should not be undervalued or dismissed.

> The absence of hope that I could recover from the severe mental illness I was experiencing or that the insurmountable problems in my life could ever be resolved was present in the attempts I made to die by suicide. Instilling hope during a crisis is vital.

Many people who die by suicide have been in contact with primary care services before death (NCISH, 2022). However,

many have had no contact with health care services or missed opportunities for this. Such findings illustrate the role of mental health, primary care, social, and voluntary services in the recognition and effective treatment of people who are suicidal. Knowing what makes a person susceptible to suicide is a fundamental part of assessing risk, as is exploring and understanding individual factors impacting a person. Assessment is not solely about what is reported or said by the individual and requires exploration and professional curiosity.

Risk assessment tools should not be used to predict future suicide or repetition of self-harm or to determine who should or should not be offered treatment. Instead, frameworks can be used as prompts or measures of change (NICE, 2022). Various factors (see below) are associated with increased suicide risk, which should be considered and explored within the assessment process. These factors and the psychology of suicide (see further below) enable an understanding of an individual's experience of suicidality to inform personalized care and safety planning. The presence of these factors does not alone provide evidence of suicidality; further context and understanding are needed. It is essential to ask questions directly, but it is also vital to ensure that the clinician does not mention other methods that have not been raised during this discussion, as this may suggest methods of harm that someone may not have previously considered.

Risk factors for suicide

The risk factors in Table 23.1 are from an overview of established demographic risk factors (NCISH, 2022) and lack a personalized context of risk; any factor that makes someone feel vulnerable or hopeless can be a risk factor for suicide. Established risk-based factors are good at describing risks in communities; however, they will not accurately describe risks for the individual without further exploration.

Essential things to explore further during risk assessment

- Significant dates and anniversaries and how these may impact risk.
- Social media and internet use in relation to suicide and self-harm, and identifying ways that someone might be seeking information, accessing methods, accessing support, and communicating with others about suicide and self-harm.

Table 23.1 Established risk factors for suicide

Sex	Being male
Age:	
Younger age group	Rising rates of suicide in young people
Middle age group	Highest number of suicides
Older age group	Risk of suicide increases in those 80+ years
Social factors	Relationship problems
	Living alone
	Isolation or loneliness
	Economic adversity
	Legal problems
	Abuse—past, present
	Bereavement (especially suicide bereavement)

(continued)

Table 23.1 Continued

Mental health history	Previous history of self-harm and suicide attempts
	Alcohol or drug misuse
	Multiple mental health diagnoses
	Family history of mental health problems
	Hopelessness
	Depression
Health	Physical health conditions and long-term medical illness (and associated risks from opioids prescribed for pain)
High or immediate intent	Method with immediate means of suicide
	Access to means of suicide and preparations
	Making plans for death (e.g. changing of will)
	Making efforts to conceal plans

Source: data from The National Confidential Inquiry into Suicide and Safety in Mental Health (2022). *Annual Report: UK Patient and General Population Data, 2009–2019, and Real-Time Surveillance Data*. University of Manchester, p. 7. Available at: https://documents.manchester.ac.uk/display.aspx?DocID=60521

There can be positive and negative uses of these, and it is essential to explore how the internet and social media are being used, particularly regarding how they might be used for research and accessing any means for self-harm or suicide.

- Immediate, short-term, and longer-term safety.
- The individual's acquired capability; it might be harder for someone the first time they act on suicidal thoughts or feelings, and the first time they self-harm. However, once a person has self-harmed or attempted suicide, a threshold has been crossed, which may make further attempts or actions more possible.
- Suicide methods and what the expected outcome was. Someone may have believed that the method they used would be lethal, even if it were not. It is essential to avoid minimizing or negating the lethality of the suicide method used.
- Address any risks to others and safeguarding concerns.
- Explore any risk-taking behaviour and ask about intent.
- Any changes observed and explore reasons for this, for example, someone appearing more optimistic may be a result of relief from having suicidal plans and intent.
- Clinicians may sometimes interpret self-harm to have other motives and gains. Clinicians should be able to reflect on context, bias, and preconceptions that may lead to assumptions and judgement.

Understanding and formulating suicidality and risk

Risk factors and contributing factors alone are not sufficient to fully explain suicidality on an individual level. Formulating risk needs to be understood in the context of the individual. There is 'art' in the skill of understanding these risk factors in the context of the individual:

- Obtain the history and the individual's story, or perspective, of what it means.
- Understand risk factors in the context of the individual.
- Remember that 'suicidal risk' is not static and suicidal ideation, plans, and associated risk are dynamic and can fluctuate and change at any time.
- Contextual risk factors need to be considered, identifying aspects that are likely to increase risks and those which may be protective factors for the individual.

An essential component of this recognizes any 'gut reaction' or when the picture does not appear to fit the information provided. This 'gut reaction' may result from non-verbal communications, veiled messages, and transferences occurring within the assessment process. Risk also changes, and there may be nuanced changes which are more accurately understood in the individual context and are needed to inform risk management and safety plans. For example, Altschul and McGovern (1985) argue that one of the most acute risk periods for suicide is when a service user just begins to recover from 'the despair that engulfed them in the acute stage of their illness. The passivity which then characterised the [service user] gives way to the first stirrings of energy which may, in [their] still very depressed state, provide [them] with the impetus to attempt to end [their] life' (p. 162). Professional curiosity and being able to explore these with the individual are essential.

Protective factors

It has long been recognized that there may be factors or identified 'reasons for living' that may appear protective but are not for the individual (Durkheim, 1951). An example may be someone indicating that they would not act on suicidal thoughts as they have children to care for but feel that they are a burden to their children. Caution should be taken not to imply explicitly or implicitly that a child has a role to protect an adult from harm. Indeed, factors that the person currently views as helping to protect, sustain, and aid them to cope could change in their influence, sometimes rapidly. This influence change may be due to a substance, new additional stressors, or overwhelming distress, causing the mitigating effects of the factor, which was previously protective, to decline. The nurse needs to be mindful of proportionality, consider the influence of those sustaining and protective factors, and be careful not to overvalue their strength and influence and remember that these factors can change.

Family involvement and collaboration with others

Involving families and other carers or supporters chosen by the individual is vital in suicide prevention. They may have important and relevant information to share. They may also be involved in care, including support in a crisis. Conflict can sometimes arise between consent, confidentiality, and capacity. The consensus statement for information sharing and suicide prevention (Department of Health and Social Care, 2021) guides clinicians in sharing information where this may help prevent suicide. A reluctance to want families or others involved in their safety plan may indicate concerns. Any reluctance requires further exploration and professional curiosity about why this is the case. Communication and collaboration should include others involved in the service user's care.

Promoting safety through safety planning

NICE (2022) recognizes the importance of developing a safety plan with people experiencing suicidality and self-harm to alleviate a crisis. Components can include recognizing warning signs, listing coping strategies, involving loved ones and trusted others, and contacting social, professional, and emergency support. They must include limiting access to methods of self-harm and suicide and promoting safety where this is not possible.

▼ Further assessment, longer-term risks, and care planning in a longer-term context

For some, suicidality and self-harm require ongoing assessment to address changes in risk and resources. Ongoing assessment does not mean repeating the same assessment repeatedly, which can be invalidating and distressing for some individuals. Instead, ongoing assessment means ensuring that the current risk assessment, care, and safety plans remain relevant and current and identify and account for changing factors and risks.

▲ Conclusion

Being able to respond to and provide care for people experiencing suicidality and self-harm is essential across all areas of healthcare. Compassionate therapeutic responses are essential, as is recognizing the individual and seeing each act of self-harm or suicidality as unique.

I am so grateful to be alive, and I love my three children so much. This chapter is so important because recovery to this better place is impossible if you have died by suicide.

✖ Tips from service users

1 'Even in extreme crisis, I could recognize when I was part of a conversation with someone who really cared and gave me hope that things could improve for me if I were able to stay safe.'

2 'Risk is dynamic. The main priority of a safety plan is to provide me with the most practical ways to stay safe in a crisis. A good safety plan feels personalized, owned by me, and does not feel like one I have been on the receiving end of.'

3 'One of the most important protective factors could be a loved one or trusted friend who plays a shared role in my safety plan.'

W Companion website

For extra resources on the topics covered in this chapter, visit the companion website at: www.oup.com/mhns

✚ References

Altschul, A. and McGovern, M. (1985). *Psychiatric Nursing. London: Bailliere Tindall.*

Bruch M. and Bond F. W. (1998). *Beyond Diagnosis: Case Formulation Approaches in CBT. London: John Wiley & Sons.*

Cerel, J., Brown, M. M., Maple, M., Singleton, M., van de Venne, J., Moore, M., and Flaherty, C. (2019). *How many people are exposed to suicide? Not six. Suicide & Life-Threatening Behavior 49(2), 529–534.*

Department of Health and Social Care (2021). *Information Sharing and Suicide Prevention: Consensus Statement. Available at: https://www.gov.uk/governm ent/publications/consensus-statement-for-information-sharing-and-suicide-prevention/information-sharing-and-suicide-prevention-consensus-statement*

Dickinson, T. and Hurley, M. A. (2012). *Exploring the antipathy of nursing staff who work within secure healthcare facilities across the United Kingdom to young people who self-harm. Journal of Advanced Nursing 68(1), 147–158.*

Durkheim, E. (1951). *Suicide: A Study in Sociology.* Glencoe, IL: The Free Press.

Geulayov, G., Casey, D., Bale, L., Brand, F., Clements, C., Farooq, B., Kapur, N., Ness, J., Waters, K., Tsiachristas, A., and Hawton, K. (2019). *Suicide following presentation to hospital for non-fatal self-harm in the Multicentre Study of Self-harm: a long-term follow-up study. Lancet Psychiatry 6(12), 1021–1030.*

Kapur, N. and Goldney, R. (2019). *Suicide Prevention.* Oxford: Oxford University Press.

McDonnell, S., Flynn, S., Shaw, J., Smith, S., McGale, B., and Hunt, I. M. (2022). *Suicide bereavement in the UK: descriptive findings from a national survey. Suicide & Life-Threatening Behavior, 52(5), 887–897.*

National Collaborating Centre for Mental Health (2018a). *Self-harm and Suicide Prevention Competence Framework: Children and Young People. Available at: https://www.ucl.ac.uk/pals/sites/pals/files/self-harm_and_suicide_prevention_competence_framewo rk_-_children_and_young_8th_oct_18.pdf*

National Collaborating Centre for Mental Health (2018b). *Self-harm and Suicide Prevention Competence Framework: Self-harm and Suicide Prevention Competence Framework: Adults and Older Adults. Available at: https://www.ucl.ac.uk/pals/sites/pals/files/ self-harm_and_suicide_prevention_competence_fra mework_-_adults_and_older_adults_8th_oct_18.pdf*

National Institute for Health and Care Excellence (2022). *Self-harm: Assessment, Management and Preventing Recurrence. NICE guideline [NG225]. Available at: https://www.nice.org.uk/guidance/ng225*

O'Connor, R. C. and Kirtley, O. J. (2018). *The integrated motivational-volitional model of suicidal behaviour. Philosophical Transactions of the Royal Society of London. Series B, Biological Sciences 373(1754), 20170268.*

Sweeney, A., Filson, B., Kennedy, A., Collinson, L., and Gillard, S. (2018). *A paradigm shift: relationships in trauma-informed mental health services. BJPsych Advances 24(5), 319–333.*

The National Confidential Inquiry into Suicide and Safety in Mental Health (2022). *Annual Report: UK Patient and General Population Data, 2009–2019, and Real-Time Surveillance Data. Manchester: University of Manchester.*

Townsend, E., Wadman, R., Sayal, K., Armstrong, M., Harroe, C., Majumder, P., Vostanis, P., and Clarke, D. (2016). *Uncovering key patterns in self-harm in adolescents: sequence analysis using the Card Sort Task for Self-harm (CaTS). Journal of Affective Disorders 206, 161–168.*

World Health Organization (2021). *Suicide: Key Facts. Available at: https://www.who.int/news-room/fact-she ets/detail/suicide*

24 Supporting people through periods of distress that may result in harm to themselves or others

Wayne Ennis
Jeanette Murray

Tommy Dickinson
Dave Riley

Learning outcomes

By the end of this chapter, you should be able to:

1 Recognize the sources of frustration and agitation for people who use mental health services, particularly in relation to the inpatient experience

2 Identify verbal interventions that reduce distress, and the personal values and human qualities that underpin successful interventions in this area

3 Recognize the harm of physical interventions and other restrictive interventions, such as seclusion

4 Examine the need to negotiate (and shape) your local culture of care within the context of continued adherence to a custodial, risk-averse approach within some areas.

▼ Introduction

When mental health nurses have been supporting people through periods of distress, the focus, and indeed the language used to describe interventions, has leaned heavily into the sense that, while the practitioner was essentially benevolent and always acting in the best interest of the person in distress, the person experiencing this acute level of disturbance has often been 'out of control', resistive to our reasoned interventions, and essentially a victim of a link between mental health challenges and propensity to 'violence and aggression'. As we moved into the last decades of the twentieth century, there was a growing sense that often our interventions (while undertaken in apparent good faith and with maintaining safety as the dominant value) were too coercive in nature and representative of a harmful power imbalance. This more enlightened perspective led to new approaches to verbal de-escalation that moved away from issuing directives and warnings towards empathic and soothing words of reassurance and support. However, despite improvements to mental health legislation and increased awareness of the potential for misuse of power within care environments, more custodial and coercive mechanisms for intervention, a relic of the old asylums, are still a source of concern.

▼ The service user experience

The traumatic source of mental health challenges and the consequent need for interventions to support periods of distress provide significant obstacles for the mental health nurse. There is an ever-increasing body of evidence that links high levels of psychological distress, mainly generated through challenging childhood experiences, to mental health challenges as a whole and, more specifically, to the behaviours of concern which can lead us to consider ethically challenging restrictive interventions, such as physical holding, seclusion, or rapid tranquillization. These interventions, while still legitimate and commonplace within clinical environments, are strongly linked to the retraumatization of people, taking them back to the horrors of previous abusive life events (Scholes et al., 2022). It is within this increasing sensitivity that UK mental health care has seen the rise in influence of 'Experts by Experience', who have used their stories of change to influence a new way of thinking and new policy direction in terms of supporting people at difficult times (Happell et al., 2020).

Experts by Experience bring a wealth of insights and a new perspective to care. Critically, they challenge our traditional assumptions about the benevolence of care environments by confronting us with their stark accounts of how significant adverse life events, in and out of services, have exposed them to increased trauma and delayed recovery (Sweeney et al., 2016). These voices can be difficult to hear, especially when they describe physical interventions used against them that they feel have been unnecessary, excessive, and potentially abusive in nature. Nonetheless, there is a sense that a more understanding, person-centred, and proportionate mode of care can be a direct consequence of empowering people to speak out honestly and openly about negative experiences of interventions employed in the name of safety. Progressive mental health services enable Experts by Experience to be at the forefront of decision-making in these areas. New mental health nurses will benefit significantly from an expanded perspective on what contributes to and ultimately alleviates fraught relationships between them and the people they serve. Box 24.1 and Box 24.2 describe Jeanette's and Wayne's lived experience of how mental health services managed their distress.

An additional layer of complexity, and acute concern, is the lived experience of people from ethnic minority backgrounds and the evidence of disproportionate use of restrictive interventions in these groups during periods of distress (Payne-Gill et al., 2021). Historical concern about 'big, black and dangerous' men (see, e.g. Blackwood Inquiry, 1993) within our services has yet to be fully overcome. It constitutes a potential for misuse of restrictions and harmful interventions. Disparities in people's care and experiences require a fundamental reassessment of our intervention and a need to address any personal and organizational bias actively. The mechanisms outlined in this chapter require mental health nurses to have an additional, heightened

Box 24.1 Practice example: my experience—Jeanette

Following an inpatient admission and my recovery, I revisited the ward with some presents for some of the girls I knew on there. I had just regained custody of my daughter from social services and was feeling very positive. I also had thank you cards for the staff, who had supported me so much on my journey. I was surprised when a staff nurse on the unit, who I had never really gotten on with, barked out an instruction to 'get her bags searched'. I tried to explain that I just wanted to share my positive experiences and some presents with people I knew that were currently in the middle of their own mental health crisis, but it became clear that I wasn't trusted by this particular nurse and was ushered towards the door.

As I stood outside the unit trying to explain my intentions, the nurse stood arrogantly at the door, asserting that there was no way I was coming in. Inevitably, I took exception to this and became physically confrontational. Before I knew it the alarms were sounded, and I was physically held on the floor by a team of staff and the nurse who didn't like me had his fingers actually in my eyes. I panicked and, feeling completely traumatized, bit his finger. In the end, I was carried off the unit by the police and ended up with a criminal record. My only intention that day was to be a positive influence on the ward. Thankfully, I now do this as a volunteer on the same ward, but that horrible event never leaves me.

Box 24.2 Practice example: my experience—Wayne

During my recovery on an inpatient unit, I witnessed a 60-year-old man threaten another service user by saying that he was going to kill him by putting a sock in his mouth. This was obviously not a nice thing for that person to hear but I had a sense that it was just words. He had zero chance of being able to carry out his threat as the person threatened had his own lockable bedroom and there were plenty of staff on duty. The service user who was threatened must have told the staff because soon afterwards several of them emerged from the office and literally grabbed the 60-year-old and bundled him to the floor. This was a total shock for me, and I discussed it with another service user, who told me, 'Oh he won't be any more trouble now, they've coshed him'. I understood this to mean that staff had administered an injection during the restraint.

The thing that struck me about all this is that this man had not been any trouble. I felt that the staff reaction was excessive and was totally overkill. It affected me badly during my recovery. I was wondering when it might be my turn to experience this if I did anything wrong, or even said the wrong thing. As my career has progressed and I have worked as a peer support worker in mental health, I remain wary of the staff who always run when the alarms go off. I am concerned they haven't sometimes got the skills to do anything but use physical force.

awareness of the potential overexposure of minority groups to restrictive interventions within local cultures. Programmes focused on reducing restrictive practices and interventions should look specifically at the needs of people from minority backgrounds and how practitioners and systems can be reformed to meet diverse needs.

▼ Understanding de-escalation

While sensitivity to the experiences of people using services should be crucial to our psychological perspective when looking to minimize the use of restrictive interventions, our direct verbal support of people during critical crisis periods—the message we send and the level of understanding we demonstrate in the face of what can sometimes be incredibly challenging circumstances—is of vital importance. There is probably no better way to frame and understand the dynamic of these fraught clinical interactions than to consider the assault cycle (Figure 24.1) (Kaplan and Wheeler, 1983).

The cycle recognizes that people in stressful inpatient environments generally function at the baseline (as illustrated), that is, people are relatively calm and composed most of the time. However, unfortunately, due to a multiplicity of potential issues related to dissatisfaction with treatment, frustration with the ward environment, symptomatic distress, or challenging family circumstances, to name but a few, a person may become distressed and challenging. As mental health nurses, we should look to be supportive as early in this cycle as possible to reduce the potential harm to all, so minimization of the initial source of stress ('the trigger') via timely interventions, for example, or ensuring treatment concerns are heard and addressed democratically.

Ideally, we strive to create calming, recovery-focused environments which eliminate or reduce the number of trigger issues identified, but this may not always be achievable. Suppose we are unable to address these issues at an early stage. In that case, a person that we are supporting may well reach a period of increased arousal (the 'escalation phase') during which frustration and agitation may manifest themselves in a more challenging way—requiring highly skilled, sensitive verbal and non-verbal interventions to facilitate a return to baseline before a 'crisis phase' is reached. Thankfully, it is one that we have every chance of undertaking successfully and safely if equipped with the correct interpersonal toolkit. In most cases, the crisis phase—representing a loss of control—is not reached; even if it is reached, it may not require the use of direct restrictive interventions. For many of us experiencing mental health challenges, a 'loss of control' may be a scream, a slammed door, or a kicked chair. Worrying, yes, but not necessarily requiring the traumatic restrictive interventions we are desperate to avoid.

Kaplan and Wheeler (1983) argue that the 'plateau' or 'recovery phase' is often where most intervention errors occur. To relieve their anxiety and conclude the assault during this phase, mental health nurses may fail to recognize the function

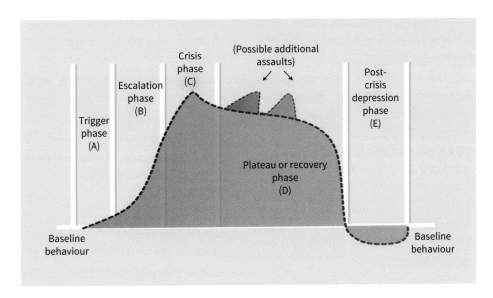

Figure 24.1 The assault cycle

Source: data from Kaplan, S. G. and Wheeler, E. G. (1983). Survival skills for working with potentially violent clients. *Journal of Contemporary Social Work* 64(6), 339–346.

of adrenaline (also known as epinephrine) and the service user's accelerated disposition to reactive assault tendencies. Adrenaline continues to serve as the principal factor long after the actual assaultive behaviour ends. Indeed, once aroused to a significant level, adrenaline will remain an active agent for 90 minutes (Kaplan and Wheeler, 1983). Therefore, failure to support the service user's recovery often leads to a return to the crisis phase. Hence, mental health nurses should use this as an opportunity to positively support a person towards returning to baseline behaviours. Supportive, friendly, relaxed interventions which understand the traumatic nature of the recent crisis phase for the person are beneficial here.

The 'post-crisis depression' phase offers an incredible opportunity to rebuild relationships and achieve critical learning. Given time, people using our services may well express regret and sadness about their loss of control—just as we all tend to do following a difficult interaction or incident. We must be realistic that people are reluctant to apologize or discuss things immediately after a loss of control. Later, however, people may express embarrassment, regret, or remorse. This provides mental health nurses with a beautiful opportunity to move on from the incident, accept any apology irrespective of harm, and take a chance to learn for the future by discussing the incident and opportunities to support the person differently moving forward.

The key to interrupting the assault cycle most commonly lies in using de-escalatory verbal and non-verbal interventions at fraught times. What has also been helpful in recent years is the arrival of materials which set out the perspective of people using services as to 'what works' for them in terms of reducing their levels of distress and a reassessment of the control/support dilemma within interactions (Price et al., 2018):

Non-verbal

- Maintain a relaxed posture with friendly open hand gestures—irrespective of the challenge.
- Intermittent eye contact—conveying interest while avoiding potentially intimidatory staring.
- Give the person in distress more space to pace and explain their position.
- Be prepared to listen silently—nodding on occasion to encourage continued dialogue.
- Make a conciliatory, submissive gesture, such as sitting down, to demonstrate your determination not to adopt a professional 'power position' within the interaction.

Verbal

- Speak clearly and calmly.
- Express regret about the person's situation—utilize apologies if possible and appropriate.

- Be authentic—acknowledge that you may not have all the solutions or that you may have contributed to the current situation somehow.

- Ask the person how they would like the situation resolved as a primary mechanism of empowerment—where the preferred resolution cannot be achieved, be willing to apologize.

- Invite the person to a quiet place to discuss issues but do not make continued dialogue conditional on a person's agreement to go somewhere else.

- Do not retaliate to personal comments—recognize them in the context of a person saying unreasonable things in a desperate situation. Be willing to even partially agree with what is being said to relieve tension.

- Be relentlessly cheerful and optimistic even in the most fraught circumstances.

- Use self-disclosure to remove boundaries and enhance your authentic appeal to the person in distress. Mental health nurses are becoming more and more willing to talk about times when they have been scared, distressed, or uncertain about the future.

- Consider service user perspectives on successful de-escalation, for example, what has worked for them in the past?

- Give more time and space.

- Make rhetorical concessions, for example, admit you are not perfect and do not know it all.

- Listen more, speak less.

- Offer an impartial investigation of the source of distress, for example, 'I know you think I have been stealing your food. Do you want the other nurses to help you with this?'

- Facilitate decisional control for service users in finding solutions—the mental health nurse does not have to have all of the answers.

- Enquire and suggest—avoid giving instructions.

▼ The drivers for change

Any mental health nurse seeking to fully employ the sort of effective interventions outlined above to resolve complex issues and support people in challenging circumstances safely would benefit from a broader sense of how the approach and culture around these issues have been shaped by landmark national guidance and significant national training developments in this area.

The abuse of vulnerable people with a learning disability at the private hospital Winterbourne View (exposed by the *Panorama* television programme in 2011) had a profound effect on the direction of care for people within inpatient services that is still hugely evident to this day and drives the focus of this chapter and the issues examined within. The excessive use of physical intervention and the cruelty which underpinned it galvanized the government to take a more robust approach to the problem and to acknowledge cultural difficulties that, of course, would not be limited to a single hospital or a particular group of vulnerable people. The fact that some staff at Winterbourne View did voice concerns, and managers at the hospital undermined these, alerted practitioners more widely to the possibility that there was a systemic issue around the care of people during periods of distress that went beyond the traditional tendency to attribute abuse to one or two 'bad apples' within an otherwise benevolent system.

Mind (2013) highlighted huge disparities around the use of restrictive physical interventions in different parts of England (once again, suggesting systemic cultural differences rather than a diversity of needs among people using services), and it called for the elimination of dangerous physical intervention positions, such as prone (face-down) positions, combined with the development of national standards for training in this area. The lack of oversight of the skills taught and the glaring lack of input from people who use our services was highlighted as an area that mainly had to change. This contributed to developing national standards for trainers and training organizations in 2019, developed by the British Institute of Learning Disabilities (BILD) and the Restraint Reduction Network.

In 2014, the Department of Health set out its comprehensive *Positive and Proactive Care: Reducing the Need for Restrictive Interventions* guidance, which committed healthcare organizations to establish an empathic person-centred culture of support for people with mental health challenges and learning disabilities that would have regulatory oversight from the Care Quality Commission to ensure progress. The guidance set out the need for greater transparency and vigour in record keeping and urged organizations to place these issues at the absolute top of their agenda moving forward. This resulted in a shift in momentum within services and the rapid development of physical intervention reduction programmes in the UK, such as 'Safewards' (Gerdtz et al., 2020), REsTRAIN YOURSELF (Duxbury et al., 2019), and 'No Force First' (Riley et al., 2018). While often distinct in their emphasis, these programmes had a common core of addressing cultural factors, particularly within inpatient institutional environments. They looked to place the voice and the needs of the people using services at the centre of any strategy to reduce restrictive interventions. While all were hugely supportive of staff teams and sensitive to the often acute challenges for them within these care environments, there was a clear challenge to all practitioners to move away from the coercive approaches of the past, grounded in risk aversion, towards a more enlightened approach which understood that the core driver for distress and subsequent conflict was very often the restrictive nature of inpatient care and a lack of personalized flexibility for people using services in challenging personal circumstances.

The long-awaited creation of national standards for training delivery to support people who may become distressed has been the most significant development in terms of cultural impact over recent years. These standards, developed by BILD and the Restraint Reduction Network (2019), have ensured that training bodies that deliver this hugely significant facet of the overall approach to interventions now reflect the national priorities in terms of ensuring that theoretical de-escalatory, preventative content is taught more within any curriculum than the last-resort, practical, physical intervention elements that have historically dominated the content delivered (Cusack et al., 2018). These national standards are now tied into regulatory oversight, which means that care providers must ensure that classroom-based content taught to staff reflects the values of compassion and sensitivity to the needs of people in distress. Alongside this is a further commitment to ensuring that the physical 'holding' content taught (if required) is only what is absolutely needed.

Within the new training requirements, the voices of people who have endured these traumatic events, and subsequent use of restrictive interventions within institutional settings, will form an ever-expanding component of any curriculum delivered. While all these national developments are helping to create and frame new, innovative approaches within clinical environments, there remains an explicit acknowledgement that there is still much more to do. Moving forward, these national changes must be driven and supported locally by people with a fresh perspective and the courage to call out individual practitioners and broader organizational systems where the aspirations of the new standards and frameworks are not reflected in the clinical reality of people in distress. Astute mental health nurses are now required to combine a high level of sensitivity to the needs of people at fraught times with a broader awareness of the impact of culture on positive outcomes, as well as a determination to act to create positive change (Bifarin and Jones, 2018).

▼ Culture and your role in shaping it

Historically, rather than developing an understanding of the source of distress and, so often, the deep scars of past traumatic events which have impacted that person's life (Muskett, 2014), some care staff have been driven by a macho ethos in which physically subduing and controlling a person who has become distressed was held as a priority. This was highlighted in seminal work by Morrison (1990), who revealed a culture of 'toughness' among predominantly unregistered support workers within the psychiatric units of a metropolitan public hospital in the southwestern US where 'control' of service user behaviour was emphasized, resulting in norms and roles that operationalized this culture. Morrison identified that staff held a 'need for physical restraint', and she labelled the nursing role as 'enforcing', which included the strategies of 'policing' and 'supermanning'. Morrison defined policing as the process of staff effectively carrying out the 'rules' aimed to control service user behaviour. She described supermanning as how a leader emerges from among the enforcers. The leader was the toughest of the enforcers and was the principal person who sanctioned the physical interventions necessary for controlling service users. Another aspect of the superman's job was to protect the remaining staff by taking the lead in potentially dangerous situations. The superman received a great deal of positive reinforcement for his behaviour from the other staff members and usually achieved high status within the organization for his 'expert' physical skills. However, enforcing the rules aimed at controlling service users inevitably leads to violence through confrontation and escalation of the violent situation. Morrison (1990) concluded that the culture of toughness was maintained in three ways. First, the leader of the enforcers was rewarded with high status and prestige. Second, staff members developed a feeling of belonging to the group when they complied with the culture of toughness. Third, the staff members promoted the culture of toughness to justify an organizational need to hire male staff members to manage violent service users. Arguably, the 'superman' role and the culture of toughness among support workers was a predominant aspect that influenced and perpetuated the abuse of vulnerable people living with a learning disability at Winterbourne View, as posited by Flynn (2012): 'over time Winterbourne View Hospital became a support worker-led hospital' (p. iii). This also chimes with Wayne's testimony in Box 24.2 whereby he refers to his wariness of the staff who always 'run when the alarms go off'.

Conflict within mental health care settings now requires mental health nurses to understand and influence how systems and cultures that develop ostensibly for the benefit of people using services may, over time, paradoxically generate environments that increase tension, frustration, and boredom, leading to fraught situations developing where harmful restrictive interventions are utilized (Paterson et al., 2013). The challenges for the mental health nurse in this context are to widen their focus from the service user, who may be highly distressed through a variety of symptoms and personal life experiences, and look at the environment (and its culture) that they are providing to ensure that it is designed to respond with maximized compassion and person-centredness. This requires us to adhere to the very core of the ethos which attracts people to these challenging roles in the first place—the need to do our absolute best for people and to put their needs and recovery ahead of our own personal and emotional priorities for the period that we engage with those we serve (Bladon, 2019). Within any commitment like this, we must explore and challenge complex issues and barriers to deliver compassionate interventions at the most fraught times. Ignoring the following questions, or not asking them of ourselves and our services in the first place, ultimately makes healthcare environments less safe:

- Do my team always talk about people using services in a positive, person-centred way, or is there a perception of a 'them and us' culture where some practitioners see their position as partly adversarial?

- Is the risk of harm to people from those living with mental health challenges analysed, debated, and examined in a way that, often unconsciously, creates a sense in the team that 'safety' for them rather than recovery is the primary consideration?

- Do your clinical managers, in both their words and actions, continually reinforce the values that will deliver less restrictive environments? Will they challenge staff whose attitudes and behaviour do not have person-centredness and which inhibit recovery?

- At the most senior levels of the organization you work for, do you sense that ending harmful restrictive interventions is a key priority and an area to establish continual improvement, with an active attempt to recruit and retain people with passion in this area?

- Does your organization support staff who have been exposed to harmful behaviours in a way that is genuinely concerned and helpful, without accepting a culture where treatment of the person who has caused this harm is not understood but challenged via the use of more restrictions, sanctions, and increased administration of medication?

- Do you feel safe enough to address and challenge the issues outlined above within an organization that recognizes improvement is delivered via openness and continual challenges to established structure, traditions, and habits?

▲ Conclusion

A new, more sophisticated nursing perspective, bringing together well-honed and proven interpersonal skills at crisis periods with an acute cultural sensitivity, while challenging to maintain, gives an incredibly rewarding avenue to increased safety and an eventual end to the interventions that have harmed vulnerable people and committed practitioners in the past. This is particularly important when a person is amid a high level of psychological distress. The recent movement towards this more humane, person-centred approach, divorced from the custodial traditions of the past, is where the new mental health nurse can potentially cement their clinical reputation from the past's custodial traditions.

✖ Service from user tips

1 Make sure the service user feels heard.
2 Hands-on intervention should be a very last resort unless someone's life is in immediate danger.

3 Challenge any ward rules that are, silly, unfair, and lead to unnecessary service user conflicts.

W   Companion website

For extra resources on the topics covered in this chapter, visit the companion website at: www.oup.com/mhns

✚   Further reading

Department of Health (2014). *Positive and Proactive Care: Reducing the Need for Restrictive Interventions. London: Department of Health.*

Restraint Reduction Network (2019). *Training Standards. Available at: https://restraintreductionnetw ork.org/training-standards/*

✚   References

Bifarin, O. O. and Jones, S. (2018). *Embedding recovery-based approaches into mental health nurse training. British Journal of Mental Health Nursing 7(5), 234–240.*

Blackwood Inquiry (1993). *Report of the Committee of Inquiry into the Death of Orville Blackwood and a Review of the Deaths of Two Other Afro-Caribbean Patients 'Big, Black, and Dangerous? London: Special Hospital Services Authority.*

Bladon, H. (2019). *Avoiding paternalism. Issues in Mental Health Nursing 40(7), 579–584.*

Cusack, P., Cusack, F. P., McAndrew, S., McKeown, M., and Duxbury, J. (2018). *An integrative review exploring the physical and psychological harm inherent in using restraint in mental health inpatient settings. International Journal of Mental Health Nursing 27(3), 1162–1176.*

Department of Health (2014). *Positive and Proactive Care: Reducing the Need for Restrictive Interventions. London: Department of Health.*

Duxbury, J., Thomson, G., Scholes, A., Jones, F., Baker, J., Downe, S., Greenwood, P., Price, O., Whittingham, R., and McKeown, M. (2019). *Staff experiences and understandings of the REsTRAIN Yourself initiative to minimise the use of physical restraint on mental health wards. International Journal of Mental Health Nursing 28(4), 845–856.*

Flynn, M. (2012). *Winterbourne View Hospital: A Serious Case Review. Gloucester: South Gloucestershire Safeguarding Adults Board.*

Gerdtz, M., Daniel, C., Jarden, R., and Kapp, S. (2020). *Use of the Safewards model in healthcare services: a mixed-method scoping review protocol. British Medical Journal Open 10(12), e039109.*

Happell, B., Waks, S., Horgan, A., Greaney, S., Manning, F., Goodwin, J., Bocking, J., Scholz, B., Hals, E., Granerud, A., Doody, R., Platania-Phung, C., Griffin, M., Russell, S., MacGabhann, L., Pulli, J., Vatula, A., Browne, G., van der Vaart, K. J., ... Biering, P. (2020). *'It is much more real if it comes from them': the role of experts by experience in the integration of mental health* theory and practice. *Perspectives in Psychiatric Care 56(4), 811–819.*

Kaplan, S. G. and Wheeler, E. G. (1983). *Survival skills for working with potentially violent clients. Journal of Contemporary Social Work 6(6), 339–346.*

Mind (2013). *Mental Health Crisis Care: Physical Restraint in Crisis. London: Mind.*

Morrison, E. F. (1990). *The tradition of toughness: a study of nonprofessional nursing care in psychiatric settings. Journal of Nursing Scholarship 22(1), 32–38.*

Muskett, C. (2014). *Trauma-informed care in inpatient mental health settings: a review of the literature. International Journal of Mental Health Nursing 23, 51–59.*

Payne-Gill, J., Whitfield, C., and Beck, A. (2021). *The relationship between ethnic background and the use of restrictive practices to manage incidents of violence or aggression in psychiatric inpatient settings. International Journal of Mental Health Nursing 30, 1221–1233.*

Paterson, B., McIntosh, I., Wilkinson, D., McComish, S., and Smith, I. (2013). *Corrupted cultures in mental health inpatient settings. is restraint reduction the answer? Journal of Psychiatric Mental Health Nursing 20(3), 228–235.*

Price, O., Baker, J., Bee, P., and Lovell, K. (2018). *The support-control continuum: an investigation of staff perspectives on factors influencing the success or failure of de-escalation techniques for the management of violence and aggression in mental health settings. International Journal of Nursing Studies 77, 197–206.*

Restraint Reduction Network (2019). *Training Standards. Available at: https://restraintreductionnetwork.org/training-standards/*

Riley, D., Benson, I., Kilcoyne, J., and Angus, D. (2018). *No force first: eliminating restraint in a mental health trust. Nursing Times 114(3), 108.*

Scholes, A., Price, O., and Berry, K. (2022). *Women's experiences of restrictive interventions within inpatient mental health services: a qualitative investigation. International Journal of Mental Health Nursing 32(2), 379–389.*

Sweeney, A., Clement, S., Filson, B., and Kennedy, A. (2016). *Trauma informed mental healthcare in the UK: what is it and how can we further its development? Mental Health Review Journal 21(3) 174–192.*

Working with people with substance misuse problems

Patrick Callaghan   Adam Sutcliffe

Learning outcomes

By the end of this chapter, you should be able to:

1 Understand the prevalence of substance misuse

2 Describe evidence- and values-based interventions that help people recover from substance misuse problems

3 Apply the skills you require to care for people with substance misuse problems

4 Demonstrate these skills in your work with service users.

▼ Introduction

Substance misuse is a growing and serious public health problem that continues to affect individuals, communities, and families. Apart from the immediate effects of substance use on health and social functioning, there are important short- and long-term psychological and psychiatric issues, physical health problems, and criminality associated with continued use.

Looking back at the training and preparation of mental health nurses over the past 20 years, substance misuse has often occupied either an 'elective' or 'specialist placement' role, and the volume of curriculum teaching on the subject has generally been low. However, there is a growing recognition that people with substance misuse problems frequently use all parts of the health and social care services, not least mental health services, which are often charged with providing 'treatment' for both people with substance misuse problems, and those with substance misuse and mental health problems. Mental health nurses working across the range of hospital-based, community, or specialist mental health services will inevitably work with people who misuse drugs or alcohol.

Working with substance misuse problems is a core skill for all mental health nurses and requires a comprehensive understanding of theoretical issues pertinent to substance misuse (e.g. development of substance use problems, drug effects, relevant legal issues, transtheoretical model of change, and physical and psychological correlates of use), alongside a set of evidence-based therapeutic working strategies (e.g. harm minimization, motivational interviewing (MI), and relapse prevention). You will encounter people with substance misuse and mental health problems in many mental health settings.

In this chapter you will learn about the prevalence of substance misuse, evidence, experience, and values-based interventions that help people recover, what skills you require to care for people you encounter, and how you can best demonstrate these skills in your work with service users.

▼ Prevalence of substance misuse in the general population

International Global Burden of Disease data for 2019 show a little over 2% of the world's population has a substance misuse problem (Institute for Health Metrics and Evaluation, 2022). Generally, it affects more men than women and, in most countries, alcohol dependency is more common. Regarding mortality rates for substance misuse, alcohol causes more deaths, and the incidence of deaths from drug misuse is around 80,000. More deaths occur in those aged 14–49. Overall, 1.5% of the global burden of disease is attributed to substance misuse. In the UK, 5.42% of the population have a substance misuse problem, 8% of who are men, and 3% women. Around 3.5% have an alcohol disorder, and approximately 2.2% have a drug disorder. Regarding UK mortality rates, 2,654 people die from illicit drug use and 1,762 die from alcohol misuse. Most deaths occur in those aged 14–49. In the UK, 63% of people being treated for substance misuse also report a mental health issue.

▼ Attitudes towards working with people with substance misuse issues

Harmful substance use is one behaviour in a spectrum of behaviours that can be understood by others as harmful: people drive too fast and people smoke cigarettes. Attempts to increase health professionals' knowledge and skills in working with people with substance use problems are a critical aspect of improving people's experiences in health care settings. However, the personal and professional attitudes of health care professionals towards drug and alcohol use (and users) are equally important as they mediate whether and how knowledge and skills are utilized by such staff. Professional attitudes in this context refers to concerns over professional and practice issues, including role legitimacy (is it appropriate to respond to drug use issues in professional health care settings?), while personal attitudes concern beliefs and feelings that originate from understandings of substance use within the popular culture (stigma, anger, and blaming) (National Council for Education and Training on Addiction, 2006). Negative attitudes towards drug users tend to be rooted in beliefs about the deservingness of substance misuse people's access to appropriate medical and psychological care and treatment and have been widely recognized as an important factor in addressing staff approaches to this group (Department of Health, 2002; National Council for Education and Training on Addiction, 2006).

From a client perspective, research evidence demonstrates that therapeutic attitude is a key indicator of effective engagement and overall 'treatment' efficacy (Albery et al., 2003).

▼ How are substance use disorders defined and categorized?

Terminology used to describe the use of, and problems relating to, substance use are manifold, and often varies from country to country, and between the general population and those where professional or family life brings them into contact with substance users. Some of the terms commonly used are based in diagnostic language (misuse, dependence), whereas others have a clearly pejorative meaning (junky, addict, misuser,). Within the two psychiatric classification systems (the International Classification of Diseases, 11th revision (ICD-11) and the *Diagnostic and Statistical Manual of Mental Disorders*, fifth edition (DSM-5)) there are two major groups of diagnoses that relate to ongoing severe and problematic drug and alcohol use; these are harmful use and dependence syndrome. The ICD-11 (World Health Organization, 2021) describes harmful use as a pattern of psychoactive substance use that is causing damage to the individual's health. The damage may relate to either physical health (as in the case of hepatitis from injection drug use behaviours) or mental health (as in depressive disorder secondary to heavy alcohol use), or indeed both.

The ICD-11 identifies four main criteria for harmful use; these are:

1 Clear evidence that the substance use was responsible for (or substantially contributed to) physical or psychological

harm, including impaired judgement or dysfunctional behaviour.

2   The nature of the harm should be clearly identifiable (and specified).

3   The pattern of use has persisted for at least 1 month or has occurred repeatedly within a 12-month period.

4   The disorder does not meet criteria for any other mental or behavioural disorder related to the same drug in the same time (except for acute intoxication).

Dependence syndrome is a cluster of behavioural, cognitive, and physiological phenomena that develop after repeated substance use, and usually includes a strong subjective desire to take the substance, difficulty in controlling its use, persisting in its use despite harmful consequences, a higher priority given to substance use than to other activities and obligations, increased tolerance, and sometimes physical withdrawal states. The dependence syndrome may be present for a specific psychoactive substance (e.g. diazepam), or for a class of substances (e.g. opiates), or for a wide range of pharmacologically different substances.

The ICD-11 (World Health Organization, 2021) identifies six main criteria in dependence, of which three must be present for a period of at least 1 month or, if persisting for periods of less than 1 month, should have occurred together repeatedly within a 12-month period:

1   A strong subjective desire or compulsion to take the substance.

2   Impaired capacities to control substance taking behaviour in terms of its onset, termination, or levels of use, as demonstrated by the substance being taken in larger amounts or over a longer period than intended, or by a persistent desire or unsuccessful efforts to reduce or control substance use.

3   A physiological withdrawal state when substance use is reduced or ceased, followed by further substance use to relieve or avoid withdrawal symptoms.

4   Evidence of tolerance to the effects of the substance(s), so there is a need for significantly increased amounts of the substance(s) to achieve intoxication or the desired effect, or a markedly diminished effect with continued use of the same amount of the substance.

5   A preoccupation with substance use, as manifest by important alternative pleasures, interests, or activities being given up or reduced because of substance use; or a great deal of time spent in obtaining, taking, or recovering from the effects of the substance.

6   Persistent substances use despite clear evidence of harmful consequences of such use of which the individual is subjectively aware.

The DSM-5 (American Psychiatric Association, 2013) also uses the same broad criteria in categorizing substance use disorders (substance dependence and substance misuse), using the term substance misuse in place of harmful use, as employed in the ICD-11. Both classification systems also have diagnoses for intoxication for each substance (e.g. in the ICD-11, acute intoxication due to use of opioids (F11.0)), and for withdrawal for each substance (e.g. in the DSM-5, alcohol withdrawal (291.8)).

▼ Step-by-step description of the skills required to care for people with substance misuse

Assessment of substance misuse problems

Comprehensive assessment of substance use problems and behaviours is an essential prerequisite in the provision of high-quality, collaborative, and patient-focused care and management. Service settings and priorities can impact the purpose and type of assessment that is provided (e.g. you may be in a setting where you see the patient only once, or you may have an ongoing relationship). Issues surrounding confidentiality are also crucial in assessing people with substance use problems. Much drug use is illegal in nature, and people may not feel comfortable in disclosing use to health service staff. This means you should be explicit with people about the parameters of confidentiality in your relationship. Thinking through under what circumstances the patient's confidence can be broken is important, as well as considering your statutory and legal duties. Discussing these issues with colleagues from substance misuse services can be helpful.

As substance use can affect all aspects of an individual's functioning, assessment must be broad and inclusive, focusing on a full range of domains. Box 25.1 shows the areas that you should cover when assessing people with substance misuse.

Box 25.1 Assessing the person with substance misuse problems

Substance use

- Full history (what used and when started, progression)
- Why? (Why do they use, what are the causes?)
- Use over past week, month, and year (what used and how: volume, frequency, and route—oral, injection, other?)
- Which is primary substance?
- Any prescribed drugs? Home storage and safety
- Urine drug screen
- Use with others or alone?
- Ever abstinent? (Why?)
- Previous treatment episodes?
- Control over use (dependent?).

Physical health

- Known medical problems
- Route related—abscesses, septicaemia, thrombosis
- History of overdose? (Circumstances? Accidental/intentional?)
- Blood-borne viruses—hepatitis A, B, C, and HIV status known?
- Respiratory and cardiac assessment
- Sexual health and contraception issues.

Psychological and psychiatric issues

- Previous or current mental health service contact?
- Evidence of current mental illness?
- Association between use and psychiatric symptoms (exacerbation or relief? Risk?)
- What do they see as their primary concerns?
- Motivation to change, and stage of change?

- Reasons/motivations for substance use.

Social and personal circumstances

- Key personal relationships—users/non-users?
- Support and social network
- Education and qualifications
- Housing
- Benefits/income
- Children—ages and location
- Employment history
- Use of time
- Interests outside substance use.

Risk issues

- Injection use ever?
- Skill in injection use?
- Ever shared injecting equipment (include partner)?
- Storage of methadone, etc. at home? Safety
- Safer sex? Condoms?
- How obtains needles?
- Use and aggression/disinhibition
- Risk of overdose?

Legal and forensic issues

- Offending history
- Outstanding charges?
- Funding of current use
- Contact (current or past) with criminal justice system?
- Types of offence (acquisitive, violent, etc.)
- Probation service involvement.

▼ Evidence-based interventions for caring for people with substance misuse problems

There are many models, interventions, and physical treatments tailored for working with people with substance use problems, ranging from harm reduction approaches and self-help to medical detoxification. The approach to everyone will depend on their needs and circumstances, and on your service setting and approach. However, without the basics of a therapeutic alliance between helper and individual, any approach is likely to be ineffective. This means offering empathy and support to people, within a professional helping relationship with clear boundaries. Responsibility for change should be left with the client, while continuing to support efficacy for change by reinforcing self-worth and self-esteem.

Success should be measured on client terms, and not by professional measures—meaning that making positive changes to substance use behaviours does not always mean complete cessation of substance use (a common goal for health professionals). For example, stabilizing substance use by not using, or reducing substance use on top of a substitution prescription (such as methadone or buprenorphine), can be as much of a success as an individual stopping all substance use. This is working on client terms.

Recommended guidelines

The National Institute for Health and Care Excellence (NICE) has published evidence-based guidelines for caring with people aged 16+ with substance misuse (NICE, 2007). Key points include:

- establish from the start whether the person is seeking abstinence, maintenance, or harm-reduction interventions

- involve partners, carers, families, and other significant others in the person's care, with the permission of the person with whom you're working

- work with families, carers, etc. should focus on information-giving, identifying sources of stress that might trigger misuse, and help understand coping mechanisms.

Regarding interventions, NICE recommends:

- opportunistic brief interventions for those with little or no contact such as needle exchange and assessing motivation for change

- self-help using a 12-steps approach

- psychosocial interventions, such as contingency management, and behavioural couples therapy, and cognitive behavioural therapy for common comorbid mental health problems such as anxiety and depression.

In 2017, the Department of Health published *Drug Misuse and Dependence: UK Guidelines on Clinical Management*. Often called the 'Orange Book', this provides the overarching guidance for clinicians treating people with drug problems. The new guidelines have a stronger emphasis on recovery and a holistic approach to the interventions that can support recovery, and includes sections on:

- essential elements of treatment provision

- psychosocial components of treatment

- pharmacological interventions

- criminal justice system

- health considerations

- specific treatment situations and populations.

▼ Understanding change in substance misuse behaviours

The Stages of Change model

Substance use behaviours develop, in most users, over a prolonged period during which they are reinforced and become part of a user's coping patterns or daily lifestyle or provide some other function to the user. Making long-lasting changes to substance use behaviours, then, is not something undertaken rapidly, but rather over a period, considering a range of psychological stages. A useful model of change has been developed by Prochaska and DiClemente (1982) which demonstrates these aspects or stages of change and is used widely in working with problem substance users, and others who want to make changes to behaviour. The chronic and relapsing nature of substance use problems are represented by the cyclical depiction of the model in Figure 25.1. Stages are not time limited, and everyone's course around the cycle may

vary enormously, taking months or years before moving from one stage to another. While helpers can assist in helping individuals to identify issues, it is important that issues and material discussed in stages of change work come from individuals themselves.

Caring for people with substance misuse problems: matching interventions to stage of change

The process of change starts in pre-contemplation, where the user has no active interest in making changes. In the context of substance use problems, the person may be aware that other people (e.g. spouse, family, employers, and medical and health care staff) feel and think their substance

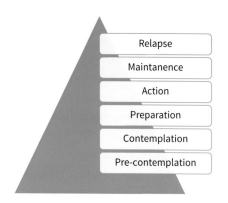

Figure 25.1 The Stages of Change model

use is problematic, but they do not understand it to be problematic themselves. This means that when you challenge the person about their substance use in a confrontational way, it has little or no effect. The skills you require in pre-contemplation are to raise concern within the individual themself as to the nature and effects of their continued substance use, and to help reduce harms of continued use. This is important in terms of the continuing relationship with the patient, and in encouraging the patient to move towards contemplation.

The skills you require during the contemplation stage are to assist the person to analyse the pros and cons of their continued substance use and weigh up the costs and benefits of change. Contemplation is not to be confused with persuasion,

and the issues raised in contemplation must be person centred, not introduced directly by the helper.

In decision, the person makes a choice to change their substance use behaviours (this does not necessarily mean stopping altogether, but could be reducing use, for example); the skills you require in this stage are to increase the person's commitment to change, and to help make a practical plan of actual change that the person will put into place.

In action, the substance use behaviours are changed, and a new pattern of behaviour emerges. The skills required in this stage are to help the person sustain the new pattern of behaviour.

Maintenance occurs when the new pattern of behaviour (in this case substance use) has been sustained for a period. The skills required during this stage are helping the person develop practical strategies to maintain the change, such as developing drug refusal skills, and awareness of environmental issues and relapse risk factors.

When relapse occurs, you require skills in helping the person to try to deconstruct what happened, using a behavioural antecedent–behaviour–consequence analysis approach, so that the individual can learn from the experience and not view it as total failure. Relapses can be helpful in identifying situations and environments that present a high risk for individuals who are attempting to stop using altogether.

▼ Motivational interviewing

MI is a style of interacting with people, as opposed to a particular set of interventions or techniques, that borrows heavily from cognitive psychology (Miller and Rollnick, 1991). The role of the helper in MI approaches is to take the lead from the individual, so that interactions are based on thoughtful, and sometimes provocative (e.g. using devil's advocate position), open-ended questions. In MI, the nurse's urge to influence, advise, and guide individuals is resisted, with the adoption of a neutral position in relation to the individual's substance use. The avoidance of lecturing, blaming, and provoking guilt is important, as these positions are likely to lead to patient defensiveness. The principles of MI involve addressing behaviours the patient wants to change to begin with, not trying to force the patient to change—and locating the responsibility for change clearly with the patient, assessing readiness and preparedness to change (using the Stages of Change

model as discussed earlier), and raising and reflecting the patient's own motivation to change. A useful way to demonstrate your skill in applying MI is to use a decision matrix by completing a cost–benefit analysis with the patient, identifying what are the costs of change and benefits of staying the same.

Demonstrating skills in using the principles of motivational interviewing with the person who misuses substances

Table 25.1 shows you how to demonstrate your skills in caring for a person who misuses substances using MI. See Box 25.2 for a practice example.

Table 25.1 How to use motivational interviewing

Principle	Rationale	Mental health nursing skills
Express empathy	Acceptance facilitates change Skilful reflective listening is fundamental (see Chapters 6 and 8). Ambivalence is normal	Be non-judgemental—do not use terms that will indicate your disapproval of the person Listen actively—do not interrupt, pay attention, be non-judgemental, do not give direct advice, clarify anything that is not clear, provide enough time, do not undermine the person's problem
Develop dissonance	Awareness of the consequences is important A discrepancy between present behaviour and important goals will motivate change Client should present the arguments for change	Use the antecedent–behaviour–consequence approach Help client to identify the discrepancies (e.g. 'There appears to be a discrepancy between what you are doing now and what your goals are. What do you think of this?') Ask the person to identify the arguments for change (e.g. 'What are the costs and benefits of change?')
Avoid arguments	Arguments are counterproductive Defending breeds defensiveness Resistance is a signal to change strategies Labelling is unnecessary	Use verbal skills—paraphrase (i.e. repeat back to the person) what they have said; reflect on the feelings that may underpin any verbal statement Be empathic—convey your understanding of the impact of what the person is saying Be non-judgemental—do not use terms that will indicate your disapproval of the person Listen actively—do not interrupt, pay attention, be non-judgemental, do not give direct advice, clarify anything that is not clear, provide enough time, do not undermine the person's problem Do a functional analysis (e.g. ask the person what their behaviour represents for them)
Roll with resistance	Momentum can be used to good advantage Perceptions can be shifted New perspectives are invited but not imposed The client is a valuable resource in finding solutions to problems	Use a collaborative problem-solving approach (e.g. ask person to state specifically the problem that is causing resistance to change) Help the person to identify all possible solutions Discuss the advantages of each solution Prioritize agreed solutions Ask the person to imagine using the solutions to deal with resistance Help the person apply the solutions

Table 25.1 Continued

Principle	Rationale	Mental health nursing skills
Support self-efficacy	Belief in the possibility of change is an important motivator	Assess level of self-efficacy using a recognized measure (e.g. https://web.uri.edu/cprc/measures/)
	The client is responsible for choosing and carrying out personal change	Ask the person to focus on those issues where their self-efficacy is particularly low
	There is hope in the range of possibilities available	Use a collaborative problem-solving approach with the person; this will help them to improve their self-efficacy levels

Box 25.2 Practice example: David

David has been using illicit substances for many years and has made several attempts to get off drugs and remain 'clean', mostly without success. After his most recent attempt he managed to get to the maintenance stage but relapsed soon afterwards. Box 25.3 shows you how to demonstrate skills in caring for David using the antecedent–behaviour–consequence approach to help David understand why he relapsed.

▼ Harm reduction approaches

Harm reduction approaches to substance use began to appear in the late 1970s and early 1980s in the Netherlands (where drug policy is based on public health and sociomedical approaches and was led by organizations such as the 'Junkie-bond') and in the UK (where they were led by health workers who established needle and syringe exchange programmes). The approach was motivated initially by the increasing numbers of people infected with the HIV virus, and the desire to prevent widespread transmission into the wider community through injecting drug users (one of the early groups infected with HIV). This was summed up by the Advisory Committee on the Misuse of Drugs, which stated that the risk to public health from HIV was greater than that posed by drug misuse.

Harm reduction approaches were initially employed with injecting drug users, although the approach can be modified to work with the full range of substances. There is no universally accepted definition of harm reduction, but Riley and O'Hare (2000) have defined it as having several main characteristics: pragmatism (accepting that substance misuse exists, and that rather than ignoring, condemning, or criminalizing individuals who use substances we should work towards minimizing their harmful effects, acknowledging that some ways of using drugs are safer than others); humanistic values (avoiding moralistic judgements about drug use, and supporting the dignity of the user); focus on harms (whether an individual uses or not is important, but harms to individual and community health, social, and economic functioning are the focus; the priority is to reduce harms of drug use to users and others, not necessarily drug use itself); and environment (acknowledging that poverty, social class, racism, social isolation, sex/gender discrimination, and inequalities affect vulnerability to and capacity for managing substance-related harms).

These approaches are manifest in needle and syringe exchange programmes, the prescribing of methadone and other opiate substitution therapies, educational and outreach programmes, and law enforcement policies that understand substance use as a health issue, and not primarily a criminal justice matter.

Box 25.3 Using the antecedent–behaviour–consequence approach

Antecedent

Ask David to list the factors that may have triggered his relapse (e.g. feeling down, having little to do, breaking up with his partner, losing his job).

Behaviour

For each of the triggers, ask David to list how he responded to these factors (e.g. went to the local bar that has a reputation for being a place to buy drugs easily).

Consequence

Ask David to discuss what were the consequences of his behaviour (e.g. met some old friends who are substance users and who sold him some drugs).

▼ Health promotion

Health promotion plays an important role in working with people who misuse substances, especially in relation to physical health. As a mental health nursing student, you are well placed to address health promotion issues with clients with substance misuse problems. The issues that you might find helpful include promoting the wider benefits of being drug-free on the client's physical, mental, and social health and well-being; promoting physical health (e.g. regular physical health check-ups, attendance at blood-borne virus services, and advice on safer injecting practices for intravenous drug users maintaining their habit); and promoting the value of social support to enable people to sustain positive changes.

▲ Conclusion

This chapter has introduced you to some of the basic issues relevant to the development of nursing skills and approaches in working with people with substance use problems. The mental health nursing skills described in this chapter can help you to enable people living with substance misuse problems to effect lasting change in their behaviour so that they may recover from their problems or manage them in a way that does not overwhelm them and allows them to lead satisfying lives.

✖ Tips from service users

The following tips are offered by a service user community group:

1 'Service users' is a debated term, some were happy with this, others found it 'unfriendly' and suggested 'inpatient' or 'client'. Be aware how language and the terms we use make people feel.

2 'We want to be treated with compassion and humanity.'

3 It is valued when professionals explain issues in more detail, and break these down to layman terms to help with understanding (i.e. around medication).

4 It is important to explain why decisions are made and the rationale for them.

W Companion website

For extra resources on the topics covered in this chapter, visit the companion website at: www.oup.com/mhns

✚ References

Albery, I. P., Heuston, J., Ward, J., Groves, P., Durand, M. A., Gossop, M., and Strang, J. (2003). *Measuring therapeutic attitude among drug workers. Addictive Behaviours 28(5), 995–1005.*

American Psychiatric Association (2013). *Diagnostic and Statistical Manual of Mental Disorders, 5th ed. Washington, DC: American Psychiatric Association.*

Department of Health (2002). *Mental Health Policy Implementation Guide: Dual Diagnosis Good Practice Guide. London: Department of Health.*

Department of Health (2017). *Drug Misuse and Dependence: UK Guidelines on Clinical Management. London: Department of Health.*

Institute for Health Metrics and Evaluation (2022). *Global Burden of Disease Study 2019 Results. Available at: http://ghdx.healthdata.org/gbd-results-tool*

Miller, W. R. and Rollnick, S. (1991). *Motivational Interviewing: Preparing People to Change Addictive Behaviours. New York: Guilford Press.*

National Council for Education and Training on Addiction (2006). *Health Professionals' Attitudes Towards Licit and Illicit Drug Users: A Training Resource. Adelaide: National Council for Education and Training on Addiction, Flinders University.*

National Institute for Health and Care Excellence (2007). *Drug Misuse for Over 16s: Psychosocial Interventions. Clinical guideline [CG51]. Available at: https://www.nice.org.uk/guidance/cg51*

Prochaska, J. O. and DiClemente, C. C. (1982). *Transtheoretical therapy: toward a more integrative model of change. Psychotherapy: Theory, Research and Practice 19, 276–88.*

Riley, D. and O'Hare, P. (2000). *Harm reduction: history, definition, and practice. In: J. A. Inciardi and L. D. Harrison, Eds., Harm Reduction: National and International Perspectives, pp. 1–26. Thousand Oaks, CA: Sage.*

World Health Organization (2021). *International Statistical Classification of Diseases and Related Health Problems, 11th ed. Available at: https://icd.who.int/en*

Skills to improve care continuity: Working in interagency and interprofessional teams

Nick Weaver   Ben Hannigan

Learning outcomes

By the end of this chapter, you should be able to:

1 Understand the prevailing policy context surrounding interagency and interprofessional working

2 Appreciate the practical significance of working across agency, professional, and organizational boundaries in improving the service user experience, as well as skills to improve care continuity

3 Be familiar with a range of organizational factors which both help and hinder effective collaboration in practice, including escalating complexity and fragmentation of services

▼ Introduction

Mental health nurses never work alone. In hospitals and in the community, nurses practise alongside psychiatrists, social workers, occupational therapists, clinical psychologists, general practitioners (GPs), and others. Practitioners will often work for different employing agencies. In the UK, many staff (including most nurses) work in the NHS, while others (including many social workers) are employed by local authorities. Contributions to care are also made by staff located in a variety of other statutory and non-statutory agencies such as the voluntary or private sector, criminal justice, housing, and service user-led organizations. In the past decade there has been an increased emphasis upon collaboration between primary care, secondary care, and the voluntary and private sectors (Baggott, 2016). This has opened up new opportunities for interagency working. However, this has also raised the potential for greater levels of complexity within services which may act as a barrier to interagency and interprofessional working.

The large number of professions and agencies sharing responsibility to provide care makes the mental health field a complex one, with implications for service users and carers. The experience of receiving interagency and interprofessional care can be a disjointed one, and service users run the risk of falling into a 'gap' between different service sectors despite the provision of various 'safety nets' in policy to guard against this possibility (Weaver, 2022; Welsh Government, 2015). This experience may be compounded where resources are scarce, where long-term deficits in financial investment into mental health services have been heightened by the impact of austerity measures and where staffing shortfalls remain (Gilburt, 2018). In this context it is vital that mental health nurses have the capabilities to provide and coordinate care across multiple agency, occupational, and organizational boundaries. This is widely recognized by national regulatory and policymaking bodies. The UK's Nursing and Midwifery Council's (NMC's) Code of Professional Conduct states that registered nurses must work cooperatively to preserve the safety of those receiving care (Standard 8; NMC, 2018). The NMC's Standards of Proficiency for Pre-Registration Nursing also determine that registrants should be able to 'Understand and apply the principles of partnership, collaboration and interagency working across all relevant sectors' (NMC, 2018, p. 25).

In addition, recent policy in England reaffirms the central importance of collaboration across organizational boundaries, and of care being planned and coordinated (NHS England et al., 2019).

▼ The evidence base

The policy context

Delivering more 'joined-up' services for the benefit of service users and carers is a long-held health and social policy aspiration in the UK and internationally. At a broad policy level, successive transformative programmes have attempted to identify and resolve key areas of disjointed or discontinuous care (Hannigan and Coffey, 2011). Actions have aimed at repeated recasting of the problem of mental health care policy through successive implementation of top-down standards, new service frameworks, and clinical guidelines (Gilburt et al., 2014). Models variously proposed in the past to integrate mental health and primary care have included enhanced community mental health teams (CMHTs) providing additional liaison and crisis intervention; shifted outpatient approaches; the attachment of mental health practitioners to primary care services; and the provision of consultation liaison care (Lester et al., 2004). Now, in England following the passing of the Health and Care Act 2022, new integrated care systems are appearing, through which integrated care boards and integrated care partnerships will be expected to work together to create and implement joined-up, cross-agency systems of care for people living in defined localities (Dunn et al., 2022). Included will be systems of care for people living with mental health difficulties.

Top-down approaches to mental health policy and services may, however, have interacted poorly with grassroots attempts at mental health recovery, leading to a proliferation of potential care pathways for service users (Weaver, 2021). Gilburt and colleagues (2014) note that, as a consequence of these policy initiatives, traditional dividing lines between various service sectors have fragmented, which may hinder interagency and interprofessional working. The need for services to be provided across multiple organizational interfaces can also contribute to care becoming disjointed. Care continuity, which may be considered to be a cornerstone of mental health care delivery, is a key concept through which to appraise and understand the nature of effective interagency or interprofessional cooperation. Where services are not joined up, however, they may be said to be characterized by discontinuities of care.

Structural barriers to joint working

Despite the long history of interorganizational working in the UK's health and social care context, relatively little is known about what helps and what hinders success in cross-agency collaboration (Aunger et al., 2021). Lack of integration between agencies may lead to unhelpful service complexity, reducing the scope for coordinated interprofessional and interagency collaboration (Hannigan, 2013; Hannigan and Coffey, 2011). For example, hospitals are a particularly expensive way of providing care, and the cost is borne by the NHS. In contrast, the cost of providing services in the community is typically shared between (health care-providing) NHS organizations and (social care-providing) local authorities. In this context, an NHS trust's wish to discharge service users into the community has the potential to conflict with a local authority's financial incentive for them to remain in hospital and thus consume scarce social care resources. Further complexities are introduced when care is provided by organizations in the private sector, where funding approaches differ from those found in the public sector. All this raises the thorny issue of health and social care integration which has been a feature of politicians' rhetoric for decades despite actual implementation being something of a chimera (Glasby, 2016).

For many years the care programme approach was the formal framework in England through which integrated care was provided to people in contact with specialist mental health services, with the current Community Mental Health Framework proposing a continuation of the care programme approach principles but a phasing out of the framework per se (NHS England et al., 2019). In Wales, the Care and Treatment Plan has been introduced as a mandatory requirement for service users treated within secondary services (Welsh Assembly Government, 2011). As the care programme approach did, Care and Treatment Plan approaches are intended to allow care coordinators to facilitate greater levels of care continuity for service users and in this way promote interagency and interprofessional working. However, discontinuity and fragmentation within services continues to be a problem and may even have been exacerbated by top-down policy implementations such as the Care and Treatment Plan approach with the Mental Health (Wales) Measure 2010 (Simpson et al., 2016; Weaver, 2022). Similarly, in Scotland, introduction of the Mental Health (Care and Treatment) (Scotland) Act 2003 and a new mental health strategy (Scottish Government, 2017) has marked out a distinct policy direction for this country's devolved administration within the UK. In Scotland, there has been greater emphasis upon increasing support for self-management and the use of new technology to deliver evidence-based services and better disseminate patient information (or achieve informational continuity, see below) (Glasby and Tew, 2015). Within Northern Ireland, the *Service Framework for Mental Health and Wellbeing* (Department of Health Social Services and Public Safety, 2011) proposes a standards-based approach related to care coordination and treatment protocols for people with specific diagnoses (Glasby and Tew, 2015).

Interprofessional barriers to joint working

Professional groups differ in significant ways. There are differences in the knowledge claimed by nurses, psychiatrists, social workers, psychologists, and others. This is important, as knowledge often underpins professional claims to control particular types of work (Abbott, 1988). In mental health care, the profession of psychiatry has been successful in advancing its biomedically based claims to identify mental illness and to oversee treatment (Hannigan and Allen, 2006). Social workers, in contrast, claim legitimacy for their work from a knowledge base derived from the social sciences, while psychologists claim a place in the mental health workforce by virtue of their knowledge of both healthy and unhealthy psychological functioning. The knowledge base of mental health nurses is a relatively broad one, borrowing from both the biomedical and the social sciences. However, the roles and responsibilities of different groups may become blurred, as professions vie for control over areas of work. Problems can arise in the contexts of team leadership, management, and accountability. Shifting of professional roles and responsibilities has created interprofessional tensions (Hannigan and Coffey, 2011), occurring in the context of a constantly changing and increasingly fragmented mental health system (Gilburt, 2015; Gilburt et al., 2014). Micro-level phenomena such as human agency, work, and responsibilities may interact with macro-level phenomena such as policies to produce unexpected and uncontrollable outcomes leading to an increasingly complex and fragmented organizational system (Hannigan, 2013; Weaver, 2021). Interprofessional barriers are therefore inextricably linked to organizational barriers to joint working at both micro- and macro-levels of health and social care services.

It is a long-standing axiom that the best way to provide joined-up services is to bring together representatives of different groups in unified teams. This thinking lay behind the establishment of interagency and interprofessional CMHTs from the mid-1980s onwards. Initially, teams of this type were intended to provide comprehensive services to all people with mental health problems living within defined localities, though since the late 1990s new mental health teams with specific functions have appeared throughout the UK. Examples include crisis resolution and home treatment services, which aim to provide care for people who might otherwise be in hospital and support for people to leave hospital at the earliest opportunity (Lloyd-Evans et al., 2018). Following on from this, collaboration between statutory, voluntary, and private sector services has been the focus of Conservative Party initiatives such as the 'Big Society' in the UK (Alcock, 2016). Although Big Society rhetoric has been largely abandoned by the current government, its legacy remains as an enduring interest in the opportunities for collaboration in healthcare and social support.

Organizational barriers to joint working

One of the features of modern systems of care is that services are typically provided across multiple sites. This can lead to fragmented service user experiences, where people with the most complex needs requiring multiple services are often most at risk. For example, people with severe and long-term mental health problems may use the services of local CMHTs; make use of new crisis resolution and home treatment teams during periods of acute illness; receive care in hospital; use NHS, private sector, local authority, or non-statutory sector day care services; and receive services in primary health care settings from GPs, and others. The potential for a disjointed experience is particularly acute when people move between different sites, as when (for example) service users cross the boundary between hospital and community, or between prison and home.

▼   Step-by-step description: skills to improve the service user
experience of care continuity

As community mental health services have become increasingly fragmented and complex, the key criterion for best quality care has become the degree to which support delivered by separate services and skilled professionals is continuous and well coordinated. Care continuity is a fundamental concept used to describe the degree to which service provision is joined up in this way. Care continuity is a cornerstone of modern mental healthcare and one of the principal aims of care coordination (Schultz and McDonald, 2014; Weaver et al., 2017). In their seminal paper, Freeman and colleagues (2002) formulated a multidimensional view of care continuity made up of various subcomponents. The essential validity of Freeman's model has been confirmed by later researchers (Burns et al., 2009; Weaver et al., 2017). The overarching component is that of 'experienced continuity', reflecting the primary concern that care be experienced by the service user as continuous, connected, and coordinated such that no detrimental gaps in provision have occurred (Freeman et al., 2002). Their recommendation was that continuity of care is best defined as 'the experience of a coordinated and smooth progression of care from the patients' point of view' (p. 91).

A number of studies have built upon this seminal view, defining experienced care continuity as the central component within this multidimensional construct (Biringer et al., 2017; D'haenens et al., 2020; Poremski et al., 2016). However, clarification of the key components of care continuity has proved challenging and a consensus has not been reached on what has proven to be a complex concept made up of various, integrated components (Weaver et al., 2017).

Alongside the overriding dimension of experienced continuity, cross-boundary and longitudinal continuity of care may be considered to be two essential dimensions of care continuity, and can be defined as follows (Ware et al., 2003):

- **Cross-boundary continuity**: effective coordination of care between professionals, services, and service users especially where this involves creating or maintaining links between different groups, caregivers, or components of care (Sweeney et al., 2016).
- **Longitudinal continuity**: care from as few professionals as possible with minimal gaps in treatment, consistent with needs being met.

These key dimensions can be considered to be the core of the care continuity phenomenon and are closely integrated. The presence of good cross-boundary links between services and professionals is vital to avoid gaps in treatment which are detrimental to longitudinal continuity. Following on from this, a variety of subdimensions of care continuity have been proposed by various researchers following the work of Freeman et al. (2002):

- **Relational continuity**: the provision of one or more named workers with whom the individual service user can establish and maintain a therapeutic relationship.
- **Informational continuity**: the degree of communication or information transfer between services, professionals, and service users including the level of consistency between care plans.
- **Flexible continuity**: care which is flexible and able to accommodate the changing needs of individuals.

Nurses, as the main profession working as care coordinators, are well placed to take action and develop skills to improve these different elements of care continuity. Care coordination can therefore be considered a key skill of mental health nurses within services promoting care continuity. The various dimensions of care continuity can be detailed as follows.

Skills to improve cross-boundary continuity

The point has been made in this chapter that the people with the most complex needs are often the people most likely to receive services from multiple professionals and organizations. Parts are typically played by NHS and local authority workers, but some service users are also likely to have their needs met by staff working in housing, employment, the third sector, criminal justice, and other agencies. Care coordinators have responsibilities to enhance continuity within and between teams, professions, and agencies. The Care and Treatment Plan approach in Wales, under the Mental Health (Wales) Measure 2010 has further enhanced opportunities for rigorous care coordination and planning within this country's devolved healthcare administration. However, while this represents a genuine attempt at improving care coordination and continuity, the policy may have led to complexity of services which in turn can act as a contributory factor for increased discontinuities of care (Weaver, 2022).

Given the increased potential for service discontinuity, mental health nurses' care coordination skills for improving cross-boundary working seem even more pertinent than ever. Skills for cross-boundary working include the demonstration of a proactive approach to coordinating care across mental health/primary care, community/hospital, health/social care, and other complex interfaces. GPs and others in primary care often complain of poor communication with mental health services, although various approaches to improving the organization of care across this boundary exist (Weaver, 2021). Simple strategies, such as convening care plan reviews at times and places accessible to busy primary care practitioners, may help to improve collaboration.

Skills to improve longitudinal continuity

Achieving longitudinal continuity of care can be a challenge in conditions of high caseloads and excessive workload pressures in the NHS (Terry and Coffey, 2019; Wilkinson, 2015). Longitudinal continuity is promoted by the policy of allocating single care coordinators to individual service users. In Wales, this approach has been implemented as a mandatory requirement of statutory legislation in the form of the Mental Health (Wales) Measure 2010. Consistent care coordination, underpinned by positive interpersonal relationships between service users and professionals, can promote continuity when the care of service users crosses multiple organizational and professional boundaries.

Skills to improve relational continuity

Care coordination, which emerges as key across many of the components contributing to continuity, involves much more than the technical organization of an individual's plan of care. Effective care coordination additionally makes demands on nurses' skills in building and maintaining a therapeutic relationship with the service user (Biringer et al., 2017; D'haenens et al., 2020; Hannigan et al., 2018). Relational or therapeutic continuity is an important dimension within a multidimensional definition of care continuity

since it is indicative of the quality and not just the frequency of care contact points.

Skills to improve continuity of information

The large number of agencies, occupations, and organizations with parts to play in the provision of mental health care to individuals makes information exchange vitally important. New technologies have the potential to improve continuity in this area. The introduction of computerized systems of recording and exchanging service user information has clear implications for nurses' technological skills. However, even the most powerful information technology systems have limitations. Systems are typically not compatible between NHS and local authority agencies, or between mental health and primary care teams. Additionally, IT systems which support care planning and risk assessment processes can be administratively burdensome and distract from face-to-face contact between nurses and service users promoting relational continuity (Coffey et al., 2017; Simpson et al., 2016). In layperson's terms this may mean that a nurse has little time for therapeutic, face-to-face contact with patients because the majority of their worktime is consumed by excessive IT documenting requirements.

Skills to improve flexible continuity

The needs of people with mental health problems vary over time. This places a premium on the capacity of nurses to modify the care they provide, and to maintain up-to-date local knowledge of the range of services available to people at different phases of their recovery. Flexibility of care is a major component of care for many of the more recent studies covering care continuity as a multidimensional phenomenon (Joyce et al., 2010; Poremski et al., 2016).

A practical example could be developing skills in evidence-based psychosocial interventions to support people with severe mental health problems and their carers. Achieving flexible care in this way means working across traditional role boundaries, provided that new ways of working do not lead to confusion or disputes over professional boundaries and subsequent erosion of service integrity.

See Box 26.1 for a practice example.

Box 26.1 Practice example: John

Here you are invited to consider the nursing actions which might be taken to improve continuity of care for a (fictitious) individual with severe mental health problems whose service use spans multiple agency, occupational, and organizational boundaries.

John is in his mid-forties and is a service user of the local CMHT. He receives care from a community mental health nurse, Patricia. Part of John's recovery is to make use of day services provided by a local voluntary sector organization, with the cost of this being borne by the local authority. This part of John's care plan was arranged by a colleague of Patricia's, a CMHT-based social worker. John also receives care and treatment from a CMHT-based psychiatrist and from his GP, who prescribes John's atypical antipsychotic medication and helps monitor John's diet-controlled diabetes.

During periods of crisis John describes the experience of hearing voices, becomes very frightened, and misperceives the actions of those around him as threatening. Over the years he has had multiple admissions to hospital as his health has deteriorated in this way.

Good practice in improving continuity of care in everyday community mental health services

Box 26.2 summarizes actions designed to promote continuity of care for John (described in Box 26.1).

Box 26.2 Continuity of care in everyday community mental health services

Promoting continuity of information

- Maintain accurate and up-to-date records using paper and/or electronic systems as per local practice, and consistent with professional standards surrounding storage and sharing of patient information.

- Care coordinator to ensure that John's care plan, once negotiated, is distributed to John and all members of his care team.

Promoting cross-boundary and team continuity

- Care coordinator to be appointed in consultation with John and with members of his care team.

- Identity and contact details of care coordinator to be clearly made known to John, his family, and other workers (including psychiatrist, social worker, GP, and day services staff).

- Consistent with local policies, care coordinator to negotiate strategies for joining up ongoing care across health–social care and mental health–primary care interfaces (e.g. by maintaining regular contact with GP, by accompanying John to primary care appointments when diabetes care is reviewed, and by convening care plan reviews in consultation with care team members).

Promoting flexible continuity

- Care coordinator to take responsibility to negotiate contingency plans with John and his care team aimed at meeting needs during periods of developing and actual crisis.

Promoting longitudinal continuity

- Once identified, care coordinator to maintain regular contact with John.

Promoting relational or therapeutic continuity

- Care coordinator to draw on personal therapeutic skills to form and maintain helpful interpersonal relationship with John and his informal carers.

For further discussion see Weaver et al. (2017).

▲ Conclusion

Mental health care is a shared responsibility. NHS, local authority, and non-statutory sector organizations have important parts to play. Nurses, while the most numerous of the groups providing specialist mental health services, always work alongside representatives of other health and social care professional groups, often fulfilling the role of care coordinators. In modern services, care is frequently fragmented across multiple teams and settings and escalating complexity is a rising phenomenon.

These factors combine to challenge the joined-up delivery and care continuity of mental health services. By drawing on personal therapeutic skills and ensuring that care is effectively coordinated across service interfaces, particularly at times of transition and scarce resources, nurses can do much to improve the service user experience and thus promote health gain.

✖ Tips from services users

1 'One thing I really struggle with is being "passed from pillar to post". I try to find the help I need from the CMHT, but then they pass me onto the GP who ends up eventually sending me back to the CMHT again. I go round in circles! The best nursing I've experienced gets beyond this sort of problem so that the right people offer me the right help at the right time.'

2 'I'm tired of having to repeat my life history whenever I meet a new professional. It would be so much easier if you were better at talking to each other.'

3 'My third sector drop-in centre has been so supportive but they don't seem to be kept in the loop with what the CMHT or my GP are doing. Is there a way that these people could work together more closely?'

W   Companion website

For extra resources on the topics covered in this chapter, visit the companion website at: www.oup.com/mhns

Glossary

Continuity of care: continuity of care is considered a cornerstone of modern healthcare including mental health care, and is one of the principal aims of care coordination. A consensus has been formed for a multidimensional understanding of care continuity whose principal dimensions are experienced care continuity, cross-boundary continuity, and longitudinal continuity.

Third sector: the third or voluntary sector (colloquially known as charities) is an umbrella term that covers a range of different organizations that occupy the 'third' sector after the public and private sectors. These organizations are non-profit-making and motivated by charitable concerns or a desire to create social impact in areas such as mental health support and recovery.

✚   Further reading

The concept of continuity of care, referred to extensively in this chapter, is comprehensively dealt with in the systematic review by the chapter co-author and associates:

Weaver, N., Coffey, M., and Hewitt, J. (2017). *Concepts, models and measurement of continuity of care in mental health services: a systematic appraisal of the literature. Journal of Psychiatric and Mental Health Nursing 24(6), 431–450.*

✚ References

Abbott, A. (1988). *The System of Professions: An Essay on the Division of Expert Labor. Chicago, IL: University of Chicago Press.*

Alcock, P. (2016). *What is social policy? In: P. Alcock, T. Haux, M. May, and S. Wright, Eds., The Student's Companion to Social Policy, 5th ed., pp. 7–13. London: Wiley-Blackwell.*

Aunger, J. A., Millar, R., Greenhalgh, J., Mannion, R., Rafferty, A. M., and McLeod, H. (2021). *Why do some inter-organisational collaborations in healthcare work when others do not? A realist review. Systematic Reviews 10, 82.*

Baggott, R. (2016). *Healthcare. In: P. Alcock, T. Haux, M. May, and S. Wright, Eds., The Student's Companion to Social Policy, 5th ed., pp. 351–357. London: Wiley-Blackwell.*

Biringer, E., Hartveit, M., Sundfør, B., Ruud, T., and Borg, M. (2017). *Continuity of care as experienced by mental health service users—a qualitative study. BMC Health Services Research 17(1), 763.*

Burns, T., Catty, J., White, S., Clement, S., Ellis, G., Jones, I. R., Lissouba, P., Mclaren, S., Rose, D., and Wykes, T. (2009). *Continuity of care in mental health: understanding and measuring a complex phenomenon. Psychological Medicine 39(2), 313–323.*

Coffey, M., Cohen, R., Faulkner, A., Hannigan, B., Simpson, A., and Barlow, S. (2017). *Ordinary risks and accepted fictions: how contrasting and competing priorities work in risk assessment and mental health care planning. Health Expectations 20(3), 471–483.*

Department of Health Social Services and Public Safety (2011). *Service Framework for Mental Health and Wellbeing. Belfast: Department of Health, Social Services and Public Safety.*

D'haenens, F., Van Rompaey, B., Swinnen, E., Dilles, T., and Beeckman, K. (2020). *The effects of continuity of care on the health of mother and child in the postnatal period: a systematic review. European Journal of Public Health 30(4), 749–760.*

Dunn, P., Fraser, C., Williamson, S., and Alderwick, H. (2022). *Integrated Care Systems: What Do They Look Like? London: The Health Foundation.*

Freeman, G., Weaver, T., Low, J., de Jonge, E., and Crawford, M. (2002). *Promoting Continuity of Care for People with Severe Mental Illness Whose Needs Span Primary, Secondary and Social Care: A Multi-Method Investigation of Relevant Mechanisms and Contexts. London: National Coordinating Centre for NHS Service Delivery and Organisation R&D.*

Gilburt, H. (2015). *Mental Health Under Pressure. London: The King's Fund.*

Gilburt, H. (2018). *Funding and Staffing of NHS Mental Health Providers: Still Waiting for Parity. The King's Fund. Available at: https://www.kingsfund.org.uk/publicati ons/funding-staffing-mental-health-providers*

Gilburt, H., Peck, E., Ashton, B., Edwards, N., and Naylor, C. (2014). *Service Transformation: Lessons from Mental Health. London: The King's Fund.*

Glasby, J. (2016). *Social care. In: P. Alcock, T. Haux, M. May, and S. Wright, Eds., The Student's Companion to Social Policy, 5th ed., pp. 387–392. London: Wiley-Blackwell.*

Glasby, J. and Tew, J. (2015). *Mental Health Policy and Practice. London: Palgrave Macmillan.*

Hannigan, B. (2013). *Connections and consequences in complex systems: insights from a case study of the emergence and local impact of crisis resolution and home treatment services. Social Science & Medicine 93, 212–219.*

Hannigan, B. and Allen, D. (2006). *Complexity and change in the United Kingdom's system of mental health care. Social Theory & Health 4, 244–263.*

Hannigan, B. and Coffey, M. (2011). *Where the wicked problems are: the case of mental health. Health Policy 101(3), 220–227.*

Hannigan, B., Simpson, A., Coffey, M., Barlow, S., and Jones, A. (2018). *Care coordination as imagined, care coordination as done: findings from a cross-national mental health systems study. International Journal of Integrated Care 18(3), 1–14.*

Joyce, A. S., Adair, C. E., Wild, T. C., McDougall, G. M., Gordon, A., Costigan, N., and Pasmeny, G. (2010). *Continuity of care: validation of a self-report measure to assess client perceptions of mental health service delivery. Community Mental Health Journal 46(2), 192–208.*

Lester, H., Glasby, J., and Tylee, A. (2004). *Integrated primary mental health care: threat or opportunity in the new NHS? British Journal of General Practice 54(501), 285–291.*

Lloyd-Evans, B., Paterson, B., Onyett, S., Brown, E., Istead, H., Gray, R., Henderson, C., and Johnson, S. (2018). *National implementation of a mental health service model: a survey of crisis resolution teams in England. International Journal of Mental Health Nursing 27(1), 214–226.*

NHS England, NHS Improvement, and the National Collaborating Central for Mental Health (2019). *The Community Mental Health Framework for Adults and Older Adults. London: NHS England.*

Nursing and Midwifery Council (2018). *The NMC Code of Professional Conduct: Standards for Conduct, Performance and Ethics. London: Nursing and Midwifery Council.*

Nursing and Midwifery Council (2018). *Future Nurse: Standards of Proficiency for Registered Nurses. London: Nursing and Midwifery Council.*

Poremski, D., Harris, D. W., Kahan, D., Pauly, D., Leszcz, M., O'Campo, P., Wasylenki, D., and Stergiopoulos, V. (2016). *Improving continuity of care for frequent users of emergency departments: service user and provider perspectives. General Hospital Psychiatry 40, 55–59.*

Schultz, E. M. and McDonald, K. M. (2014). *What is care coordination? International Journal of Care Coordination 17(1–2), 5–24.*

Scottish Government (2017). *Mental Health Strategy: 2017–2027. Edinburgh: Scottish Government.*

Simpson, A., Hannigan, B., Coffey, M., Jones, A., Barlow, S., Cohen, R., Všetečková, J., and Faulkner, A. (2016). *Cross-national comparative mixed-methods case study of recovery-focused mental health care planning*

and coordination: Collaborative Care Planning Project (COCAPP). Health Services and Delivery Research 4(5).

Sweeney, A., Davies, J., McLaren, S., Whittock, M., Lemma, F., Belling, R., Clement, S., Burns, T., Catty, J., Jones, I. R., and Rose, D. (2016). *Defining continuity of care from the perspectives of mental health service users and professionals: an exploratory, comparative study. Health Expectations 19(4), 973–987.*

Terry, J. and Coffey, M. (2019). *Too busy to talk: examining service user involvement in nursing work. Issues in Mental Health Nursing 40(11), 957–965.*

Ware, N. C., Dickey, B., Tugenberg, T., and McHorney, C. A. (2003). *CONNECT: a measure of continuity of care in mental health services. Mental Health Services Research 5(4), 209–221.*

Weaver, N. (2021). *Recovery and care continuity experiences of people in mental health care: a conciliatory approach to the challenge of implementing recovery-based services. Sociology of Health and Illness 43(9), 1996–2014.*

Weaver, N. (2022). *Escalating complexity and fragmentation of mental health service systems: the role of recovery as a form of moral communication. Kybernetes 51(5), 1800–1813.*

Weaver, N., Coffey, M., and Hewitt, J. (2017). *Concepts, models and measurement of continuity of care in mental health services: a systematic appraisal of the literature. Journal of Psychiatric and Mental Health Nursing 24(6), 431–450.*

Welsh Assembly Government (2011). *Implementing the Mental Health (Wales) Measure 2010: Guidance for Local Health Boards and Local Authorities. Cardiff: Welsh Assembly Government.*

Welsh Government (2015). *The Duty to Review Final Report: Post-Legislative Assessment of the Mental Health (Wales) Measure 2010. Cardiff: Welsh Government.*

Wilkinson, E. (2015). *UK NHS staff: stressed, exhausted, burnt out. Lancet 385(9971), 841–843.*

Leadership and management in mental health nursing

Emma Wadey

Learning outcomes

By the end of this chapter, you should be able to:

1 Discuss the difference between leadership and management

2 Describe how leadership and management roles are central to safe and therapeutic mental health nursing practice

3 Define the key skills/competencies required to lead successfully.

▼ Introduction

Throughout our careers, all registered mental health nurses require leadership and management skills. This chapter discusses the key leadership and management activities undertaken by mental health nurses and the critical skills that are needed to be most effective in the delivery of safe and therapeutic care to service users and their families.

The aims of this chapter are to enable readers to understand the definitions of leadership and management within healthcare, to be able to identify the skills needed to be a nurse leader and manager, and to be able to reflect on their strengths and areas of improvement in these areas.

▼ What is leadership and management?

> Management is doing things right; leadership is doing the right things.
>
> Peter F. Drucker

Leadership and management are terms which are often used interchangeably within healthcare. In nursing practice, we can differentiate between management and leadership in the following way. Management is usually linked with an assigned authority and associated with directing a team or group to achieve a desired outcome. Leadership can include this function but also refers to an individual's ability to influence, motivate, and enable others to contribute towards success and is not associated with a particular job role or banding.

▼ Why leadership is important in mental health nursing

All registered mental health nurses regardless of role or practice setting require the ability to utilize leadership skills. The concept of leadership in nursing has traditionally been associated with senior nurses in matron and management roles.

However, from the very beginning of your career, leadership qualities are a fundamental component of the mental health nursing role. Effective leadership qualities are intrinsic to the Nursing and Midwifery Council's Code of Practice, which reinforces the importance of all nurses demonstrating leadership behaviours regardless of whether they occupy formal leadership positions. Therefore, everybody who enters mental health nursing should acknowledge their leadership role and understand how to develop leadership skills and behaviours. Nurse leaders should also acknowledge that all mental health nurses should have the support and ongoing education to be a nurse leader, irrespective of role.

When do mental health nurses lead?

As described previously, all mental health nurses are required to use leadership skills in their practice, although this may not be formally recognized in their job descriptions. A couple of examples of roles which definitely require leadership skills and activity as integral to their role, without being linked to a management role are nurse consultants and the more recent edition of professional nurse advocates. Professional nurse advocates are registered nurses who have undertaken an accredited programme of professional and clinical leadership training to enable them to support healthcare colleagues by delivering restorative clinical supervision and improve care to service users and their families by using quality improvement activities to create cultures of learning and development (NHS England, 2021). Nurse consultants have advanced and specialist knowledge and skills underpinned by academic achievements and research to enable them to provide clinical expertise, leadership, and critical thinking in the mental health setting. They do not usually manage staff but have the responsibility to lead, influence, and provide expert professional practice across professionals and potentially across systems.

Values and leadership

Effective leadership and indeed management need to reflect our values in mental health nursing. Therefore, mental health nurses need to constantly reflect on their leadership style to ensure it matches with these. Models of collaborative and inclusive leadership are found to be highly congruent with mental health nursing values and contribute not only to better service user experience and care but also to improved staff experience and retention.

The importance of leadership skills

The importance of leadership within contemporary mental health nursing practice is well documented and has been recognized in the recently published *The Mental Health Nurse's Handbook* (NHS England, 2022) and in Baroness Watkins of Tavistock's review of mental health nursing: *Commitment and Growth: Advancing Mental Health Nursing Now and in the Future* (Health Education England, 2022). Both documents acknowledge that leadership skills are required throughout the mental health nurse's career and are integral to the delivery of effective and safe therapeutic care. The Nursing and Midwifery Council guide nurses to lead and promote care provision that is person-centred, anti-discriminatory, culturally competent, and inclusive.

It is of note that all recent mental health nursing-specific good practice guidance refers to leadership skills and activities rather than management.

For a practice example, see Box 27.1.

Box 27.1 Practice example 1

Leadership in clinical roles

Ahmed is a recently qualified community mental health nurse working in a community mental health team. He is the care coordinator for Mark who has recently been referred following discharge from an acute admission ward after experiencing a psychotic episode. During admission, Mark was reported as being distressed, suspicious, and consequently was at times aggressive and hostile towards staff.

Ahmed's leadership role includes overseeing and ensuring the delivery of a multidisciplinary care plan within the community setting, which includes support from the clinical psychologist and community healthcare support worker. He leads by raising and resolving issues that might arise day to day and which may need

to be addressed by the wider multidisciplinary team. Ahmed also leads by ensuring that Mark's view and opinions are heard and considered, role modelling a collaborative approach to care. Ahmed also leads and manages by providing clinical supervision and support to the healthcare care support worker.

Ahmed must also manage his own professional boundaries, time management, and the organizational aspects of providing community support and treatment to Mark. These tasks include ensuring medication is administered correctly, providing psychosocial interventions, and ensuring Mark receives ongoing care and treatment when Ahmed is on leave. Ahmed also leads by role modelling reflection in practice by utilizing clinical supervision and asking Mark and his family for feedback.

▼ Skills for successful leadership

Collaborative and inclusive leadership versus transactional leadership skills

Transactional leadership refers to leadership through management, where given the authority to issue instructions directly to staff. Typically, this approach is linked with formal management relationships and can also be called 'top-down' management. However, within mental health nursing settings, certain roles can still at times be assumed to have authority to provide instruction even in the absence of a formal management relationship. For example, this can be seen in relationships between medical and other allied health professions and nursing. This approach can often also be seen in practice at times of crisis or emergency such as most recently during the response to the COVID-19 pandemic. However, this approach is not seen as the most helpful or effective at other times. Instead, a more collaborative and inclusive leadership approach

is seen as more conducive to effective and safe therapeutic care.

Collaborative and inclusive leadership

A **collaborative leadership** style is one in which the leader asks for input from their team before embarking on a new change or process. Being **inclusive** in your leadership style is taking this approach one step further to ensure every member of your team or work area is expected to contribute and is made to feel comfortable and can contribute. This style of leadership matches the values which underpin mental health nursing and is important and effective as it brings more ideas to the table to help with problem-solving, helps people learn from each other, boosts morale and retention, and is more likely to have a positive impact.

For a practice example, see Box 27.2.

Box 27.2 Practice example 2

A new ward manager, Pauline, has recently started working in a child and young person's acute admission ward. She immediately had concerns about the quality of safety planning and a lack of clear boundaries for services users. Pauline felt that immediate change was essential and shared her concerns with all service users and all the staff group, seeking their feedback, ideas, and engagement in changing practice. However, when they did not seem to understand the urgency of the situation and the action required, she decided to issue clear instructions about safety planning processes and set out what behaviours by staff and service users were not acceptable, together with a clear explanation of why this action was required.

Once the new process had been put in place, Pauline set up a series of community meetings which included staff and service users to discuss and measure the impact of the changes. She also facilitated restorative clinical supervision with staff to hear how the impact of the changes and the work made them feel and set up an innovation forum for all staff and service users so that future ideas for change and improvement could be discussed and agreed.

Pauline started with a collaborative and inclusive leadership approach to management of change by trying to engage staff and service users in understanding the urgency of the problems. However, when this approach did not elicit the pace of change required, she used her managerial authority as ward manager and adopted a transactional leadership approach.

▼ Key messages for successful mental health nursing leadership

The following key messages for mental health nursing leadership were reflected in *The Mental Health Nurse's Handbook* published by NHS England (2022). This handbook was co-produced by service users, mental health nurses, mental health nurse academics, and mental health nurse leaders.

- Being an effective leader in mental health care means the patient's voice is always heard. This is the focus of decision-making and intervention.

- Effective communication skills support teams to work together and contribute to improved collaboration in care while leading other professionals and healthcare teams.

- Embodying professionalism and role modelling appropriate ways to work with others enables shared understanding of expected standards and empowers teams and individuals to influence outcomes in care.

- Be visible, sharing expert knowledge at individual, team, and system levels.

- Innovation, technology, and developing new ways of delivering mental health nursing care are vital to the sustainability of the mental health nursing profession. Get involved in transformation at an individual, team, and system level.

- Taking time to understand research and current evidence for best practice is necessary and will ensure continued advancement of the mental health nursing profession.

- Have an awareness and understanding of the political and organizational context in which they are practising in.

- Strive for integrity, honesty, and humility to underpin all of your behaviours.

So how do we learn and develop such leadership skills in practice? The next section sets out the skills required and how these can be developed and improved over time.

▼ How to develop key nursing leadership skills

Leaders are not born with leader skills—all of us have the ability and opportunity to develop and improve leadership skills and techniques over time through experiential learning in practice, mentorship, and clinical supervision. These skills include the following:

- **Communication skills**: an ability to convey ideas and concepts clearly both informally and in professional meetings and in documentation and report writing.

- **Personal resilience**: due to the nature of mental health care, all mental health nurses will be exposed to trauma either through the life experiences and adverse events of service users, and/or the complexity of organizational demands. Therefore, leadership requires the ability to manage this by being aware of one's own feelings, recognizing when to seek support, and accessing restorative clinical supervision on a regular basis.

- **Maintaining professional boundaries**: to always act appropriately, professionally and in accordance with the Nursing and Midwifery Council's Code of Practice at all times. Set an example to others and address non-adherence to this from others.

- **Empathy**: an ability to understand the viewpoint of others is essential as only by doing so will the mental health nurse leader be able to recognize and respond to the needs and fears of others, especially when negotiating change.

- **Flexibility**: an ability to adapt and change at pace as required given the constant change in acuity and demands within the mental health care setting.

- **Inclusiveness**: ensuring in practice that all policies, access to care and treatment, and staff development opportunities are equally accessible for people who might otherwise be marginalized or excluded.

- **Integrity**: be honest and ensure that as a leader you adhere to your moral and ethical principles; in practice, this would look like taking personal responsibility for your actions and omissions and treating others with respect.

- **Commitment to continued professional development**: leadership skills are improved and developed over time, therefore effective nurse leaders attend to their continued professional development and learning and support a culture of learning in their practice setting.

In addition to these skills, successful leaders need to be aware of and understand the political and organizational context in which they work and be able to adjust and flex their leadership style in response. While those with one leadership style can be successful in some circumstances, this may cease to be the case should the situation change.

The following activities will help with developing and improving the above-listed skills. They can be applied in all student placements and can continue after qualifying within your practice setting.

▼ Activities to develop nursing leadership skills

Communication skills

Undertake a presentation to the multidisciplinary team setting out a proposed change or innovation and ask for feedback, specifically focused on what went well and what could be improved to improve your communication skills.

Personal resilience

Identify a time in practice when you felt demoralized or when something you did had not gone well. Use restorative clinical supervision to reflect on how you felt, acknowledging that its normal to feel like this and then focus on what positive learning can be gained. If the events that led to you feeling like that were out of your control, identify strategies you used to recognize the impact on how you felt and what helped you move on which could be used in future.

Maintaining professional boundaries

The very nature of mental health nursing and its use of the therapeutic relationship as the main vehicle for the delivery of effective care and treatment can mean that it can be difficult to always maintain professional boundaries. Indeed, it should be acknowledged that it is likely to be a frequent tension which needs attention. Equally, the environment in which care is provided, especially if within a long-term patient setting such as a forensic setting, can mean that professional boundaries can be prone to drift over time. It is therefore vital that you engage in regular clinical supervision and can reflect on and hear feedback from others on your practice and therapeutic relationships. Use reflective accounts and your clinical supervision to discuss a recent time that you felt your boundaries were challenged; this could be a service user asking personal information or trying to add you on Facebook. What did you do? How did you raise this with the service user, what did you learn, and how can this be shared to help others?

Empathy

Identify a time when you had a very strong but different opinion to a colleague. Spend time in clinical supervision thinking about their perspective and what may have led them to that view. The aim is not to decide if they were right or wrong but to appreciate their perspective.

Flexibility

Undertake an audit in practice or evaluate a change that has occurred, and seek feedback on what worked and what didn't. Ask what has been learnt and what can be done differently as a result. Adapt your response and enact change accordingly.

Inclusiveness

Practise inclusive meetings, ensuring everyone is invited and able to contribute, by considering the time of the meeting, meeting format, purpose, and who should be there. Provide space for those who are quiet to contribute, invite comments in the chat box if the meeting is virtual and attendees don't feel able to contribute verbally, don't allow interruptions, and consider how to engage those who were unable to contribute. Give credit and recognition and follow up meetings with written notes which can be accessed afterwards.

Integrity

Demonstrate the principles of courage, transparency, and the professional duty of candour; recognize that we all make mistakes and that it is important to take responsibility. Reflect in supervision on a time that you made a mistake—what have you learnt and what would you do differently? Would you be comfortable sharing your learning from a mistake with colleagues so that they too could learn?

Commitment to continual professional development

Be open to learning and development opportunities. Take time to shadow a nursing leader who demonstrates the leadership skills you would like to improve on. Ask them how they continue to learn and develop and ask for feedback on your leadership style, including asking what your strengths are as well as areas for improvement.

▼ What is mental health nursing management?

So far, this chapter has focused on leadership skills, highlighting that all registered mental health nurses, regardless of role or setting, will need to learn and use these skills in practice to be most effective. However, management skills are also important in practice, although the scope of these will vary dependent on role. Mental health nurses are expected to manage service user care and treatment, ensure family involvement where appropriate, and coordinate care from wider health and social care stakeholders. Most mental health nurses will also manage a clinical case load, or inpatient setting. In addition, all mental health nurses will need to learn to manage their own time, professional boundaries, and emotions, while for some their role will include the management of others, including wider multidisciplinary team members, the physical environment, and financial resources.

▼ Values in mental health nursing management

Management tasks are often associated with performance and the management of change; as with values in leadership, it is vital that management activities align with mental health nursing values. In practice, this will mean that nurses must continually reflect and challenge themselves to consider 'Is the change necessary?', and 'Why is the change happening?' Central to reflection and decision-making will be to consider 'Is the change in the best interests of service users, their families, and the healthcare team?' Some key questions to ask yourself to assist in this are:

• Have we engaged with staff, service users, and their families to hear their views and ideas?

- Is there evidence and/or research to support that the change and/or actions are necessary, reflect best practice, and would be beneficial?

- Is it in line with both organizational values and vision and/or national policy and vision? For example, service user and carer involvement in care planning.

▼ Key skills and competencies of nursing management

Like leadership skills, management skills too can be learnt and developed and are often focused on the completion of specific tasks associated with the role. For a ward manager or community team leader, the management activities to be completed would include the following:

- Management of staff, including safer staffing, duty roster, training, supervision, appraisal, performance and annual leave/sickness absence

- Recruitment of new staff

- Finance, ensuring the service remains in budget
- Communication
- Audit and analysis
- Setting standards/maintaining professional boundaries
- Management of environment—cleaning, repairs equipment, supplies
- Management of risk, incident reporting, learning from incidents, and maintaining risk register.

▼ Combining good leadership and good management

Shirey (2006) provides a useful list of five practices that are described as essential for both good leadership and good management:

1 Balancing the tension between productivity and efficiency

2 Creating and sustaining trust throughout the organization

3 Actively managing the process of change

4 Involving the team in decision-making pertaining to workflow and work design

5 Using knowledge to establish a culture of learning.

For a practice example, see Box 27.3.

Box 27.3 Practice example 3

Patience is a community mental health nurse working in an older person's team. Although she does not line mange anyone, she still has several line management functions that are core to her role. These include:

- managing the placements of nursing students, arranging preceptorship for newly qualified staff, negotiating how to spend time, and providing professional advice, guidance, and instruction

- managing her own time, prioritizing the diverse needs of her clinical case load while balancing the wider organizational demands of undertaking new assessments, attendance at professional and team meetings, keeping cotemporaneous clinical records, and maintaining continual professional development

- supporting service users with the management of personal budgets and in negotiating care packages with wider system leaders and the multidisciplinary team.

▲ Conclusion

This chapter emphasizes that all mental health nurses throughout their career need both leadership and management skills. Different roles and functions will require mental health nurses to utilize these leadership and management skills to a greater or lesser extent at different times and in response to differing organizational and system demands. Skills for both are learnt and developed over time and so to continually improve, nurses must engage in continual professional development. It is the combination of both good leadership and management skills that ensures that service users and their families receive excellent care and treatment. It should also be noted that effective leadership and management also supports healthcare staff to thrive and can increase morale and improve retention.

✖ Tips from service users

1 Work in partnership with us and our families.
2 Take your time to make a judgement—gather all facts first.
3 Listen and seek feedback.
4 Be visible.

W   Companion website

For extra resources on the topics covered in this chapter, visit the companion website at: www.oup.com/mhns

✚   References

Health Education England (2022). *Commitment and Growth: Advancing Mental Health Nursing Now and in the Future: Baroness Watkins of Tavistock Review of Mental Health Nursing in England. Available at: https://www.hee.nhs.uk/sites/default/files/documents/Commitment%20and%20Growth%20Advancing%20Mental%20Health%20Nursing%20Now%20and%20for%20the%20Future.pdf*

NHS England (2021). *Professional Nurse Advocate A-EQUIP Model: A Model of Clinical Supervision for Nurses. Available at: https://www.england.nhs.uk/publication/professional-nurse-advocate-a-equip-model-a-model-of-clinical-supervision-for-nurses/*

NHS England (2022). *The Mental Health Nurse's Handbook. Available at: https://www.england.nhs.uk/publication/the-mental-health-nurses-handbook/*

Shirey, M. R. (2006). *Authentic leaders creating healthy work environments for nursing practice. American Journal of Critical Care 15(3), 256–267.*

(28) Health behaviour change theories

Opeyemi Atanda
Patrick Callaghan

Eleni Vangeli
Paula Reavey

Learning outcomes

By the end of this chapter, you should be able to:

1 Understand the development of evidence-based behaviour change theories

2 Examine the components of various behaviour change theories

3 Apply behaviour change theories to mental health nursing practice

4 Evaluate the application of behaviour change theories.

▼ Introduction

Several theories or models can explain or understand health behaviour change. While it is beyond the scope of this chapter to examine all theories or models, the authors will focus on those for which there is a robust evidence base. The authors will evaluate these theories further, using Brawley's model for what makes a good theory, illustrate the components of each theory, and show how mental health nurses can adapt theories in their everyday practice working with those with lived experience of mental distress.

The value of health behaviour change theories to mental health nursing is that they can be used with ease in practice. Brawley (1993) and Callaghan (2014) reported helpful methods for assessing the practical value of theories with the latter showcasing how mental health nurses can apply these to practice. In assessing the value of different theories, Brawley suggests the following:

- **Description of the relationship between each of the theories components**: the relationship between the theory's components allows the person using the theory to better understand how each of the components of the theory relate to each other. This is important as it may be that some components of theory may have more explanatory value in achieving a particular

outcome than others, and this may reduce wasted effort.

- **Guidance on assessing the different components of the theory**: if mental health nurses wish to use the theory to apply to an element of their practice, helping service users lose weight, for example, they need guidance on how to assess the different components of the theory.

- **Design interventions to change behaviour**: while the purpose of health behaviour change theories is to predict and explain how behaviour change occurs, mental health nurses also need to understand how to design interventions to achieve behaviour change.

- **Predictive utility**: this is concerned with how well the theory can predict a particular outcome. For example, if mental health nurses apply the components of a health behaviour change theory to develop interventions to reduce disruptive behaviour, they must be assured that the interventions they use will lead to the desired outcome, that is, reduce disruptive behaviour.

- **Explain why an intervention succeeds or fails**: when mental health nurses use the theory as prescribed, they

Table 28.1 Selected health behaviour change theories and models

Behaviour change theories	Description
Health belief model (HBM; Becker et al., 1974)	Beliefs primarily determine the likelihood of preventative action: perceived susceptibility to the disease, perceived severity, perceived benefits, and perceived barriers
Andersen' behavioural model[1] (Andersen, 1995)	The model recognizes three predictors to health service utilization namely: predisposing factors, enabling factors, and needs
Theory of planned behaviour (TPB; Ajzen, 1991)	The theory acknowledges intentions to be critical in undertaking any given action. Intentions are influenced by attitude to behaviour, subjective norm—the influence others have on the person, and perceived behavioural control—a person's perception of the control they have over behaviour change
COM-B model (Michie et al., 2011)	In the execution of any intended behaviour (B), there is usually an interaction between three essential components, which are Capability, Opportunity, and Motivation (COM)

[1] Strictly speaking, not a health behaviour change in the traditional sense, but help-seeking is a health-related behaviour.

should evaluate its use and find out which components have had the greatest impact. Put simply: did it work, if not, why not?

Table 28.1 describes briefly the theories of interest in this chapter. We then we examine them in more detail and assess them against Brawley's criteria.

▼ Health belief model

The health belief model (HBM) was the first conceptualized model for understanding health behaviours on a large scale; the model has been utilized in several ways in understanding some healthy behaviours like healthy eating (Webb et al., 2010) and screening uptake in the general population (Lau et al., 2020; Ritchie et al., 2021). The HBM posits that specific beliefs primarily determine the likelihood of preventative action: perceived susceptibility to the disease, perceived severity, perceived benefits, and perceived barriers (Michie et al., 2014).

With Brawley's criteria for the theory's applicability (see below), the HBM has been reported to have moderately performed on the predictive utility criteria. The theory has been reported elsewhere to have a low predictive capability as it predicts only 20% of the variance in healthy behaviour (Orji et al., 2012). Also, the theory is notably weak in describing the relationships between its variables as some of the variables are not directly related to health behaviour. However, the lack of a description of the relationship between the variables allows for flexibility in using the HBM across several healthy behaviours; there is less knowledge on the model's validity in predicting mental

health behaviour. In a meta-analysis by Carpenter (2010), only perceived barriers and perceived benefits were the strongest predictors of behaviour. The usefulness of the HBM in predicting mental health service utilization remains an emerging area addressed in help-seeking literature (Henshaw and Freedman-Doan, 2009). An earlier study by O'Connor et al. (2014) examined the aspects of the HBM that explains the predictors for mental health help-seeking. The study reported that high perceived benefits, low perceived barriers, high extraversion, and low social support were indicated of likelihood to seek help while level of perceived treatment benefits predicted the likelihood to seek help despite perceived barriers identified (Langley et al., 2021). The utility of the HBM has been used in predicting help-seeking intentions for depressive symptoms and anxiety disorder (Langley et al., 2018, 2021). Perceived treatment benefits were reported as the most significant predictors of intentions to seek help (Langley et al., 2018). Despite the ability of the HBM to predict help-seeking intentions, these intentions do not necessarily translate to actual behaviour. This is an area that is still lacking across current literature.

▼ Andersen's behavioural model

Andersen's behavioural model has also been applied to predicting help-seeking behaviour for mental health difficulties (Goodwin and Andersen, 2002; Portes et al., 1992). The model explains incorporating both individual and contextual determinants of health services use. In doing so, it 'divides the major components of contextual characteristics in the same way as individual characteristics have traditionally divided—those that predispose …, enable …, or suggest a need for individual use of health services' (Andersen, 2008, p. 652).

The model recognizes three predictors to health service utilization, **predisposing factors** which are not limited to demographic variables like age, sex, and race, and attitudes and beliefs about seeking help (Andersen, 1995). The **enabling factors** refer to resources that support access to formal support, including an individual's support system and structural resources like income. The third predictor is **needs**, how symptoms are perceived and experienced, which predisposes an individual to use services.

Cairney et al. (2004) utilized Andersen's model to examine whether mental health service utilization among single-parent mothers was due to need factors (as defined based on diagnostic criteria reported in the *Diagnostic and Statistical Manual of Mental Disorders*, third edition, revised (DSM-III-R) and International Classification of Disease, tenth revision (ICD-10)) compared to the other variable as predictors of service utilization. The study utilized data from two large surveys in Canada to test this assumption. The study findings revealed that single-parent mothers were more likely than married mothers to have sought professional help for mental health issues, mainly due to the need factors and no other variable.

In a systematic review exploring the factors associated with health service utilization for mental health difficulties (Roberts et al., 2018), needs factors were the most associated with treatment-seeking for mental health difficulties. The review also highlighted the lack of evidence linking psychological and health system factors to predict treatment-seeking. In contrast to the review, a study by Simo et al. (2018) reported having a family doctor, previous experience of mental health services, and being employed were the three main enabling factors predictive of the use of services. The study also reported three non-clinical needs variables to predict mental health service use. The needs factors included individual perception about mental health, unmet needs, and stressful events. Although this finding adds to the current literature on predictors of mental health service use, data utilized for this conclusion were from self-reported measures. The study relied on the participant's ability to recall past events predisposes the finding to report bias.

With Brawley's framework, the model has a low to moderate predictive utility in explaining help-seeking behaviour. The predictive utility has been shown in studies across various populations (Roh et al., 2017; Simo et al., 2018). In assessing key variables on a general basis, the model has explained the key variables quite well. Although observed in a few studies identified in a systematic review by Babitsch et al. (2012), variables were merged. The relationships between the variables were sufficiently described within this model (Andersen and Davidson, 2007), with some variables like socioeconomic factors playing a dual role in explaining health service use. However, a significant criticism of Andersen's model is the lack of emphasis on health beliefs and social structures' influence on individual needs, particularly service utilization (Babitsch et al., 2012).

▼ Theory of planned behaviour

Ajzen's theory of planned behaviour (TPB) (1991) has been applied to improve help-seeking behaviour (Gulliver et al., 2012). Compared to other psychological models, it is regarded as the only model that addresses all aspects of help-seeking intentions (White et al., 2018). Help-seeking intentions are defined as 'a conscious plan to exert effort to communicate about a problem, emotional pain or psychological issue where that communication is an attempt to obtain perceived support, advice or assistance that will reduce personal distress' (White et al., 2018, p. 65).

The theory acknowledges intentions to be critical in undertaking any given action. It is also understood to 'capture the motivational factors that influence a behaviour; they are indications of how hard people are willing to try, of how much of an effort they are planning to exert, performing the behaviour' (Ajzen, 1991, p. 181).

TPB components have also been linked to the various stages of help-seeking (Tomczyk et al., 2020), subjective norms that are regarded as beliefs about what others think about the behaviour that links to recognition and awareness of social support available to deal with a mental health concern. The attitudes element appraises behaviour, weighing its benefits linked to an individual's readiness/willingness to seek help. The last component of the TPB, which is perceived behavioural control, focuses on an individual's confidence and control over performing any behaviour and is linked to an individual's ability to seek help for their mental health difficulty.

A range of studies has investigated TPB components in help-seeking for mental health concerns (Hui et al., 2015; Mak and Davis, 2014; Schomerus et al., 2009; Tomczyk et al., 2020). Previously identified studies have examined the predictors of help-seeking intentions using TPB apart from the study by Tomczyk et al. (2020) that aimed at addressing the help-intentions and behaviour gap commonly not addressed by previous studies. The study examined the prediction of actual help-seeking behaviour from help-seeking intentions, although they reported a strong prediction 54% of the participants examined in the study has previously received some form of therapeutic support for a mental health difficulty. Therefore, expectancies about actual help-seeking behaviour might be misunderstood. Mak and Davis (2014) reported perceived behavioural control as the strongest predictor of help-seeking intention. Schomerus et al. (2009) reported a slightly different result where attitudes and subjective control were regarded as the strongest predictors of intention. In contrast, the study by Hui et al. (2015) reported no significant changes to help-seeking intentions. However, their lack of adequate statistical power might have accounted for the non-significant result.

With Brawley's framework, the TPB fulfils two of the five criteria. The two criteria include its ability to explain why an intervention succeeds or fails and the possibility of designing interventions to change the variables. The former could be due to a lack of an explanation of the theoretical basis for the intervention by the developers. The TPB, among other theories designed to predict health behaviour, interprets goal intention as a willingness to perform the behaviour. Gollwitzer (1999) developed the implementation intentions model to address the misinterpretation of a goal intention. Based on the model of action phases developed by Heckhausen and Gollwitzer (1987), intention alongside steps taken to implement intentions complement each other to ensure goal attainment. The concept has been utilized in smoking cessation (McWilliams et al., 2019).

In mental health help-seeking, implementation intention formation involves overcoming limitations to help-seeking by coming up with active responses referred to as 'variable[s] that determine effective goal pursuit' by Gollwitzer (1999, p. 493) that are accessible to carry out the intended action.

▼ COM-B model

The development of theory-based interventions requires an understanding of the critical elements of the intervention and its mechanisms of action. The mechanisms of action provide a more comprehensive understanding of how theory-based interventions achieve their predicted outcomes (Carey et al., 2018).

Behavioural interventions are commonly delivered as part of a complex system that includes behavioural change techniques that serve as active ingredients designed to alter or redirect causal processes that effect a change in health behaviour (Carey et al., 2018). To develop an effective intervention, there is a need to understand the mechanisms through which various 'active ingredients' of an intervention achieve their predicted outcomes. The mechanisms of action are referred to as theoretical constructs through which behavioural change technique alters a behaviour (Michie et al., 2018).

Michie and colleagues also developed the COM-B model (Figure 28.1) as a response to the failings of the prominent theories to provide strategies to change behaviour and as a means of describing interventions and linking them to addressing targeted behaviours (Michie et al., 2011). Embedded into COM-B is a psychological model that explains how human behaviour interacts through various mechanisms to achieve a behavioural change. The model assumption is that for the execution of any intended behaviour (B), there is usually an interaction between three essential components: Capability, Opportunity, and Motivation (COM). Each of the components is understood to directly influence behavioural change, whereas capability and opportunity might also influence motivation to change behaviour.

Capability can be 'psychological', knowledge and psychological skills involved in undertaking the behaviour, or 'physical', physical skills involved in undertaking any behaviour. Opportunity can be either 'social', for example, social influences and cultural norms that influence behaviour, or 'physical', resources needed to enact the behaviour. Motivation could be conscious or 'automatic', that is, emotions and impulses at play while performing any behaviour (Michie et al.,

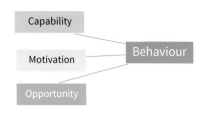

Figure 28.1 COM- B Model

Reproduced from Michie, S., van Stralen, M. M., and West, R. (2011). The behaviour change wheel: a new method for characterising and designing behaviour change interventions. *Implementation Science*, 6(1), 42 under a Creative Commons Attribution License (http://creative commons.org/licenses/by/2.0).

2014). The six-item self-evaluation questionnaire (Keyworth et al., 2020) can be used to measure the components of the COM-B model.

The lack of a comprehensive theoretical assessment of the implementation of behavioural change interventions and the overlapping nature of the constructs used in developing these interventions (Nigg et al., 2002) has also been highlighted as a concern in the behaviour change field. An integrative framework of behaviour change theories was developed using a six-step consensus process (Michie et al., 2005). Further development has mapped a Theoretical Domains Framework onto the COM-B model, showing the relationship between domains in the three components of the COM-B model (Michie et al., 2014).

The Theoretical Domains Framework has been utilized across several studies internationally, and in the UK, including studies related to hand hygiene (Dyson et al., 2011), it has also been utilized successfully to identify theories that guide decision-making and implementing guidelines relating to

working with people diagnosed with schizophrenia within mental health (Michie et al., 2007).

The COM-B model can also be used to account for the barriers and facilitators to help-seeking behaviour for mental health issues. Reluctance to seek help for mental health difficulty among young adults and adolescents has been investigated (Barker, 2007; Gulliver et al., 2012; Rickwood et al., 2005). In a key review of barriers and facilitators to help-seeking among young people reported by Rickwood et al. (2005), the review identified three barriers to help-seeking: the inability to identify, understand, and describe emotions effectively; the lack of utilizing available help when needed, especially in suicidal ideation; and negative attitudes and beliefs to seeking professional help due to negative past experiences engaging with services.

Facilitators to help-seeking identified in the review include higher emotional competence levels, positive attitudes and mental health literacy, and social influences on help-seeking. In relation to the COM-B components, mental health literacy relates to psychological capability; a lack of emotional competence and perceived stigma could relate to reflective motivation; negative attitudes towards seeking professional relate to automatic motivation; and social support from family relates to social opportunity on the COM-B model.

The COM-B model, and the extensive research that followed its introduction meets Brawley's criteria overall: the relationships between components are explicit, likewise for guidance in assessing each component. It is particularly strong on the issue of designing interventions to change behaviour, and in its predictive utility. Explaining why an intervention succeeds, or fails, will require additional research methods, mixed method studies, for example, but these have been used in research into the model.

▼ Applying a health behaviour change theory to mental health nursing practice

The final section of this chapter illustrates how health behaviour change theories can be used in mental health nursing practice (see the practice example in Box 28.1). It is important to emphasize that little or no additional training is needed to apply these to practice.

Box 28.1 Practice example: Tim

Tim is a 17-year-old living with moderate mental distress which has caused him to have suicidal thoughts, which he has acted upon occasionally by harming himself. On one occasion, he may have died but for the swift actions of a passing stranger. Tim has been admitted to your child and adolescent mental health ward. Following an assessment, he has been diagnosed with depression. Tim dislikes taking medication, but he recognizes it may improve his feelings if taken for a while, but, as a keen exerciser he worries the medication may blunt his volition to exercise, which he enjoyed. As part of his care plan which he helped develop and agreed with you as his named nurse, Tim would like to get back to exercising, but he has lost the will. You are familiar with research that shows exercise is beneficial for people diagnosed with depression, and with Tim's agreement you decide to help Tim re-start his

exercise activity using an evidence-based behavioural change technique developed from the COM-B model. The following points outline how you might help Tim through goal setting, graded tasks, adding objects to the environment, and providing feedback through self-monitoring (Samdal et al., 2018).

1 Work with Tim to agree a goal he wishes to achieve, for example, running 45 minutes each week as part of his local parkrun at weekends.

2 Agree graded tasks with Tim and help him implement them towards achieving the end goal. For example, each day prior to the weekend parkrun Tim can run around 10 minutes at his preferred pace.

3 Add objects to the environment: suggest Tim uses a timer to check his progress while running.

4 At the session's end, ask Tim to report on his progress.

▲ Conclusion

Health behaviour change theories are evidence-based models designed to enable behaviour change through the application of evidence-based interventions arising from the theories. They are a useful tool in helping

mental health nurses work with people seeking to change their behaviour, where their existing behaviour may be harmful, or to enhance their overall mental health and well-being.

✖ Tips from service users

1 Is your patient ready for change?
2 Ensure you are honest with your patient that the treatment you and the clinical team are providing will help bring about some change to their behaviour. It is difficult to know when to start the change but be posi-

tive with your patients on how the change will relieve some of their difficulties.

3 Be honest that it will not happen overnight, there will be ups and downs. Take one step at a time and deal with any challenges as just a setback.

W   Companion website

For extra resources on the topics covered in this chapter, visit the companion website at: www.oup.com/mhns

✛ References

Ajzen, I. (1991). *The theory of planned behavior. Organizational Behavior and Human Decision Processes 50(2), 179–211.*

Andersen, R. M. (1995). *Revisiting the behavioral model and access to medical care: does it matter? Journal of Health and Social Behavior 36(1), 1–10. https://10.2307/2137284*

Andersen, R. M. (2008). *National health surveys and the behavioral model of health services use. Medical Care 46(7), 647–653.*

Andersen, R. M. and Davidson, P. L. (2007). *Improving access to care in America: individual and contextual indicators. In: R. M. Andersen, T. H. Rice, and G. F. Kominski, Eds., Changing the US Health Care System: Key Issues in Health Services Policy and Management, 3rd ed., pp. 3–31. San Francisco, CA: Jossey-Bass.*

Babitsch, B., Gohl, D., and von Lengerke, T. (2012). *Re-revisiting Andersen's behavioral model of health services use: a systematic review of studies from 1998–2011. Psycho-Social Medicine 9, 11.*

Barker, G. (2007). *Adolescents, Social Support and Help-Seeking Behaviour: An International Literature Review and Programme Consultation with Recommendations for Action. World Health Organization. Available at: https://www.who.int/publications/i/item/9789241595711*

Becker, M. H. (1974). *The health belief model and sick role behavior. Health Education Monographs 2(4), 409–419. doi:10.1177/109019817400200407*

Brawley, L. R. (1993). *The practicality of using social psychological theories for exercise and health research and intervention. Journal of Applied Sport Psychology 5(2), 99–115. https://10.1080/10413209308411309*

Cairney, J., Boyle, M. H., Lipman, E. L., and Racine, Y. (2004). *Single mothers and the use of professionals for mental health care reasons. Social Science & Medicine 59(12), 2535–2546.*

Callaghan, P. (2014). *Behavior change theories. In: T. Stickley and N. Wright, Eds., Theories for Mental Health Nursing: A Guide for Practice, pp. 324–343. London: SAGE Publications.*

Carey, R. N., Connell, L. E., Johnston, M., Rothman, A. J., De Bruin, M., Kelly, M. P., and Michie, S. (2018). *Behavior change techniques and their mechanisms of action: a synthesis of links described in published intervention literature. Annals of Behavioral Medicine 53(8), 693–707.*

Carpenter C. J. (2010). *A meta-analysis of the effectiveness of health belief model variables in predicting behavior. Health Communication 25(8), 661–669.*

Dyson, J., Lawton, R., Jackson, C., and Cheater, F. (2011). *Does the use of a theoretical approach tell us more about hand hygiene behaviour? The barriers and levers to hand hygiene. Journal of Infection Prevention. https://10.1177/1757177410384300*

Gollwitzer, P. M. (1999). *Implementation intentions: strong effects of simple plans. American Psychologist 54(7), 493–503.*

Goodwin, R. and Andersen, R. M. (2002). *Use of the behavioral model of health care use to identify correlates of use of treatment for panic attacks in the community. Social Psychiatry and Psychiatric Epidemiology 37(5), 212–219.*

Gulliver, A., Griffiths, K. M., Christensen, H., and Brewer, J. L. (2012). *A systematic review of help-seeking interventions for depression, anxiety and general psychological distress. BMC Psychiatry 12, 81.*

Heckhausen, H. and Gollwitzer, P. M. (1987). *Thought contents and cognitive functioning in motivational versus volitional states of mind. Motivation and Emotion 11(2), 101–120.*

Henshaw, E. J. and Freedman-Doan, C. R. (2009). *Conceptualizing mental health care utilization using the health belief model. Clinical Psychology: Science and Practice 16(4), 420–439.*

Hui, A., Wong, P. W.-C., and Fu, K.-W. (2015). *Evaluation of an online campaign for promoting help-seeking attitudes for depression using a Facebook advertisement: an online randomized controlled experiment. JMIR Mental Health 2(1), 1–11.*

Keyworth, C., Epton, T., Goldthorpe, J., Calam, R. and Armitage, C.J. (2020). *Acceptability, reliability, and* validity of a brief measure of capabilities, opportunities, and motivations ('COM-B'). British Journal of Health Psychology 25, 474–501.

Langley, E. L., Clark, G., Murray, C., and Wootton, B. M. (2021). The utility of the health belief model variables in predicting help-seeking intention for depressive symptoms. Australian Psychologist 56(3), 233–244.

Langley, E. L., Wootton, B. M., and Grieve, R. (2018). The utility of the health belief model variables in predicting help-seeking intention for anxiety disorders. Australian Psychologist 53(4), 291–301.

Lau, J., Lim, T. Z., Jianlin Wong, G., and Tan, K. K. (2020). The health belief model and colorectal cancer screening in the general population: a systematic review. Preventive Medicine Reports 20, 101223.

Mak, H. W. and Davis, J. M. (2014). The application of the theory of planned behavior to help-seeking intention in a Chinese society. Social Psychiatry & Psychiatric Epidemiology 49, 1501–1515.

McWilliams, L., Bellhouse, S., Yorke, J., Lloyd, K., and Armitage, C. J. (2019). Beyond 'planning': a meta-analysis of implementation intentions to support smoking cessation. Health Psychology 38(12), 1059–1068.

Michie, S., Carey, R. N., Johnston, M., Rothman, A. J., De Bruin, M., Kelly, M. P., and Connell, L. E. (2018). From theory-inspired to theory-based interventions: a protocol for developing and testing a methodology for linking behaviour change techniques to theoretical mechanisms of action. Annals of Behavioral Medicine 52(6), 501–512.

Michie, S., Johnston, M., Abraham, C., Lawton, R., Parker, D., and Walker, A. (2005). Making psychological theory useful for implementing evidence based practice: a consensus approach. Quality & Safety in Health Care 14(1), 26–33. https://10.1136/qshc.2004.011155

Michie, S., Pilling, S., Garety, P., Whitty, P., Eccles, M. P., Johnston, M., and Simmons, J. (2007). Difficulties implementing a mental health guideline: an exploratory investigation using psychological theory. Implementation Science 2, 8.

Michie, S., van Stralen, M. M., and West, R. (2011). The behaviour change wheel: a new method for characterising and designing behaviour change interventions. Implementation Science 6(1), 42.

Michie, S., West, R., Campbell, R., Brown, J., and Gainforth, H. (2014). ABC of Behaviour Change Theories Book: An Essential Resource for Researchers, Policy Makers and Practitioners. Silverback Publishing. Available at: http://www.behaviourchangetheories.com/online-book#1

Nigg, C. R., Allegrante, J. P., and Ory, M. (2002). Theory-comparison and multiple-behavior research: common themes advancing health behavior research. Health Education Research 17(5), 670–679.

O'Connor, P. J., Martin, B., Weeks, C. S., and Ong, L. (2014). Factors that influence young people's mental health help-seeking behaviour: a study based on the health belief model. Journal of Advanced Nursing 70(11), 2577–2587.

Orji, R., Vassileva, J., and Mandryk, R. (2012). Towards an effective health interventions design: an extension of the health belief model. Online Journal of Public Health Informatics 4(3), ojphi.v4i3.4321.

Portes, A., Kyle, D., and Eaton, W. W. (1992). Mental illness and help-seeking behavior among Mariel Cuban and Haitian refugees in south Florida. Journal of Health and Social Behavior 33(4), 283–298.

Rickwood, D., Deane, F. P., Wilson, C. J., and Ciarrochi, J. (2005). Young people's help-seeking for mental health problems. Australian E-Journal for the Advancement of Mental Health 4(3), 218–251.

Ritchie, D., Van den Broucke, S., and Van Hal, G. (2021). The health belief model and theory of planned behavior applied to mammography screening: a systematic review and meta-analysis. Public Health Nursing 38(3), 482–492.

Roberts, T., Miguel Esponda, G., Krupchanka, D., Shidhaye, R., Patel, V., and Rathod, S. (2018). Factors associated with health service utilisation for common mental disorders: a systematic review. BMC Psychiatry 18(1), 262.

Roh, S., Burnette, C. E., Lee, K. H., Lee, Y. S., Martin, J. I., and Lawler, M. J. (2017). Predicting help-seeking attitudes toward mental health services among American Indian older adults: is Andersen's behavioral model a good fit? Journal of Applied Gerontology 36(1), 94–115.

Samdal, G. B., Eide, G. E., Barth, T., Williams, G., and Meland, E. (2017). Effective behaviour change techniques for physical activity and healthy eating in overweight and obese adults; systematic review and meta-regression analyses. *Journal of Behavioral Nutrition and Physical Activity 14, 42. https://doi.org/10.1186/s12966-017-0494-y*

Schomerus, G., Herbert, A. E., Ae, M., and Angermeyer, M. C. (2009). *The stigma of psychiatric treatment and help-seeking intentions for depression. European Archives of Psychiatry and Clinical Neuroscience 259, 298–306.*

Simo, B., Bamvita, J. M., Caron, J., and Fleury, M. J. (2018). *Predictors of mental health service use among individuals with high psychological distress and mental disorders. Psychiatry Research 270, 1122–1130.*

Tomczyk, S., Schomerus, G., Stolzenburg, S., Muehlan, H., and Schmidt, S. (2020). *Ready, willing and able? An investigation of the theory of planned behaviour in help-seeking for a community sample with current untreated depressive symptoms. Prevention Science 21(6), 749–760.*

Webb, T. L., Joseph, J., Yardley, L., and Michie, S. (2010). *Using the internet to promote health behavior change: a systematic review and meta-analysis of the impact of theoretical basis, use of behavior change techniques, and mode of delivery on efficacy. Journal of Medical Internet Research 12(1), e4.*

White, M. M., Clough, B. A., and Casey, L. M. (2018). *What do help-seeking measures assess? Building a conceptualization framework for help-seeking intentions through a systematic review of measure content. Clinical Psychology Review 59, 61–77.*

Index

For the benefit of digital users, indexed terms that span two pages (e.g., 52–53) may, on occasion, appear on only one of those pages.

Tables, and boxes are indicated by an italic *t*, and *b* following the page number.